FIRST AID FOR THE® USMLE Step 3

Third Edition

TAO LE, MD, MHS
Assistant Clinical Professor of Medicine and Pediatrics
Chief, Section of Allergy and Immunology
Department of Medicine
University of Louisville

VIKAS BHUSHAN, MD
Diagnostic Radiologist

HERMAN SINGH BAGGA, MD
Resident, Department of Urology
University of California, San Francisco

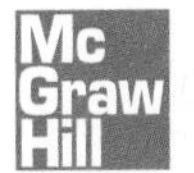

Medical

New York Chicago San Francisco Lisbon London Madrid Mexico City
Milan New Delhi San Juan Seoul Singapore Sydney Toronto

The McGraw-Hill Companies

First Aid for the® USMLE Step 3, Third Edition

Copyright © 2011, 2008, 2005 by The McGraw-Hill Companies, Inc. All rights reserved. Printed in the United States of America. Except as permitted under the United States Copyright Act of 1976, no part of this publication may be reproduced or distributed in any form or by any means, or stored in a data base or retrieval system, without the prior written permission of the publisher.

1 2 3 4 5 6 7 8 9 0 QDB/QDB 14 13 12 11 10

ISBN 978-0-07-171297-2
MHID 0-07-171297-6
ISSN 1554-1363

NOTICE

Medicine is an ever-changing science. As new research and clinical experience broaden our knowledge, changes in treatment and drug therapy are required. The authors and the publisher of this work have checked with sources believed to be reliable in their efforts to provide information that is complete and generally in accord with the standards accepted at the time of publication. However, in view of the possibility of human error or changes in medical sciences, neither the authors nor the publisher nor any other party who has been involved in the preparation or publication of this work warrants that the information contained herein is in every respect accurate or complete, and they disclaim all responsibility for any errors or omissions or for the results obtained from use of the information contained in this work. Readers are encouraged to confirm the information contained herein with other sources. For example and in particular, readers are advised to check the product information sheet included in the package of each drug they plan to administer to be certain that the information contained in this work is accurate and that changes have not been made in the recommended dose or in the contraindications for administration. This recommendation is of particular importance in connection with new or infrequently used drugs.

This book was set in Electra LH by Rainbow Graphics.
The editors were Catherine A. Johnson and Christine Diedrich.
The production supervisor was Phil Galea.
Project management was provided by Rainbow Graphics.
The designer was Alan Barnett.
Quad/Graphics was printer and binder.

This book is printed on acid-free paper.

McGraw-Hill books are available at special quantity discounts to use as premiums and sales promotions, or for use in corporate training programs. To contact a representative please e-mail us at bulksales@mcgraw-hill.com.

DEDICATION

To the contributors to this and future editions, who took time to share their experience, advice, and humor for the benefit of students.

and

To our families, friends, and loved ones, who endured and assisted in the task of assembling this guide.

Contents

AUTHORS

Clarissa Barnes, MD
Resident, Department of Internal Medicine
Johns Hopkins Hospital

Jonathan Day, MD
Resident, Department of Internal Medicine
Saint Vincent Hospital

Amar Dhand, MD, DPhil
Resident, Department of Neurology
University of California, San Francisco

Catherine R. Harris, MD
Resident, Department of Urology
University of California, San Francisco

Sandarsh Kancherla, MD
Fellow, Department of Gastroenterology
St. Luke's-Roosevelt Hospital

Nilay Kavathia, MD
Resident, Department of Internal Medicine
Thomas Jefferson University

K. Pallav Kolli, MD
Imaging Editor
Resident, Department of Radiology and Biomedical Imaging
University of California, San Francisco

Heidi Reetz, MD
Resident, Family Medicine
Santa Rosa Family Medicine Residency

Sapna Shah, MD
Resident, Department of Internal Medicine
University Hospitals Case Medical Center

Shannon Shea, MD, MPH
Resident, Department of Pediatrics
University of California, San Francisco

Benjamin Silverberg, MD, MS
Resident, Department of Family Medicine
University of Virginia

Alex Wu, MD
Resident, Department of Urology
University of California, San Francisco

FACULTY REVIEWERS

Charles Angell, MD
Assistant Professor of Medicine
Johns Hopkins University

Rizwan Aslam, MD
Associate Clinical Professor, Department of Radiology and Biomedical Imaging
University of California, San Francisco

Mitchell Conn, MD
Associate Professor of Medicine, Department of Gastroenterology
Thomas Jefferson University Hospital

Vanja Douglas, MD
Assistant Clinical Professor, Department of Neurology
University of California, San Francisco

Aleksandr Gorenbeyn, MD, FACEP
Assistant Professor, Department of Traumatology and Emergency Medicine
University of Connecticut

Sharad Jain, MD
Professor, Department of Clinical Medicine
University of California, San Francisco

Gregory S. Janis, MD
Associate Director, CCU
St. Luke's-Roosevelt Hospital Center

Gregory C. Kane, MD
Professor of Medicine, Vice-Chairman, Education
Jefferson Medical College

Armand Krikorian, MD
Assistant Professor, Division of Clinical and Molecular Endocrinology
Case Western Reserve University

Lowell Lo, MD
Assistant Professor, Department of Medicine
University of California, San Francisco

Andrea Marmor, MD, MSEd
Assistant Clinical Professor, Department of Pediatrics
University of California, San Francisco

Charles J. Nock, MD
Assistant Professor, Department of Medical Oncology
University Hospitals Case Medical Center

Maria Isabel Rodriguez, MD
Clinical Instructor, Department of Obstetrics and Gynecology
University of California, San Francisco

David Schneider, MD
Faculty, Santa Rosa Family Medicine Residency
Associate Clinical Professor, Department of Family and Community Medicine
University of California, San Francisco

Preface

With *First Aid for the USMLE Step 3*, we continue our commitment to providing residents and international medical graduates with the most useful and up-to-date preparation guides for the USMLE exams. This third edition represents a thorough review in many ways and includes the following:

- An updated review of hundreds of high-yield Step 3 topics with full-color images, presented in a format designed to encourage easier learning.
- An exam preparation guide for the computerized USMLE Step 3 with test-taking strategies for the FRED v2 format.
- A high-yield guide to the CCS that includes invaluable tips and shortcuts.
- One hundred minicases with presentations and management strategies similar to those of the actual CCS cases.

We invite you to share your thoughts and ideas to help us improve *First Aid for the USMLE Step 3*. See How to Contribute, p. xiii.

Tao Le
Louisville

Vikas Bhushan
Los Angeles

Herman Singh Bagga
San Francisco

Acknowledgments

This has been a collaborative project from the start. We gratefully acknowledge the thoughtful comments, corrections, and advice of the residents, international medical graduates, and faculty who have supported the authors in the development of *First Aid for the USMLE Step 3*.

For support and encouragement throughout the process, we are grateful to Thao Pham, Selina Franklin, and Louise Petersen.

Thanks to our publisher, McGraw-Hill, for the valuable assistance of their staff. For enthusiasm, support, and commitment to this challenging project, thanks to our editor, Catherine Johnson. For outstanding editorial work, we thank Andrea Fellows. A special thanks to Rainbow Graphics—especially David Hommel, Tina Castle, and Susan Cooper—for remarkable editorial and production work.

Thank you to Leighton Huey, MD, for his great feedback.

Tao Le
Louisville

Vikas Bhushan
Los Angeles

Herman Singh Bagga
San Francisco

How to Contribute

To help us continue to produce a high-yield review source for the USMLE Step 3 exam, you are invited to submit any suggestions or corrections. We also offer **paid internships** in medical education and publishing ranging from three months to one year (see below for details).

Please send us your suggestions for:

- Study and test-taking strategies for the computerized USMLE Step 3.
- New facts, mnemonics, diagrams, and illustrations.
- CCS-style cases.
- Low-yield topics to remove.

For each entry incorporated into the next edition, you will receive a $10 gift certificate as well as personal acknowledgment in the next edition. Diagrams, tables, partial entries, updates, corrections, and study hints are also appreciated, and significant contributions will be compensated at the discretion of the authors. Also let us know about material in this edition that you feel is low yield and should be deleted.

The preferred way to submit entries, suggestions, or corrections is via the First Aid Team's blog at:

www.firstaidteam.com.

Please include name, address, school affiliation, phone number, and e-mail address (if different from the address of origin).

NOTE TO CONTRIBUTORS

All entries become property of the authors and are subject to editing and reviewing. Please verify all data and spellings carefully. In the event that similar or duplicate entries are received, only the first entry received will be used. Include a reference to a standard textbook to facilitate verification of the fact. Please follow the style, punctuation, and format of this edition if possible.

INTERNSHIP OPPORTUNITIES

The author team is pleased to offer part-time and full-time paid internships in medical education and publishing to motivated physicians. Internships may range from three months (eg, a summer) up to a full year. Participants will have an opportunity to author, edit, and earn academic credit on a wide variety of projects, including the popular First Aid series. Writing/editing experience, familiarity with Microsoft Word, and Internet access are desired. For more information, e-mail a résumé or a short description of your experience along with a cover letter to the authors at **firstaidteam@yahoo.com.**

CHAPTER 1

GUIDE TO THE USMLE STEP 3

Introduction

For house officers, the USMLE Step 3 constitutes the last step one must take toward becoming a licensed physician. For international medical graduates (IMGs) applying for residency training in the United States, it represents an opportunity to strengthen the residency application and to obtain an H1B visa. Regardless of who you are, however, do **not** make the mistake of assuming that the Step 3 exam is just like Step 2. Whereas Step 2 focuses on clinical diagnosis, disease pathogenesis, and basic management, Step 3 emphasizes initial and **long-term** management of **common** clinical problems in **outpatient** settings. Indeed, part of the exam includes **computerized patient simulations** in addition to the traditional multiple-choice questions.

KEY FACT

Step 3 is not a retread of Step 2.

In this section, we will provide an overview of the Step 3 exam and will offer you proven approaches toward conquering the exam. For a high-yield guide to the Computer-Based Clinical Simulations (CCS), go to **Section I Supplement: Guide to the CCS.** For a detailed description of Step 3, visit **www.usmle.org** or refer to the *USMLE Step 3 Content Description and Sample Test Materials* booklet that you will receive upon registering for the exam.

USMLE Step 3—Computer-Based Testing Basics

HOW IS STEP 3 STRUCTURED?

The Step 3 exam is a two-day computer-based test (CBT) administered by Prometric, Inc. The USMLE is now using updated testing software called **FRED v2.** FRED v2 allows you to **highlight text** and **strike out** test choices as well as make **brief notes** to yourself.

Day 1 of Step 3 consists of seven 60-minute blocks of 48 multiple-choice questions for a total of 336 questions over seven hours. You get a minimum of 45 minutes of break time and 15 minutes for an optional tutorial. During the time allotted for each block, you can answer test questions in any order as well as review responses and change answers. Examinees cannot, however, go back and change answers from previous blocks. Once an examinee finishes a block, he or she must click on a screen icon to continue to the next block. Time not used during a testing block will be added to your overall break time, but it cannot be used to complete other testing blocks. Expect to spend up to nine hours at the test center.

Day 2 consists of four 45-minute blocks of 36 multiple-choice questions for a total of 144 questions over three hours. This is followed by **nine interactive case simulations** over four hours using the Primum CCS format. There is a 15-minute CCS tutorial as well as 45 minutes of allotted break time.

WHAT IS STEP 3 LIKE?

Even if you're familiar with the CBT and the Prometric test centers, FRED v2 is a relatively new testing format that you should access from the USMLE CD-ROM or Web site and try out prior to the exam. In addition, the CCS format definitely requires practice.

If you familiarize yourself with the FRED v2 testing interface ahead of time, you can skip the 15-minute tutorial offered on exam day and add those minutes to your allotted break time of 45 minutes.

For security reasons, examinees are not allowed to bring personal electronic equipment into the testing area, including watches of any kind (digital or analog), cellular telephones, and electronic paging devices. Food and beverages are also prohibited in the testing area. For note-taking purposes, examinees are given laminated writing surfaces that must be returned after the examination. The testing centers are monitored by audio and video surveillance equipment.

You should become familiar with a typical question screen. A window to the left displays all the questions in the block and shows you the incomplete questions (marked with an "*i*"). Some questions will contain figures or color illustrations adjacent to the question. Although the contrast and brightness of the screen can be adjusted, there are no other ways to manipulate the picture (eg, zooming or panning). You can also call up a window displaying normal **lab** values. You may mark questions to review at a later time by clicking the check mark at the top of the screen. The **annotation** feature functions like the provided erasable dryboards and allows you to jot down notes during the exam. Play with the **highlighting/strike-through** and annotation features with the vignettes and multiple-choice questions.

If you find that you are not using the marking, annotation, or highlighting tools, the available keyboard shortcuts can save you time over using the mouse.

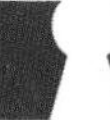

KEY FACT

Keyboard shortcuts:

- A–E—Letter choices.
- Enter or Spacebar—Move to the next question.
- Esc—Exit pop-up Lab and Exhibit windows.
- Alt-T—Countdown and time-elapsed clocks for current session and overall test.

The Primum CCS software is a patient simulation in which you are **completely** in charge of the patient's management regardless of the setting. You obtain a selected history and physical, develop a short differential, order diagnostics, and implement treatment and monitoring. CCS cases feature simulated time (a case can play out over hours, days, or months), **different locations** from outpatient to ER to ICU settings, free-text entry of orders (no multiple choice here!), and patient responses to your actions over simulated time (patients can get well, worsen, or even die depending on your actions or inaction). Please see **Section I Supplement: Guide to the CCS** for a practical guide to acing the CCS.

The USMLE also offers an opportunity to take a simulated test, or "Practice Session," at a Prometric center in the United States or Canada for about $50. You may register for a practice session online at the USMLE Web site.

WHAT TYPES OF QUESTIONS ARE ASKED?

Virtually all questions on Step 3 are vignette based. A substantial amount of extraneous information may be given, or a clinical scenario may be followed by a question that could be answered without actually necessitating that you read the case. It is your job to determine which information is superfluous and which is pertinent to the case at hand. There are three question formats:

- **Single items.** This is the **most frequent** question type. It consists of the traditional single-best-answer question with 4–5 choices.
- **Multiple-item sets.** This consists of a clinical vignette followed by 2–3 questions regarding that case. These questions can be answered **independently** of each other. Again, there is only one best answer.

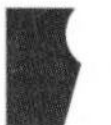

KEY FACT

For long vignettes, skip to the question stem first, and then read the case.

- **Cases.** This is a clinical vignette followed by 2–5 questions. You actually receive additional information as you answer questions, so it is important that you answer questions sequentially without skipping. As a result, once you proceed to the next question in the case, you cannot change the answer to the previous question.

The questions are organized by clinical **settings,** including an outpatient clinic, an inpatient hospital, and an emergency department. According to the USMLE, the clinical care **situations** you will encounter in these settings include the following:

- **Initial Workup:** 20–30%.
- **Continued Care:** 50–60%.
- **Urgent Intervention:** 15–25%.

The clinical tasks that you will be tested on are as follows:

- **History and Physical:** 8–12%.
- **Diagnostic Studies:** 8–12%.
- **Diagnosis:** 8–12%.
- **Prognosis:** 8–12%.
- **Applying Basic Concepts:** 8–12%.
- **Managing Patients:** 39–55%.
    - **Health Maintenance:** 5–9%.
    - **Clinical Intervention:** 18–22%.
    - **Clinical Therapeutics:** 12–16%.
    - **Legal and Ethical Issues:** 4–8%.

When approaching the vignette questions, you should keep a few things in mind:

KEY FACT

Remember that Step 3 tends to focus on outpatient continuing management scenarios.

- Note the age and race of the patient in each clinical scenario. When ethnicity is given, it is often relevant. Know these associations well (see high-yield facts), especially for more common diagnoses.
- Be able to recognize key facts that distinguish major diagnoses.
- Questions often describe clinical findings rather than naming eponyms (eg, they cite "audible hip click" instead of "positive Ortolani's sign").

HOW ARE THE SCORES REPORTED?

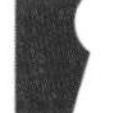

KEY FACT

Check the USMLE Web site for the latest passing requirements.

Like the Step 1 and 2 score reports, your Step 3 report includes your pass/fail status, two numeric scores, and a performance profile organized by discipline and disease process. The first score is a three-digit scaled score based on a predefined proficiency standard. A three-digit score of **184** is required for passing. The second score scale, the two-digit score, defines 75 as the minimum passing score (equivalent to a score of 184 on the first scale). This score is not a percentile. A score of 82 is equivalent to a score of 200 on the first scale. Approximately **95%** of graduates from U.S. and Canadian medical schools pass Step 3 on their first try (see Table 1-1). Approximately **two-thirds of IMGs** pass on their first attempt.

HOW DO I REGISTER TO TAKE THE EXAM?

To register for the Step 3 exam in the United States and Canada, apply online at the Federation of State Medical Boards (FSMB) Web site **(www.fsmb.org).** A printable version of the application is also available on this site. Note that some states require you to apply for licensure when you register for Step 3. A

TABLE 1-1. Recent Step 3 Examination Results

	2007		2008[a]	
	# Tested	% Passing	# Tested	% Passing
Examinees from U.S./Canadian schools				
MD degree	17,570	95	18,241	94
First-time takers	16,633	96	17,245	95
Repeaters	937	72	996	67
DO degree	21	86	21	90
First-time takers	20	85	19	95
Repeaters	1	Not reported	2	Not reported
Total U.S./Canadian	17,591	95	18,262	94
Examinees from non-U.S./Canadian schools				
First-time takers	9,384	79	9,376	78
Repeaters	3,537	60	3,293	54
Total non-U.S./Canadian	12,921	73	12,669	71

[a]Source: www.usmle.org/Scores_Transcripts/performance/2008.html.

list of those states can be found on the FSMB Web site. The registration fee varies and was $705 or higher in 2010.

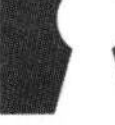

KEY FACT

Because the exam is scheduled on a "first-come, first-served" basis, you should contact Prometric as soon as you receive your scheduling permit!

Your scheduling permit is sent via e-mail to the e-mail address provided on the application materials. Once you have received your scheduling permit, it is your responsibility to print it and decide when and where you would like to take the exam. For a list of Prometric locations nearest you, visit **www.prometric.com.** Call Prometric's toll-free number or visit www.prometric.com to arrange a time to take the exam.

The electronic scheduling permit you receive will contain the following important information:

- Your USMLE identification number.
- The eligibility period in which you may take the exam.
- Your "scheduling number," which you will need to make your exam appointment with Prometric.
- Your "Candidate Identification Number," or CIN, which you must enter at your Prometric workstation in order to access the exam.

Prometric has no access to these codes or your scheduling permit and will not be able to supply these for you. You will not be allowed to take Step 3 unless you present your permit, printed by you ahead of time, along with an unexpired, government-issued photo identification that contains your signature (eg, a driver's license or passport). Make sure the name on your photo ID exactly matches the name that appears on your scheduling permit.

WHAT IF I NEED TO RESCHEDULE THE EXAM?

You can change your date and/or center within your three-month eligibility period without charge by contacting Prometric. If space is available, you may reschedule up to five days before your test date. If you reschedule within five days of your test date, Prometric will charge a rescheduling fee. If you need to reschedule outside your initial three-month period, you can apply for a single three-month extension (e.g., April/May/June can be extended through July/August/September) after your eligibility period has begun (go to **www.nbme.org** for more information). For other rescheduling needs, you must submit a new application along with another application fee.

WHAT ABOUT TIME?

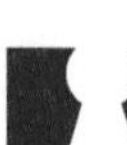

KEY FACT

Never, ever leave a question blank! You can always mark it and come back later.

Time is of special interest on the CBT exam. The computer will keep track of how much time has elapsed. However, the computer will show you only how much time you have remaining in a given block (unless you look at the full clock with **Alt-T**). Therefore, it is up to you to determine if you are pacing yourself properly. Note that on both day 1 and day 2 of testing, you have approximately **75 seconds** per multiple-choice question. If you recognize that a question is not solvable in a reasonable period of time, move on after making an educated guess; there are **no penalties** for wrong answers.

It should be noted that 45 minutes is allowed for break time. However, you can elect not to use all of your break time, or you can gain extra break time either by skipping the tutorial or by finishing a block ahead of the allotted time. The computer **will not warn you** if you are spending more than your allotted break time.

IF I LEAVE DURING THE EXAM, WHAT HAPPENS TO MY SCORE?

You are considered to have started the exam once you have entered your CIN onto the computer screen. In order to receive an official score, however, you must finish the entire exam. This means that you must start and either finish or run out of time for each block of the exam. If you do **not** complete all the blocks, your exam will be documented on your USMLE score transcript as an incomplete attempt, but no actual score will be reported.

The exam ends when all blocks have been completed or time has expired. As you leave the testing center, you will receive a written test-completion notice to document your completion of the exam.

HOW LONG WILL I HAVE TO WAIT BEFORE I GET MY SCORES?

The USMLE typically reports scores 3–4 weeks after the examinee's test date. During peak periods, however, it may take **up to six weeks** for scores to be made available. Official information concerning the time required for score reporting is posted on the USMLE Web site.

USMLE/NBME Resources

We strongly encourage you to use the free materials provided by the testing agencies and to study the following NBME publications:

- ***USMLE Bulletin of Information.*** This publication provides you with nuts-and-bolts details about the exam (included on the USMLE Web site; free to all examinees).
- ***USMLE Step 3 Content Description and Sample Test Materials.*** This is a hard copy of test questions and test content also found on the CD-ROM.
- **NBME Test Delivery Software (FRED v2) and Tutorial.** This includes 168 valuable practice questions. The questions are available on the USMLE CD-ROM and Web site. Make sure you are using the new FRED v2 version and not the older Prometric version.
- **USMLE Web site (www.usmle.org).** In addition to allowing you to become familiar with the CBT format, the sample items on the USMLE Web site provide the only questions that are available directly from the test makers. Student feedback varies as to the similarity of these questions to those on the actual exam, but they are nonetheless worthwhile to know.

Testing Agencies

National Board of Medical Examiners (NBME)
Department of Licensing Examination Services
3750 Market Street
Philadelphia, PA 19104-3102
215-590-9500
Fax: 215-590-9457
www.nbme.org

Educational Commission for Foreign Medical Graduates (ECFMG)
3624 Market Street, Fourth Floor
Philadelphia, PA 19104-2685
215-386-5900
Fax: 215-386-9196
www.ecfmg.org

Federation of State Medical Boards (FSMB)
P.O. Box 619850
Dallas, TX 75261-9850
817-868-4000
Fax: 817-868-4099
www.fsmb.org

USMLE Secretariat
3750 Market Street
Philadelphia, PA 19104-3190
215-590-9700
www.usmle.org

NOTES

SUPPLEMENT

GUIDE TO THE CCS

Introduction

The Primum CCS is a computerized patient simulation that is administered on the second day of Step 3. You will be given nine cases over four hours and will have up to 25 minutes per case. As with the rest of the Step 3 exam, the CCS is meant to test your ability to properly diagnose and manage common conditions in a variety of patient-care settings. Many of these conditions are obvious or easily diagnosed. Clinical problems range from acute to chronic and from mundane to life-threatening. A case may last from a few minutes to a few months in terms of **simulated time,** even though you will be allotted only 25 minutes of real time per case. Cases can, and frequently do, end in less than 25 minutes. No matter where the patient is situated during the case (ie, office, ER, or ICU), you will serve as the patient's **primary** physician and will bear **complete** responsibility for his or her care.

KEY FACT

The focus is management, management, management. You will see few diagnostic zebras in the CCS.

What Is the CCS Like?

For the CCS, there is **no substitute** for trying out the cases on the USMLE CD-ROM or downloading the software from the USMLE Web site. If you spend at least a few hours doing the sample cases and familiarizing yourself with the interface, you **will do better** on the actual exam, regardless of your prior computer experience.

KEY FACT

Do all the sample CCS cases prior to the actual exam.

For each case, you will be presented with a chief complaint, vital signs, and the history of present illness (HPI). At that point, you will initiate patient management, continue care, and advance the case by taking one of the following four actions that are represented on the computer screen.

1. GET INTERVAL HISTORY OR PHYSICAL EXAM

You can obtain a focused or full physical exam. You can also get interval history to see how a patient is doing. Getting interval history or doing a physical exam will **automatically** advance the clock in simulated time.

Quick tips and shortcuts:

- If the vital signs are unstable, you may be forced to write some orders (eg, IV fluids, oxygen, type and cross-match) even **before** you perform the exam.
- Keep the physical exam **focused.** A full physical and exam is often wasteful and can cost you valuable simulated time in an emergency. You can always do additional physical exam components as necessary.

2. WRITE ORDER OR REVIEW CHART

You can manage the patient by typing orders. As part of your management, for example, you can order tests, monitoring, treatments, procedures, consultations, and counseling. The order sheet format is free-text entry, so you can type whatever you choose; the computer has a 12,000-term vocabulary that can accommodate approximately 2,500 orders or actions. If you order a medication, you will also need to specify the **route** and **frequency.** If a patient comes into a case with preexisting medications, these meds will appear on the order sheet with an order time of "Day 1 @00:00." The medications will continue unless you decide to cancel them. Unlike interval history or PE, you must **manually** advance simulated time to see the results of your orders (see the next page).

KEY FACT

The orders require free-text entry. There is no multiple choice here!

Quick tips and shortcuts:

- As long as the computer can recognize the **first three characters** of your order, it can provide a list of orders from which to choose.
- Simply type the test, therapy, or procedure you want. Don't type verbs such as "get," "administer," or "do."
- Do the sample cases to get a sense of the common abbreviations the computer will recognize (eg, CBC, CXR, ECG).
- Familiarize yourself with routes and dosing frequencies for common medications. You do not need to know dosages or drip rates.
- Never assume that other health care staff or consultants will write orders for you. Even routine actions such as IV fluids, oxygen, monitoring, and diabetic diet must be ordered by you. If a patient is preop, don't forget NPO, type and cross-match, and antibiotics.
- You can always change your mind and cancel an order as long as the clock has not been advanced.
- Review any preexisting medications on the order sheet. Sometimes the patient's problem may be due to a preexisting medication **side effect** or a drug-drug interaction!

3. OBTAIN RESULTS OR SEE PATIENT LATER

To see how the case evolves after you have entered your orders, you must advance the clock. You can specify a time to see the patient either in the future or when the next results become available. When you advance the clock, you may receive messages from the patient, the patient's family, or the health care staff updating you on the patient's status prior to the specified time or result availability. If you stop a clock advance to a future time (such as a follow-up appointment) to review results from previous orders, that future appointment will be canceled.

Quick tips and shortcuts:

- Before advancing the clock, ask yourself whether the patient will be okay during that time period.
- Before advancing the clock, ask yourself whether the patient is in the appropriate location or should be transferred to a new location.
- If you receive an update while the clock is advancing, especially if the patient is **worsening,** you should review your current management.

4. CHANGE LOCATION

According to the USMLE, you have an outpatient office with admitting privileges to a 400-bed tertiary-care facility. As in real life, the patient typically presents to you in an office or ER setting. Once you've done all you can, you can transfer the patient to another setting to receive appropriate care. This may include the **ward** or the **ICU.** Note that in this context, the ICU represents all types of ICUs, including medical, surgical, pediatric, obstetrics, and neonatal. When appropriate, the patient may be discharged **home** with follow-up.

Quick tips and shortcuts:

- Always ask yourself if the patient is in the right location to receive optimal management.
- Remember that you remain the **primary physician** wherever the patient goes.

NOTES

CHAPTER 2

AMBULATORY MEDICINE

Ophthalmology

GLAUCOMA

A form of optic neuropathy that is caused by elevated intraocular pressure (defined as > 20 mm Hg) and that results in loss of vision.

Open-Angle Glaucoma

- The most common type of glaucoma. More common in African Americans.
- **Sx/Dx:** Diagnosis is made in patients who are **losing peripheral vision** and who have high intraocular pressures and an abnormal cup-to-disk ratio (> 50%) (see Figure 2-1).
- **Tx:** Treat with the following:
  - Nonselective topical β-blockers (eg, timolol, levobunolol).
  - Topical adrenergic agonists (eg, epinephrine).
  - Topical cholinergic agonists (eg, pilocarpine, carbachol).
  - Topical carbonic anhydrase inhibitors (eg, dorzolamide, brinzolamide).

Closed-Angle Glaucoma

A 42-year-old woman presents with headache, nausea, vomiting, and a red eye that has progressively worsened since this morning. She also notes vision changes. Exam reveals conjunctival injection; moderately fixed, dilated pupils; and no focal weaknesses in the extremities. What should you do next?

Use tonometry to check intraocular pressures. A pressure of ≥ 30 mm Hg confirms the diagnosis. Refer to ophthalmology. Initial treatments include timolol, acetazolamide, and topical pilocarpine.

- **An emergency!**
- A result of the anterior chamber angle impairing drainage of aqueous humor and increasing intraocular pressure. Normal pressure is 8–21 mm Hg, whereas pressures in closed-angle glaucoma can be ≥ 30 mm Hg.
- Anatomic predisposition is a 1° cause; 2° causes include fibrovascular membrane formation and hemorrhage. Risk factors include a family history, female gender, age > 40–50, and Asian ethnicity.
- **Sx/Exam:** Presents with eye pain, headache, nausea, conjunctival injection, halos around lights, and fixed, moderately dilated pupils. Check intraocular pressure.
- **Tx:**
  - Contact an ophthalmologist immediately!
  - Treatment consists of topical pilocarpine for pupillary constriction, timolol and acetazolamide to ↓ intraocular pressure, and laser iridotomy. Systemic treatments include acetazolamide and mannitol.

KEY FACT

Do not confuse closed-angle glaucoma with a simple headache!

DIABETIC RETINOPATHY

- Asymptomatic, gradual vision loss in patients with diabetes. The leading cause of blindness in the United States.

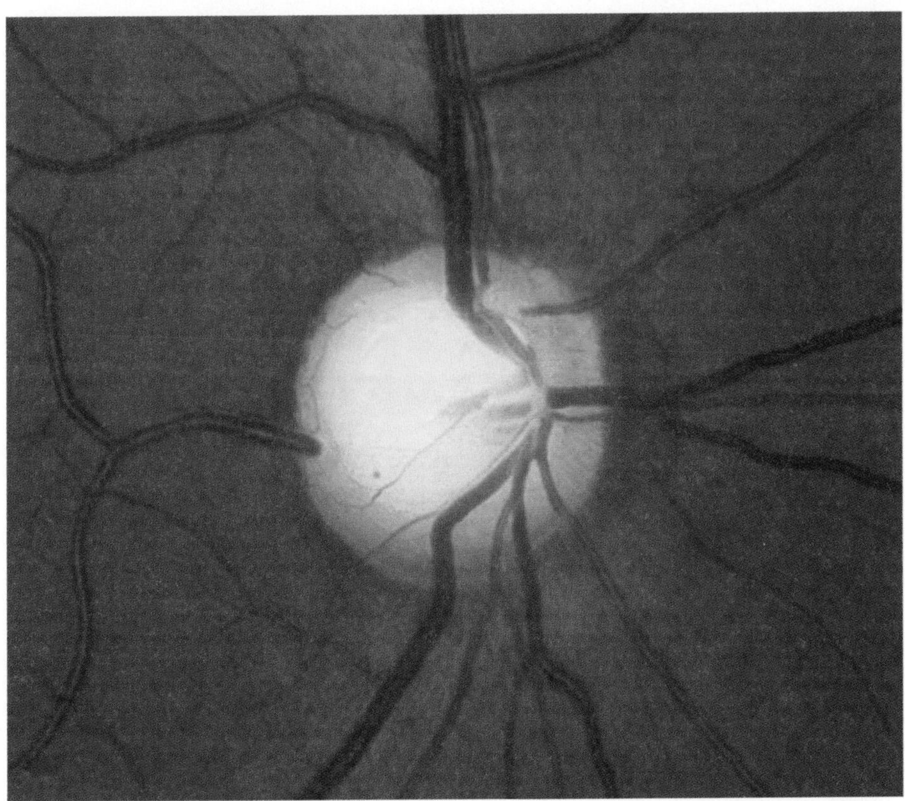

FIGURE 2-1. Open-angle glaucoma. Note the change in the cup-to-disk ratio. (Reproduced with permission from USMLERx.com.)

- **Sx/Exam: Funduscopic findings** include neovascularization, microaneurysms, flame hemorrhages, and macular edema.
- **Tx:** Proliferative retinopathy may be treated, and progression slowed, by laser photocoagulation surgery or vitrectomy.
- **Prevention:**
  - Patients with diabetes should have a comprehensive ophthalmologic exam at least annually to screen for signs of retinopathy.
  - Progression can be slowed with tight glucose and BP control.

Ear, Nose, and Throat (ENT)

INFLUENZA

- An acute respiratory illness that is caused by influenza A or B and occurs primarily during the winter.
- **Sx/Exam:** Generally presents following an incubation period of 1–2 days with acute-onset upper and lower respiratory tract symptoms, myalgias, fevers, and weakness.
- **Dx:** Rapid antigen tests have a sensitivity of only 40–60%. Diagnosis may be established through PCR testing or viral culture.
- **Tx:** The antiviral drugs zanamivir and oseltamivir can be used as prophylaxis against or to treat infection in at-risk individuals; these drugs are most effective when given within 48 hours of exposure or at symptom onset. Most influenza strains have become resistant to amantadine and rimantadine.

- **Cx:**
  - Pneumonia is the 1° complication of influenza. Those who are predisposed to it usually have an underlying condition such as diabetes mellitus (DM) or cardiopulmonary disease. Patients > 50 years of age and residents of nursing homes are also at risk.
  - 2° bacterial pneumonia, often from *Streptococcus pneumoniae*, is an important complication and is responsible for one-quarter of influenza-related deaths.
  - Other complications of influenza include myositis, rhabdomyolysis, CNS involvement, myocarditis, and pericarditis.

HEARING LOSS

Common in the elderly. Principal causes are as follows:

- **External canal:** Cerumen impaction, foreign bodies in the ear canal, otitis externa, new growth/mass.
- **Internal canal:** Otitis media, barotrauma, perforation of the tympanic membrane.

Additional causes include the following:

- **Presbycusis:** Age-related hearing loss. High-pitched sounds are lost first, so speak loudly in a low-pitched voice.
- **Otosclerosis:** Progressive fixation of the stapes, leading to bilateral progressive conductive hearing loss. Begins in the second or third decade of life, and may advance in pregnancy. Exam is normal; surgery with stapedectomy or stapedotomy yields excellent results.
- **Other:** Drug-induced loss (eg, from aminoglycosides); noise-induced loss.

DIAGNOSIS

Distinguish conductive from sensorineural hearing loss via the Weber and Rinne tests:

- **Weber test:** Press a vibrating tuning fork in the middle of the patient's forehead and ask in which ear it sounds louder.
  - **Conductive hearing loss:** The sound will be louder in the affected ear.
  - **Sensorineural hearing loss:** The sound will be louder in the normal ear.
- **Rinne test:** Place a vibrating tuning fork against the patient's mastoid bone, and once it is no longer audible, immediately reposition it near the external meatus.
  - **Conductive hearing loss:** Bone conduction is audible longer than air conduction.
  - **Sensorineural hearing loss:** Air conduction is audible longer than bone conduction.

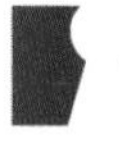

KEY FACT

Otosclerosis is the most common cause of conductive hearing loss in young adults.

ALLERGIC RHINITIS

Affects up to 20% of the adult population. Patients may also have asthma and atopic dermatitis.

SYMPTOMS/EXAM

- Presents with congestion, rhinorrhea, sneezing, eye irritation, and postnasal drip.
- Generally, one can readily identify exposure to environmental allergens such as pollens, animal dander, dust mites, and mold spores. May be seasonal.

- Exam reveals edematous, pale mucosa; cobblestoning in the pharynx; scleral injection; and blue, boggy turbinates.

Diagnosis

- Often based on clinical impression given the signs and symptoms.
- Skin testing to a standard panel of antigens can be performed, or blood testing can be conducted to look for specific IgE antibodies via radioallergosorbent testing (RAST).

Treatment

- **Allergen avoidance:** Use dust mite–proof covers on bedding and remove carpeting. Keep the home dry and avoid pets.
- **Drugs:**
  - **Antihistamines (diphenhydramine, fexofenadine):** Block the effects of histamine released by mast cells. Selective antihistamines such as fexofenadine may cause less drowsiness than nonselective agents such as diphenhydramine.
  - **Intranasal corticosteroids:** Anti-inflammatory properties lead to excellent symptom control.
  - **Sympathomimetics (pseudoephedrine):** α-adrenergic agonist effects result in vasoconstriction.
  - **Intranasal anticholinergics (ipratropium):** ↓ mucous membrane secretions.
  - **Immunotherapy ("allergy shots"):** Slow to take effect, but useful for difficult-to-control symptoms.

EPISTAXIS

Bleeding from the nose or nasopharynx. Roughly 90% of cases are anterior nasal septum bleeds (at Kiesselbach's plexus). The most common etiology is local trauma 2° to digital manipulation. Other causes include dryness of the nasal mucosa, nasal septal deviation, use of antiplatelet medications, bone abnormalities in the nares, rhinitis, and bleeding diatheses.

Symptoms/Exam

- **Posterior bleeds:** More brisk and less common; blood is swallowed and may not be seen.
- **Anterior bleeds:** Usually less severe; bleeding is visible as it exits the nares.

Treatment

- Treat with prolonged and sustained direct pressure and topical nasal vasoconstrictors (phenylephrine or oxymetazoline).
- If bleeding does not stop, cauterize with silver nitrate or insert nasal packing (with antibiotics to prevent toxic shock syndrome, covering for *S aureus*).
- If severe, type and screen, obtain IV access, and consult an ENT surgeon.

LEUKOPLAKIA

White patches or plaques in the oral mucosa that are considered precancerous and cannot be removed by rubbing the mucosal surface. However, if these white lesions are easily removed, think of *Candida*. Lesions can occur in response to chronic irritation and can represent either dysplasia or early invasive squamous cell carcinoma. Common among those who use chewing tobacco.

Dermatology

"DERM TERMS"

The following terms describe common dermatologic lesions:

- **Macule:** A flat, circumscribed, nonpalpable lesion usually < 0.5 cm in diameter. Examples include flat nevi and café-au-lait spots.
- **Patch:** A flat, nonpalpable lesion > 0.5 cm in diameter. Examples include large café-au-lait spots and vitiligo.
- **Papule:** An elevated, palpable lesion < 0.5 cm in diameter. Examples include elevated nevi and molluscum contagiosum.
- **Plaque:** An elevated, palpable lesion > 0.5 cm in diameter. Often formed by a confluence of papules. Examples include psoriasis and lichen simplex chronicus.
- **Nodule:** A circumscribed, elevated, solid lesion measuring between 0.5 and 2.0 cm in diameter. May be in the epidermis or in deeper tissue. Examples include fibromas and xanthomas.
- **Tumors:** Larger and more deeply circumscribed, solid lesions. Examples include lipomas and various neoplastic growths.
- **Vesicles:** Circumscribed, elevated, fluid-containing lesions measuring ≤ 0.5 cm in diameter. Examples include HSV and VZV lesions.
- **Bullae:** Circumscribed, elevated, fluid-containing lesions measuring > 0.5 cm in diameter. Examples include burns, pemphigus, and epidermolysis bullosa.
- **Pustules:** Circumscribed elevations that contain purulent exudate.

ATOPIC DERMATITIS (ECZEMA)

Pruritic, lichenified eruptions that are classically found in the antecubital fossa but may also appear on the neck, face, wrists, and upper trunk.

- Has a chronic course with remissions.
- Characterized by an early age of onset (often in childhood).
- Associated with a ⊕ family history and a personal history of atopy.
- Patients tend to have ↑ serum IgE and repeated skin infections.

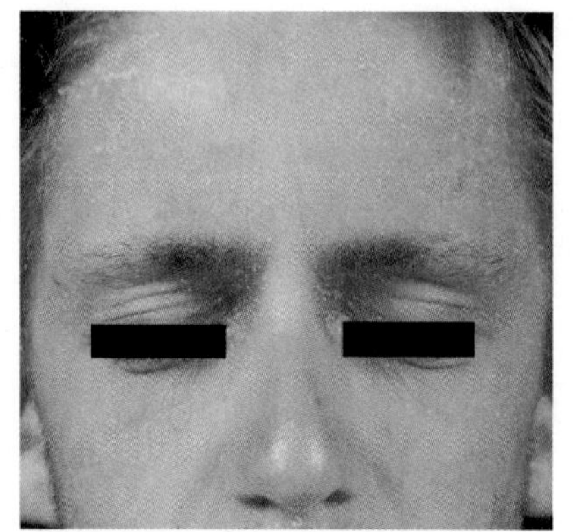

FIGURE 2-2. Atopic dermatitis. Infiltrated, erythematous facial skin with scaliness in an adolescent with atopic dermatitis. (Reproduced with permission from Wolff K et al. *Fitzpatrick's Dermatology in General Medicine*, 7th ed. New York: McGraw-Hill, 2008, Fig. 14-6.)

SYMPTOMS/EXAM

Presents with severe pruritus, with distribution generally in the face, neck, upper trunk, and bends of the elbows and knees. The skin is dry, leathery, and lichenified (see Figure 2-2). The condition usually worsens in the winter and in low-humidity environments. Often known as "the itch that rashes."

DIFFERENTIAL

Seborrheic dermatitis, contact dermatitis, impetigo.

DIAGNOSIS

Diagnosis is clinical.

TREATMENT

Keep skin moisturized. **Topical steroid creams should be used sparingly** and should be tapered off once flares resolve. The first-line steroid-sparing agent is tacrolimus ointment.

CONTACT DERMATITIS

Caused by exposure to certain substances in the environment. Allergens may lead to acute, subacute, or chronic eczematous inflammation.

KEY FACT

Common causes of contact dermatitis include leather, nickel (earrings, watches, necklaces), and poison ivy.

Symptoms

Patients present with itching, burning, and an intensely pruritic rash.

Exam

- **Acute:** Presents with papular erythematous lesions and sometimes with vesicles, weeping erosions where vesicles have ruptured, crusting, and excoriations. The pattern of lesions often reflects the mechanism of exposure (eg, a line of vesicles or lesions under a watchband; see Figure 2-3).
- **Chronic:** Characterized by hyperkeratosis and lichenification.

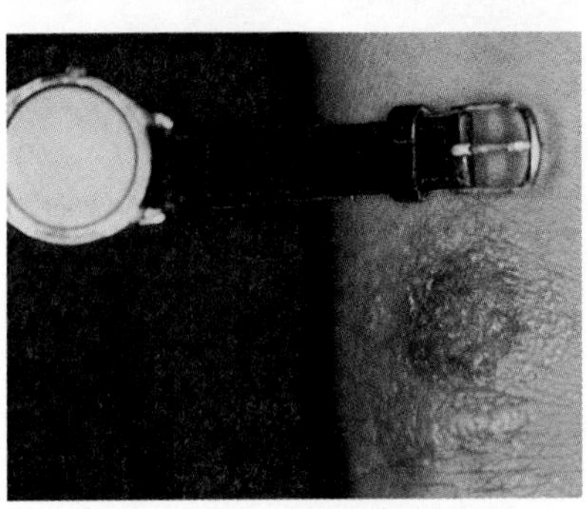

FIGURE 2-3. Contact dermatitis. The erythematous, edematous base of the eruption corresponds to the posterior surface of the watch. (Courtesy of the Department of Dermatology, Wilford Hall USAF Medical Center and Brooke Army Medical Center, San Antonio, TX, as published in Knoop KJ et al. *Atlas of Emergency Medicine,* 2nd ed. New York: McGraw-Hill, 2002, Fig. 13-56.)

Diagnosis

- Usually a clinical diagnosis that is made in the setting of a possible exposure.
- A detailed history for exposures is essential.
- In the case of leather, patch testing can be used to elicit the reaction with the exact agent that caused the dermatitis.
- Consider the occupation of the individual and the exposure area of the body to determine if they suggest a diagnosis.

Treatment

- Avoid causative agents.
- Cold compresses and oatmeal baths help soothe the area.
- Administer topical steroids. A short course of oral steroids may be needed if a large region of the body is involved.

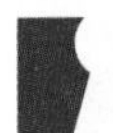

KEY FACT

Psoriatic arthritis characteristically involves the DIP joints.

PSORIASIS

An immune-mediated skin disease characterized by silver plaques with an erythematous base and sharply defined margins. The condition is common and is generally chronic with a probable genetic predisposition.

Symptoms/Exam

Presents with well-demarcated, silvery, scaly plaques (the most common type) on the knees, elbows, gluteal cleft, and scalp (see Figure 2-4). **Nails may show pitting** and onycholysis.

Treatment

- **Limited disease:** Topical steroids, occlusive dressings, topical vitamin D analogs, topical retinoids.
- **Generalized disease (involving > 30% of the body):** UVB light exposure three times per week; PUVA (psoralen and UVA) if UVB is not effective. Methotrexate may also be used for severe cases.

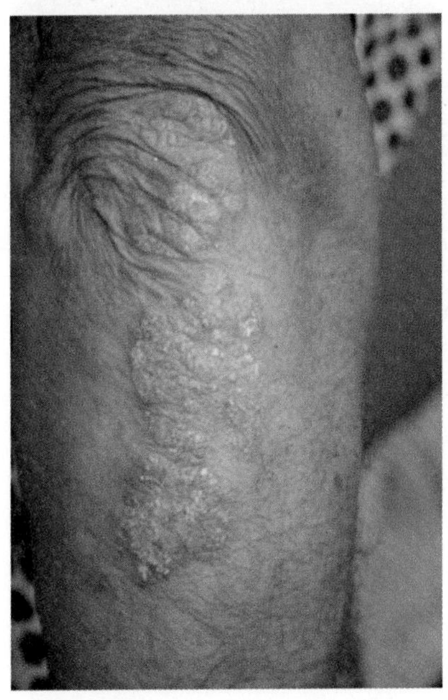

FIGURE 2-4. Psoriasis. Note the well-demarcated, erythematous plaque with micaceous scale of the elbow. (Reproduced with permission from USMLERx.com.)

ERYTHEMA NODOSUM

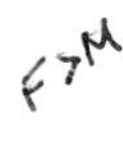

An inflammatory lesion that is characterized by red or violet nodules and is more common in women than in men. Although the condition is often idiopathic, it may also occur 2° to sarcoidosis, IBD, or conditions such as streptococcal infection, coccidioidomycosis, and TB.

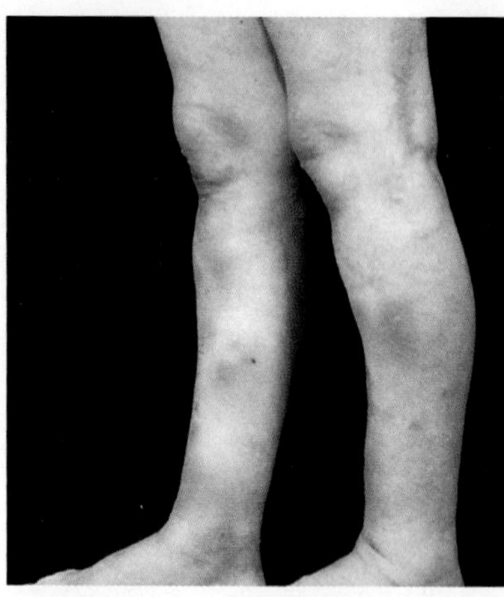

FIGURE 2-5. Erythema nodosum. Note the bilateral erythematous nodules localized over the shins. (Reproduced with permission from Wolff K et al. *Fitzpatrick's Dermatology in General Medicine,* 7th ed. New York: McGraw-Hill, 2008, Fig. 68-4.)

Symptoms/Exam

- Lesions are painful and may be preceded by fever, malaise, and arthralgias. Recent URI or diarrheal illness may suggest a cause.
- Exam reveals deep-seated, poorly demarcated, painful red nodules without ulceration on the extensor surfaces of the lower legs (see Figure 2-5).

Differential

Cellulitis, trauma, thrombophlebitis.

Treatment

Treat the underlying disease. The condition is usually self-limited, but NSAIDs are helpful for pain. In more persistent cases, potassium iodide drops and systemic corticosteroids may be of benefit.

ROSACEA

A chronic condition that occurs in patients 30–60 years of age. Most commonly affects people with fair skin, those with light hair and eyes, and those who have frequent flushing.

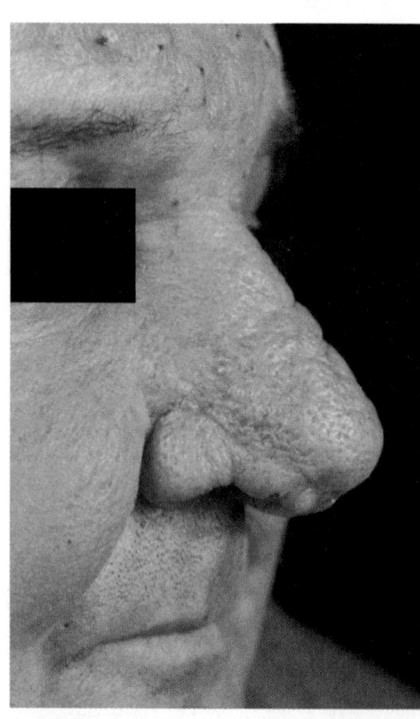

FIGURE 2-6. Rhinophyma. (Reproduced with permission from Wolff K et al. *Fitzpatrick's Color Atlas & Synopsis of Clinical Dermatology,* 5th ed. New York: McGraw-Hill, 2005: 11.)

Symptoms/Exam

- Presents with erythema and with inflammatory papules that mimic acne and appear on the cheeks, forehead, nose, and chin.
- Open and closed comedones (whiteheads and blackheads) are not present.
- Recurrent flushing may be elicited by spicy foods, alcohol, or emotional reactions.
- Rhinophyma (thickened, lumpy skin on the nose) occurs late in the course of the disease and is a result of sebaceous gland hyperplasia (see Figure 2-6).

Differential

The absence of comedones in rosacea and the patient's age help distinguish the condition from acne vulgaris.

Treatment

- **Initial therapy:** The goal is to control rather than cure the chronic disease. Use mild cleansers (Dove, Cetaphil), benzoyl peroxide, and/or metronidazole topical gel with or without oral antibiotics as initial therapy.
- **Persistent symptoms:** Treat with oral antibiotics (tetracycline, minocycline) and tretinoin cream.
- **Maintenance therapy:**
  - Topical metronidazole may be used once daily.
  - Clonidine or α-blockers may be effective in the management of flushing, and patients should avoid triggers.
  - Consider referral for surgical evaluation if rhinophyma is present and is not responding to treatment.

ERYTHEMA MULTIFORME (EM)

An acute inflammatory disease that is sometimes recurrent. EM is probably a distinct disease entity from Stevens-Johnson syndrome and toxic epidermal necrolysis. **Many causative factors** are linked with EM, such as infectious agents (especially HSV and *Mycoplasma*), drugs, connective tissue disorders, physical agents, radiotherapy, pregnancy, and internal malignancies. Many cases are idiopathic and recurrent.

SYMPTOMS/EXAM

- May be preceded by malaise, fever, or itching and burning at the site where the eruptions will occur.
- Presents with sudden onset of rapidly progressive, symmetrical lesions.
- Target lesions and papules are typically located on the back of the hands and on the palms, soles, and limbs but can be found anywhere (see Figure 2-7). Lesions recur in crops for 2–3 weeks.

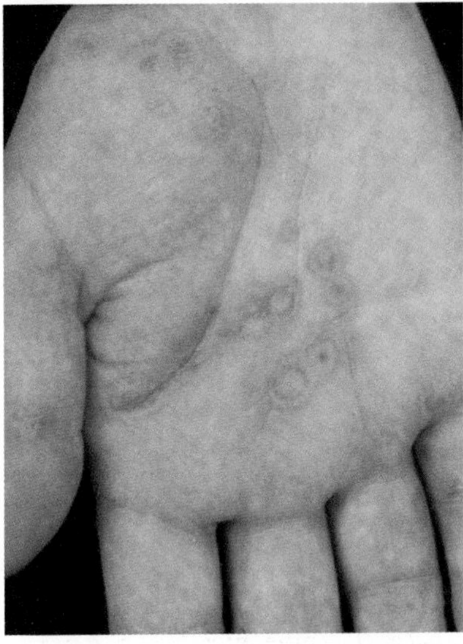

FIGURE 2-7. Erythema multiforme. Note the typical target lesions on the palm. (Reproduced with permission from Wolff K et al. *Fitzpatrick's Dermatology in General Medicine,* 7th ed. New York: McGraw-Hill, 2008, Fig. 38-2.)

DIAGNOSIS

Typically a clinical diagnosis. Biopsy can help in uncertain cases.

TREATMENT

- Mild cases can be treated symptomatically with histamine blockers for pruritus.
- If many target lesions are present, patients usually respond to prednisone for 1–3 weeks.
- Azathioprine has been helpful in cases that are unresponsive to other treatments. Levamisole has also been successfully used in patients with chronic or recurrent oral lesions.
- When HSV causes recurrent EM, maintenance acyclovir or valacyclovir can ↓ recurrences of both.

PEMPHIGUS VULGARIS

A rare autoimmune disease in which blisters are formed as **autoantibodies destroy intracellular adhesions between epithelial cells** in the skin. Pemphigus vulgaris is the most common subtype of pemphigus.

SYMPTOMS/EXAM

- Presents with **flaccid bullae** and with **erosions** where bullae have been unroofed (see Figure 2-8). Oral lesions usually precede skin lesions.
- If it is not treated early, the disease usually generalizes and can affect the esophagus.
- Nikolsky's sign is elicited when gentle lateral traction on the skin separates the epidermis from underlying tissue.

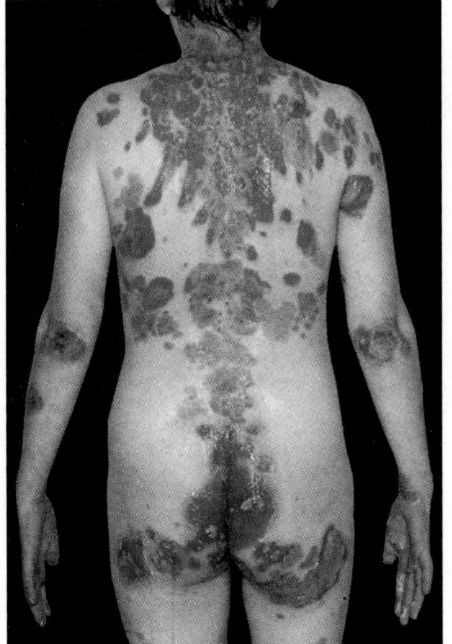

FIGURE 2-8. Pemphigus vulgaris. Note the extensive erosions due to blistering and the intact, flaccid blisters at the lower border of the eroded lesions. (Reproduced with permission from Wolff K et al. *Fitzpatrick's Dermatology in General Medicine,* 7th ed. New York: McGraw-Hill, 2008, Fig. 52-4.)

DIAGNOSIS

Skin biopsy shows acantholysis (separation of epidermal cells from each other); immunofluorescence reveals antibodies in the epidermis.

TREATMENT

Corticosteroids and immunosuppressive agents.

BULLOUS PEMPHIGOID

- An autoimmune disease characterized by **antibodies against basement membrane that lead to subepidermal bullae.** More common than pemphigus vulgaris, and typically occurs in those > 60 years of age (the median age at onset is 80 years).
- **Sx/Exam:** Presents as large, tense bullae with few other symptoms.
- **DDx:** Pemphigus vulgaris, dermatitis herpetiformis.

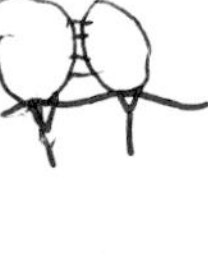

- **Dx:** Diagnosis is made with skin biopsy, with confirmation via immuno- and histopathology.
- **Tx:** Topical corticosteroids.

ACNE VULGARIS (COMMON ACNE)

A common skin disease that primarily affects adolescents. Results from ↑ pilosebaceous gland activity, *Propionibacterium acnes*, and plugging of follicles.

SYMPTOMS/EXAM

Characterized by a variety of lesions, including closed comedones (whiteheads), open comedones (blackheads), papules, nodules, and scars. Lesions are typically seen over the face, back, and chest.

DIFFERENTIAL

Rosacea, folliculitis.

DIAGNOSIS

Diagnosis is clinical.

TREATMENT

- Begin with topical antibiotics such as erythromycin, benzoyl peroxide gels, and topical retinoids.
- A 2° line of treatment includes addition of oral antibiotics such as minocycline and tetracycline.
- Isotretinoin (Accutane) can be used but is teratogenic and should be prescribed with caution in women of childbearing age. Concomitant contraception and pregnancy tests are necessary.

HERPES ZOSTER

A 71-year-old man presents to urgent care complaining of a lesion on his right flank. He states that the appearance of this lesion was preceded by some tingling in the same area one day ago. Exam reveals a four-inch band of painful vesicles with 2° crusting and a clear midline border. How do you evaluate this patient?

The patient's presentation is highly suspicious for herpes zoster. Although a clinical exam is typically sufficient for diagnosis, a PCR of fluid from the lesion or a Tzanck smear can be confirmatory. NSAIDs may be useful for pain control, and antiviral therapy may ↓ the likelihood of postherpetic neuralgia and speed resolution of the lesion.

A disease caused by reactivated varicella-zoster virus (VZV), which remains dormant in the dorsal roots of nerves. Risk factors include ↑ age and immunosuppression. Patients can develop postherpetic neuralgia, a painful disorder, after the eruption.

SYMPTOMS/EXAM

Presents with the cutaneous finding of **painful vesicles evolving into crusted lesions in a dermatomal distribution.** Lesions are typically preceded by paresthesias in the area of distribution.

DIFFERENTIAL

Contact dermatitis.

DIAGNOSIS

Diagnosis is largely clinical. Giant cells may be seen on Tzanck smear of fluid.

TREATMENT

- Pain management.
- If initiated within 72 hours of rash onset, antiviral treatment with acyclovir, valacyclovir, or famciclovir can ↓ the duration of illness and may also ↓ the occurrence of postherpetic neuralgia. Use of glucocorticoids is controversial and is usually not recommended.
- Vaccination to help prevent recurrence is becoming more popular in select patients.

DERMATOPHYTOSES

Dermatophytes attach to and proliferate on the superficial layers of the epidermis, nails, and hair. Typically, they form a red and scaly lesion. Examples include the following:

- **Tinea capitis:** Erythema and scaling under the scalp with thickened and broken-off hairs. Common organisms are *Trichophyton tonsurans* and *Microsporum canis*. Treatment includes griseofulvin, itraconazole, and selenium sulfide shampoo.
- **Tinea corporis:** Presents as annular, marginated plaques with a thin scale and a clear center. Common organisms include *Trichophyton mentagrophytes* and *M canis*. Treatment includes griseofulvin, itraconazole, and clotrimazole cream.
- **Tinea pedis:** Presents with red, scaly soles; maceration and fissuring and occasionally with blisters between the toes. Treatment includes griseofulvin, terbinafine, itraconazole, and antifungal foot powder.
- **Onychomycosis:** Initially presents with a loosened nail plate, yellow discoloration, and thickening of the distal nail plate. This is followed by scaling of the nail plate. *Trichophyton rubrum* and *T mentagrophytes* are the most common causes. Treatment includes terbinafine and itraconazole.
- **Tinea versicolor:** Hypopigmented macules in areas of sun-induced pigmentation. During winter, the macules appear reddish-brown. Treatment includes griseofulvin, topical selenium sulfide, and topical ketoconazole.

Genitourinary Disorders

ERECTILE DYSFUNCTION (ED)

Inability to achieve or maintain an erection sufficient to effect penetration and ejaculation. Affects 30 million men. Associated with age; some degree of ED is seen in 40% of 40-year-olds and in 70% of 70-year-olds. Etiologies are as follows:

- **Psychological:**
  - Symptoms often have a sudden onset.
  - Patients are unable to sustain or sometimes even obtain an erection.
  - Patients have normal nocturnal penile tumescence (those with organic causes do not).

- **Organic:**
  - **Endocrine:** DM, hypothyroidism or thyrotoxicosis, pituitary or gonadal disorders, ↑ prolactin.
  - **Vascular:** Atherosclerosis of penile arteries or venous leaks.
  - **Neurologic:** Stroke, DM, temporal lobe seizure, MS, spinal surgery, neuropathy.
- **Exogenous:** Drugs that cause ED include β-blockers, SSRIs, α-blockers, clonidine, CNS depressants, anticholinergics, chronic opioids, and TCAs.

> **KEY FACT**
>
> DM is associated with both vascular and neurologic causes of ED.

EXAM

- Look for exam findings suggesting an organic cause—eg, small testes, evidence of Peyronie's disease, perineal sensation/cremaster reflex, evidence of peripheral neuropathy, or galactorrhea.
- Assess peripheral pulses; look for skin atrophy, hair loss, and low skin temperature.

DIAGNOSIS

Assess **TSH, prolactin, and testosterone**; order a fasting glucose to assess for diabetes.

TREATMENT

- PDE-5a inhibitors (sildenafil [Viagra], tadalafil, vardenafil) inhibit cGMP-specific phosphodiesterase type 5a, thereby improving relaxation of smooth muscle in the corpora cavernosa. Side effects include flushing, headache, and ↓ BP. Patients cannot be on nitrates or α-blockers.
- Injectable therapies such as alprostadil are also available.
- An external penile pump in combination with a PDE-5a inhibitor may be useful.
- For those who fail medical therapy, an inflatable penile prosthesis is available.
- Give testosterone for hypogonadism; behavioral treatment is appropriate for depression and anxiety. A PDE-5a inhibitor may be effective for patients with psychogenic causes.
- Vascular surgery if indicated.

BENIGN PROSTATIC HYPERPLASIA (BPH)

Hyperplasia of the prostate that leads to bladder outlet obstruction. Incidence ↑ with age. Common in patients > 45 years of age. In patients < 45 years of age with urinary retention, consider an alternative diagnosis such as a urethral stricture or a neuropathic etiology.

SYMPTOMS/EXAM

- Patients complain of frequency, urgency, nocturia, ↓ force and size of the urine stream, and incomplete emptying leading to overflow incontinence.
- Exam reveals a firm, rubbery, smooth prostatic surface (versus the rock-hard areas that suggest prostate cancer).

DIAGNOSIS

Diagnosed by an appropriate history and exam. Check a UA for infection or hematuria, both of which should prompt further evaluation. PSA is elevated in up to 50% of patients but is not diagnostically useful.

TREATMENT

- α-blockers (terazosin), 5α-reductase inhibitors (finasteride).
- Avoid anticholinergics, antihistamines, or narcotics.
- If the condition is refractory to medications, consider surgical options such as transurethral resection of the prostate (TURP). An open procedure is appropriate if gland size is > 75 g. In general, indications for TURP include recurrent UTIs, bladder stones, hematuria, episodes of acute urinary retention, and renal failure 2° to obstruction.

WORKUP OF PROSTATIC NODULES AND ABNORMAL PSA

- Significant controversy surrounds prostate cancer screening, with different groups offering varying recommendations ranging from no screening at all to a yearly rectal exam and PSA testing (see Table 2-1).
- If an abnormality is found on exam, proceed to prostatic biopsy.
- The PSA may be used as a marker to follow the response to prostate cancer treatment. With successful cancer treatments, PSA falls to undetectable levels.

Health Care Maintenance

A 41-year-old woman who recently acquired health insurance comes to your primary care clinic for the first checkup in her life. She has no current complaints and no known past medical history, and she doesn't smoke, drink, or use drugs. She has never had children. She has a stable partner with whom she has been in a monogamous relationship for 20 years. Her mother had type 2 DM. Her physical exam is within normal limits, and she is not overweight. Which screening tests might you recommend?

An otherwise healthy 41-year-old woman would be well served by a Pap smear, a breast exam, and hypertension screening. Given her family history of DM, a fasting glucose test or a two-hour glucose tolerance test would be considered appropriate as well. Given her age, a screening mammogram is controversial. It is important to discuss the risks, benefits, and alternatives of screening before proceeding.

CANCER SCREENING

Table 2-1 outlines recommended guidelines for the screening of common forms of cancer.

TABLE 2-1. Recommended Cancer Screening Guidelines

TYPE OF CANCER	RECOMMENDATIONS
Cervical cancer	An annual Pap smear is recommended starting at age 21 or within three years of onset of sexual activity. Patients should be screened annually until three consecutive normal results, after which the frequency of screening may be ↓ to every three years.
Breast cancer	Monthly self-examination and an annual exam by a physician. Mammography should be conducted every two years after age 50 (may start earlier if there is a ⊕ family history at a young age). The age at which mammographic screening should begin is the subject of controversy. The USPSTF recommends biennial screening mammography for women 50–74 years of age. For patients in their 40s, it is recommended that the decision to begin screening be thoroughly discussed with their doctors.
Colon cancer	Hemoccult annually (especially in patients > 50 years of age); flex sigmoidoscopy (every 3–5 years in those > 50) or colonoscopy (every 10 years in those > 50). If a first-degree relative has colon cancer, begin screening at age 40 or when the patient is 10 years younger than the age at which that relative was diagnosed, whichever comes first.
Prostate cancer	Controversial. Some groups recommend no screening; others recommend a yearly rectal exam and PSA beginning at age 45, especially for African Americans and for patients with a strong family history.

OTHER ROUTINE SCREENING

- **Hypertension:** BP screening should be done at every clinic visit. For young patients (age < 50) with elevated BP, look for 2° causes of hypertension, such as chronic kidney disease, pheochromocytoma, thyroid/parathyroid disease, sleep apnea, renovascular disease, Cushing's syndrome, coarctation of the aorta, and 1° hyperaldosteronism.
- **Hyperlipidemia:** The U.S. Preventive Services Task Force (USPSTF) strongly recommends screening men ≥ 35 years of age and women ≥ 45 years of age for lipid disorders. Treatment goals vary depending on risk factors (see Table 2-2). However, some people suggest that statins should be put in drinking water along with fluoride. Risk factors that modify LDL goals include the following:
  - Cigarette smoking.
  - Hypertension (BP ≥ 140/90 mm Hg or on antihypertensive medication).
  - Low HDL cholesterol (< 40 mg/dL).
  - A family history of premature CAD (CAD in a male first-degree relative < 55 years of age; CAD in a female first-degree relative < 65 years of age).
  - Age (men ≥ 45 years; women ≥ 55 years).

- The Framingham risk calculator may be used to determine the 10-year risk of developing CAD and includes age, gender, total cholesterol, HDL, smoking status, and systolic BP.
- **Diabetes:** The ADA recommends testing for diabetes or prediabetes in all adults with a BMI ≥ 25 kg/m² and one or more additional risk factors for diabetes (see below). In individuals without risk factors, testing should begin at age 45. Either fasting plasma glucose or a two-hour oral glucose tolerance test is appropriate. Additional risk factors for diabetes are as follows:
  - A family history of DM in a first-degree relative.
  - Habitual physical inactivity.
  - Belonging to a high-risk ethnic or racial group (eg, African American, Hispanic, Native American, Asian American, Pacific Islander).
  - A history of delivering a baby weighing > 4.1 kg (9 lbs) or of gestational diabetes.
  - Hypertension (BP ≥ 140/90 mm Hg).
  - Dyslipidemia.
  - Polycystic ovary syndrome.
  - A history of vascular disease.
- **Osteoporosis:** The USPSTF recommends that women ≥ 65 years of age be screened routinely for osteoporosis. Screening should begin at age 60 for women at ↑ risk for osteoporotic fractures (eg, low weight, low estrogen state). DEXA is the screening test of choice.
- **Abdominal aortic aneurysm (AAA):** The USPSTF recommends one-time screening for AAA in men 65–75 years of age who have smoked at any time. Abdominal ultrasound is the screening test of choice.

TABLE 2-2. Treatment of Hyperlipidemia

Risk Category	LDL Treatment Goal (mg/dL)
High risk (CAD or CAD equivalent)	< 100 to < 70
Moderate risk (2+ risk factors)	< 130
Low risk (< 2 risk factors)	< 160

IMMUNIZATIONS

Table 2-3 lists indications for adult immunizations.

TABLE 2-3. Indications for Immunization in Adults

IMMUNIZATION	INDICATION/RECOMMENDATION
Tetanus	Give 1° series in childhood, then boosters every 10 years.
Hepatitis B	Administer to all young adults and to patients at ↑ risk (eg, IV drug users, health care providers, those with chronic liver disease).
Pneumococcal	Give to those > 65 years of age or to any patient at ↑ risk (eg, splenectomy, HIV, or immunocompromised patients on chemo or posttransplant).
Influenza	Give annually to all patients > 50 years of age and to high-risk patients.
Hepatitis A	Give to those traveling to endemic areas, those with chronic liver disease (hepatitis B or C), and IV drug abusers.
Zoster	Recommended for all patients ≥ 60 years of age who have no contraindications, including those who report a previous episode of zoster or who have chronic medical conditions.
Smallpox	Currently recommended only for those working in laboratories in which they are exposed to the virus.
Meningococcal	Not recommended for routine use. Used in outbreaks. There is an ↑ risk of disease in college students, but the vaccine is only suggested and is not mandatory in this group.

CHAPTER 3

CARDIOVASCULAR

Ischemic Heart Disease

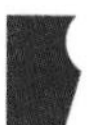

KEY FACT

Major risk factors for ischemic heart disease:

- Age > 65
- Male gender
- Family history
- Smoking
- Hypertension
- Hyperlipidemia
- Diabetes mellitus

KEY FACT

Unstable angina is any new angina or accelerating stable angina.

KEY FACT

Watch out for diabetics! They often present with ischemic disease with highly atypical symptoms. Diabetes is considered a CAD equivalent.

The 1° cause of ischemic heart disease is atherosclerotic occlusion of the coronary arteries. **Major risk factors** include age, family history, smoking, diabetes, hypertension, and hyperlipidemia.

Symptoms

- **May be asymptomatic.**
- **Stable angina** presents with substernal chest tightness/pain or shortness of breath with a consistent amount of exertion; relief is obtained with rest or nitroglycerin. Reflects a stable, flow-limiting plaque.
- **Unstable angina (acute coronary syndrome)** presents with chest tightness/pain and/or shortness of breath, typically at rest, that does not totally improve with nitroglycerin or recurs soon after nitroglycerin. Reflects plaque rupture with formation of a clot in the lumen of the blood vessel.

Exam

- Exam can be normal when the patient is asymptomatic. During episodes of angina, an S4 or a mitral regurgitation murmur may occasionally be heard.
- Look for signs of heart failure (eg, ↑ JVD, bibasilar crackles, lower extremity edema) from prior MI causing left ventricular dysfunction.
- Look for vascular disease elsewhere—eg, bruits, asymmetric or diminished pulses, and lower extremity ischemic ulcers.

Differential

Consider pericarditis, pulmonary embolism, pneumothorax, aortic dissection, peptic ulcer, esophageal disease (including diffuse esophageal spasm), GERD, and musculoskeletal causes.

Diagnosis

- **Initial workup:** Elevated cardiac biomarkers (troponin, CK, CK-MB) +/– ECG changes (ST elevation/depression/Q waves); CXR to rule out dissection.
- **Stress testing:** Exercise or dobutamine to ↑ HR; ECG, echocardiography, or radionuclide imaging to assess perfusion (see the discussion of advanced cardiac evaluation below).
- **Cardiac catheterization:** Defines the location and severity of lesions.

Treatment

- **Acute coronary syndrome:** Initial treatment includes heparin (frequently LMWH), aspirin, nitroglycerin, oxygen, morphine, and an ACEI. GPIIb/IIIa antagonists (abciximab, eptifibatide, tirofiban) and angioplasty are also employed.
- **To slow progression: Control diabetes,** ↓ BP, ↓ cholesterol (**goal for low-density cholesterol < 70 mg/dL**), and encourage **smoking cessation.**
- **To prevent angina:** β-blockers ↓ HR, ↑ myocardial perfusion time, and ↓ cardiac workload, which ↓ exertional angina. If symptoms arise on a β-blocker, a long-acting nitrate or calcium channel blocker (CCB) can be added.
- **To prevent MI: Aspirin;** clopidogrel can be given to aspirin-sensitive patients.
- **Drugs that have been shown to improve mortality after MI:** Aspirin, β-blockers, ACEIs (or angiotensin receptor blockers [ARBs] in ACEI-intolerant patients), and HMG-CoA reductase inhibitors.

Valvular Disease

Table 3-1 describes the clinical characteristics and treatment of common valvular lesions.

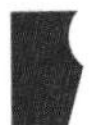

KEY FACT

Ventricular septal defects are holosystolic murmurs that radiate all over the precordium with a thrill. They are the most common cardiac malformation at birth.

TABLE 3-1. Presentation and Treatment of Select Valvular Lesions

Lesion	Symptoms	Exam	Treatment	Comments
Mitral stenosis	Symptoms of heart failure; hemoptysis; atrial fibrillation (AF).	Diastolic murmur best heard at the apex; opening snap; usually does not radiate.	HR control, balloon valvuloplasty, valve replacement.	Usually caused by **rheumatic fever.**
Mitral regurgitation	Has a long asymptomatic period; when severe or acute, presents with symptoms of heart failure.	**Blowing** systolic murmur at the apex, **radiating to the axillae.** The posterior leaflet may lead to a murmur along the sternal border.	If acute, surgery is always required. For chronic mitral regurgitation, repair or replace the valve when symptomatic or if the ejection fraction (EF) is < 60%.	Long-standing regurgitation dilates the atrium, increasing the chance of AF.
Mitral valve prolapse	Asymptomatic.	Midsystolic click; also murmur if mitral regurgitation is present.	Endocarditis prophylaxis is not required.	Questionable association with palpitations and panic attacks. The most common cause of mitral regurgitation.
Aortic stenosis	Chest pain, syncope, heart failure, shortness of breath.	Harsh systolic crescendo-decrescendo murmur radiating to the carotids and right sternal border. **A small and slow carotid upstroke** (parvus et tardus) is seen with severe stenosis.	**Avoid overdiuresis; avoid vasodilators** such as nitrates and ACEIs. Surgery for all symptomatic patients.	Once symptoms appear, mortality is 50% at three years.
Aortic regurgitation	Usually asymptomatic until advanced; then presents with symptoms of heart failure.	**Wide pulse pressure;** soft, high-pitched diastolic murmur along the left sternal border. Radiates toward the apex.	**Afterload reduction** with ACEIs, hydralazine; valve replacement if symptomatic or in the setting of a ↓ EF.	Many cases are associated with aortic root disease, dissection, syphilis, ankylosing spondylitis, and Marfan's syndrome.

Heart Failure (Congestive Heart Failure)

A 58-year-old man with long-standing hypertension is admitted to the hospital with dyspnea on exertion and bibasilar crackles, and you suspect CHF as the cause of his symptoms. Which imaging modality would you order to confirm your diagnosis?

Echocardiography.

Defined as inability of the heart to pump adequate blood to meet the demands of the body. Can be categorized in different ways. One such categorization scheme includes the following:

- Systolic dysfunction
- Diastolic dysfunction
- Valvular dysfunction
- Arrhythmia causing heart failure

SYSTOLIC HEART FAILURE

Weakened pumping function of the heart. Common causes include **ischemic heart disease, long-standing hypertension,** and viral or idiopathic cardiomyopathy in younger patients.

Symptoms

- Patients present with poor exercise tolerance, exertional dyspnea, and easy fatigability.
- If patients are volume overloaded, they may present with **orthopnea,** paroxysmal nocturnal dyspnea, and ankle swelling.

Exam

Exam will reveal bibasilar crackles, a diffuse PMI that is displaced to the left (reflects cardiomegaly), an **S3 gallop,** JVD (normal is about 0–2 cm vertical elevation above the sternomanubrial junction), and lower extremity edema.

Differential

Deconditioning, lung disease (eg, COPD), other categories of heart failure (eg, diastolic dysfunction), other causes of edema (eg, vascular incompetence, low albumin, nephrotic syndrome).

Diagnosis

- The history and exam are suggestive, but determination of the EF via an imaging study (eg, **echocardiography,** radionuclide imaging, cardiac MRI) confirms the diagnosis.
- **Look for the cause of the low EF:**
  - Perform a stress test or cardiac catheterization to look for CAD; obtain TSH levels.
  - Look for a history of alcohol use or exposure to offending medications such as **doxorubicin.**
  - Dilated cardiomyopathy is seen in postpartum females.
  - A myocardial biopsy may be performed in selected cases.

Treatment

- **Maintenance medications** include the following:
  - **β-blockers:** Metoprolol, bisoprolol, **carvedilol.**
  - **Afterload reduction:** Ideally an **ACEI** or an ARB.
  - **Other:** Give spironolactone if the potassium level is not high and the patient is on optimal dosages of β-blockers and ACEIs/ARBs. Digoxin may lower the frequency of hospitalizations and improve symptoms but does not ↓ mortality. Hydralazine and long-acting nitrates may be used in African Americans.
- **Exacerbations:** Give **loop diuretics** such as furosemide when the patient is volume overloaded.
- **Automatic implantable cardiac defibrillators (AICDs)** are associated with ↓ mortality from VT/VF when the EF is < 35%.
- Treat the cause of the systolic heart failure (eg, CAD).

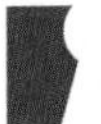

KEY FACT

ACEIs, ARBs, and spironolactone all cause hyperkalemia.

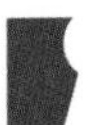

KEY FACT

Ventricular tachycardia leading to ventricular fibrillation is a common cause of death in patients with a ↓ ejection fraction. For this reason, AICD placement is indicated for patients with an EF < 35%.

DIASTOLIC HEART FAILURE

During diastole, the heart is **stiff** and does not relax well, resulting in ↑ diastolic filling pressure. **Hypertension with left ventricular hypertrophy** (LVH) is the most common cause; other causes include hypertrophic cardiomyopathy and infiltrative diseases such as amyloidosis and sarcoidosis.

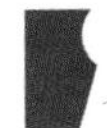

KEY FACT

Important 2° causes of diastolic heart failure:

- Sarcoidosis
- Amyloidosis
- Hemochromatosis
- Scleroderma
- Fibrosis (radiation, surgery)

Symptoms/Exam

- Symptoms are the same as those of systolic heart failure.
- Exam findings are similar to those of systolic failure. Listen for an **S4** rather than an S3.

Differential

The same as that for systolic heart failure.

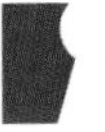

KEY FACT

Don't forget—systolic heart failure is associated with a low ejection fraction, whereas diastolic heart failure often has a normal-to-elevated ejection fraction.

Diagnosis

- Presents with symptoms of heart failure with a normal EF on echocardiogram.
- Echocardiography usually shows ventricular hypertrophy. Biopsy may be needed to establish the underlying diagnosis if infiltrative disease is suspected. MRI is becoming increasingly popular.

Treatment

- Control hypertension.
- Give diuretics to control volume overload and symptoms, but **avoid overdiuresis,** which ↓ preload and cardiac output.

KEY FACT

Active ischemia can acutely worsen diastolic dysfunction, so treat any coexisting CAD!

CARDIOMYOPATHIES

- **Dilated cardiomyopathy:** Frequently caused by ischemia, tachycardia, hypertension, alcohol, and Chagas' disease (in South America). Echocardiography is useful for diagnosis. Treat with ACEIs, ARBs, β-blockers, and spironolactone. Digoxin can improve symptoms but does not improve mortality.
- **Restrictive cardiomyopathy:** Associated with sarcoid, amyloid, hemochromatosis, cancer, and glycogen storage disease. ECG shows low voltage. Echocardiography is useful for diagnosis and shows LVH, but biopsy is occasionally required to determine the underlying cause. Treatment is directed at the underlying cause and also involves diuretics.

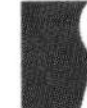

KEY FACT

Alcoholic and tachycardia-induced cardiomyopathy are almost completely reversible through removal of the offending source.

- **Hypertrophic cardiomyopathy:** Genetically inherited in an autosomal dominant pattern; associated with sudden death. Echocardiography is useful for diagnosis and may reveal a normal EF and an asymmetrically thickened ventricle. Treat with β-blockers, CCBs, or disopyramide. Inotropes (eg, digoxin), vasodilators, and excessive diuresis should be avoided.

VALVULAR CAUSES OF HEART FAILURE

- Right-sided valvular lesions do not typically cause heart failure but can cause profound edema that is refractory to diuresis.
- Left-sided valvular lesions can produce heart failure.

ARRHYTHMIA CAUSING HEART FAILURE

- This cause of heart failure is generally apparent from palpitations or ECG.
- Rhythms that can cause symptoms of heart failure include rapid **AF** and bradyarrhythmias. Others present abruptly with palpitations, shortness of breath, or even syncope.

Pericardial Disease

PERICARDITIS

A 54-year-old business executive develops chest pain while at work. His vital signs remain stable. The chest pain is partially relieved by nitroglycerin but worsens with cough and deep inspiration. He is brought to the ER, where his ECG reveals diffuse ST-T elevations. His cardiac enzymes are normal. What is the appropriate treatment?

NSAIDs for pericarditis.

Inflammation of the pericardial sac. May be acute (< 6 weeks; most common), subacute (6 weeks to 6 months), or chronic (> 6 months). Causes include viral infection (especially enterovirus), mediastinal radiation, post-MI (Dressler's syndrome), cancer, rheumatologic diseases (SLE, RA), uremia, TB, and prior cardiac surgery. May also be idiopathic.

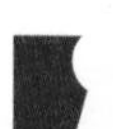

KEY FACT

Remember, chest pain that is improved by sitting up or leaning forward and diffuse ST-segment elevation with PR depression are frequently associated with pericarditis.

SYMPTOMS/EXAM

- Presents with **chest pain** that is often improved by sitting up or leaning forward. The pain may radiate to the back and to the left trapezial ridge.
- If a large effusion is present, the patient may be short of breath.
- Exam may reveal a pericardial friction rub (a leathery sound that is inconstant).

DIFFERENTIAL

Myocardial ischemia, aortic dissection, pneumonia, pulmonary embolism, pneumothorax.

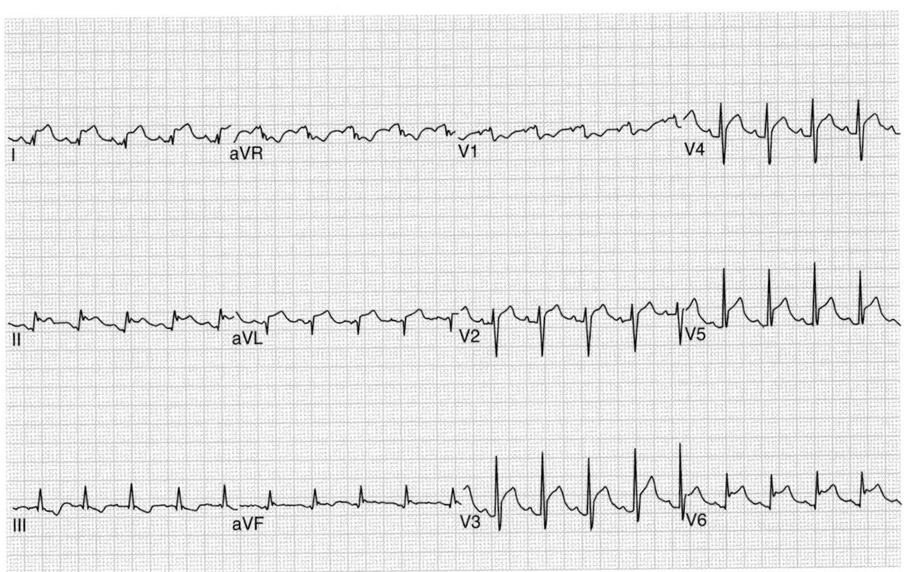

FIGURE 3-1. Pericarditis. Note diffuse ST-segment elevation.

DIAGNOSIS

- Look for diffuse ST-segment elevation (often with upward concavity) on ECG (see Figure 3-1) and PR-segment depression. ECG changes in pericarditis tend to be more generalized. Sequential ECGs are helpful in distinguishing pericarditis from MI, as in the latter, ECG changes tend to normalize more rapidly.
- Echocardiography may reveal an associated effusion.
- Search for an underlying cause—ie, take a history for viral illness, radiation exposure, and malignancy. Check ANA, PPD, blood cultures if febrile, and renal function.
- In North America, TB is an uncommon cause of chronic constrictive pericarditis that presents with ascites, hepatomegaly, and distended neck veins. A chest CT or cardiac MRI will be needed for diagnosis, and pericardial resection may be required. Prior pericardiotomy for cardiac surgery is a more common cause of chronic constrictive pericarditis in North America.

TREATMENT

- Where possible, treat the underlying disorder, such as SLE or advanced renal failure.
- For viral or idiopathic pericarditis, give NSAIDs, colchicine, or aspirin. Avoid NSAIDs in post-MI pericarditis, as they may interfere with scar formation.

COMPLICATIONS

Patients may develop a clinically significant pericardial effusion and **tamponade** (see below).

PERICARDIAL EFFUSION AND CARDIAC TAMPONADE

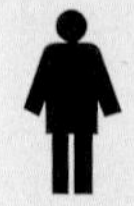

A 62-year-old man suddenly develops hypotension and shortness of breath one day after CABG surgery. Exam reveals JVD and muffled heart sounds. Echocardiography reveals tamponade physiology. What is your next step?

Pericardiocentesis.

Accumulation of fluid (usually chronic) or blood (usually acute and posttraumatic/postsurgical) in the pericardial cavity surrounding the heart.

SYMPTOMS/EXAM

- If **acute,** patients may present with **shock.** If **chronic,** patients may present with **shortness of breath and heart failure. One to two liters of fluid may gradually accumulate.**
- Exam reveals distant heart sounds, elevated JVP, and pulsus paradoxus (more than a 10-mm Hg drop in systolic BP during inspiration).

DIFFERENTIAL

Pneumothorax, MI, cardiac failure.

KEY FACT

Echocardiography is the diagnostic procedure of choice when tamponade is suspected.

DIAGNOSIS

Echocardiography is needed to confirm the diagnosis. CXR may show a large cardiac silhouette (see Figure 3-2), and ECG may show low voltages and electrical alternans.

TREATMENT

Consider emergent pericardiocentesis for patients with post–chest trauma shock as well as for those in whom echocardiography shows evidence of tamponade physiology. Also consider a pericardial window for those with recurrent or malignant effusions.

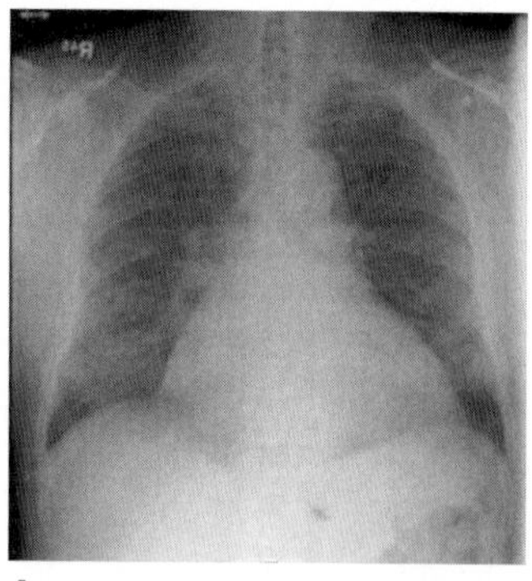

A

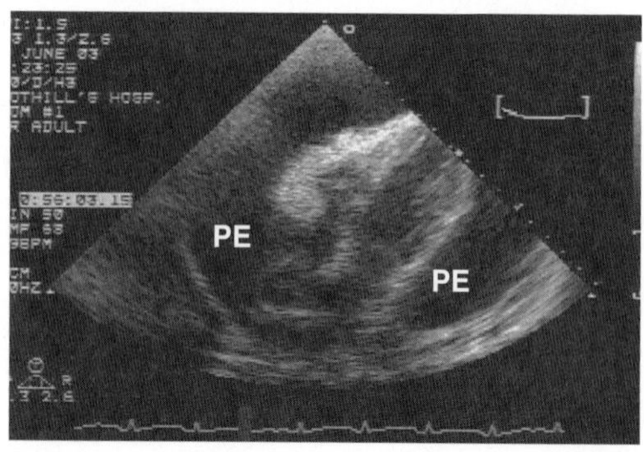

B

FIGURE 3-2. Pericardial effusion and tamponade. (**A**) CXR with enlargement of the cardiac silhouette ("water-bottle heart") in a patient with a pericardial effusion. (**B**) Apical four-chamber transthoracic echocardiogram with a large pericardial effusion (PE) and collapse of the right atrium and right ventricle during diastole in a patient with cardiac tamponade. (Image A reproduced with permission from USMLERx.com. Image B reproduced with permission from Hall JB et al. *Principles of Critical Care,* 3rd ed. New York: McGraw-Hill, 2005, Fig. 28-7A.)

TABLE 3-2. Stressing Modalities in Cardiac Testing

Stressing Modality	Pros	Cons
Treadmill	Good for patients who can walk.	–
Dobutamine	Good for patients who cannot exercise.	–
Adenosine or dipyridamole (with nuclear imaging)	Good for patients who cannot exercise.	Can cause bronchospasm—be cautious in patients with asthma/COPD.

Advanced Cardiac Evaluation

- **Indications for stress testing** include the following (not exhaustive):
  - Diagnosis of CAD/evaluation of symptoms.
  - Preoperative evaluation.
  - Risk stratification in patients with known disease.
  - Decision making about the need for revascularization.
- **Contraindications** include severe aortic stenosis, acute coronary syndrome, and decompensated heart failure.
- Testing consists of a stressing modality and an evaluating modality (see Tables 3-2 and 3-3).
  - The stressor can be walking on a treadmill or IV dobutamine.
  - Evaluating modalities are ECG, echocardiography, and nuclear imaging such as thallium.

TABLE 3-3. Evaluating Modalities in Cardiac Testing

Evaluating Modality	Pros	Cons
ECG	Inexpensive.	Cannot localize the lesion; cannot use with baseline ST-segment abnormalities or left bundle branch block (LBBB); cannot use if the patient is on digoxin.
Echocardiography	Good in patients with LBBB; cheaper than nuclear imaging.	Technically limited echo images or resting wall motion abnormalities can limit usefulness.
Radionuclide tracer (thallium or technetium)	Localizes ischemia; localizes infarcted tissue.	Expensive.

- An additional testing method combines adenosine or dipyridamole with nuclear imaging.
  - These agents dilate the coronary arteries, but areas with plaque cannot vasodilate.
  - Such agents thus ↑ blood flow in healthy arteries but cause no change in diseased arteries, thereby creating a differential flow that is detected on nuclear imaging.

Hypertension

A 40-year-old patient with a history of diabetes and hypertension who is currently on a thiazide and metformin has BP readings of 150/90 and 140/95 on multiple office visits. In the past you have tried adding an ACEI, but the patient developed a cough with the medication. What class of antihypertensive would you start next?

Discontinue the ACEI and start the patient on an ARB.

A major contributor to cardiovascular disease; more common with increasing age and among African Americans.

Symptoms

Asymptomatic unless severe. If severe, patients may complain of chest tightness, shortness of breath, headache, or visual disturbances.

Exam

- BP > 140/90.
- A displaced PMI or an **S4** indicates LVH.
- Fundi show **AV nicking** and "copper-wire" changes to the arterioles. Listen for bruits, which indicate peripheral vascular disease.
- In severe hypertension, look for papilledema and retinal hemorrhages.

Differential

Most cases are essential hypertension, but consider causes of 2° hypertension:

- **Endocrine causes:** Cushing's syndrome, Conn's syndrome (aldosterone-producing tumor), hyperthyroidism, pheochromocytoma.
- **Renal causes:** Chronic kidney disease; renal artery stenosis (listen for an abdominal bruit).
- **Young patients: Fibromuscular dysplasia** of the renal arteries; aortic coarctation.
- **Medications:** OCPs, NSAIDs.
- **Other:** Obstructive sleep apnea, alcohol.

Diagnosis

- Diagnosed in the setting of a **BP > 140/90** on two separate occasions (elevation of either systolic or diastolic BP).
- A systolic BP of 120–139 or a diastolic BP of 80–89 is considered "prehypertension" and predicts the development of hypertension.

TABLE 3-4. Antihypertensive Medications

Commonly Used Classes	Optimal Use	Main Side Effects
Thiazide diuretics	First-line treatment if there is no indication for other agents.	↓ excretion of calcium and uric acid; hyponatremia.
β-blockers	Low EF, **angina, CAD.**	Bradycardia, erectile dysfunction, bronchospasm in asthmatics.
ACEIs	Low EF, chronic kidney disease, diabetes with **microalbuminuria.**	**Cough,** angioedema, hyperkalemia.
ARBs	Same as ACEIs; cough with ACEIs.	Hyperkalemia.
CCBs	Second-line agents.	Lower extremity edema.

Treatment

- The **goal BP** is < 140/90. In diabetics and those with renal insufficiency, the goal is < 130/80.
- **Interventions** include the following:
  - **Step 1—lifestyle modification:** Weight loss, exercise, ↓ sodium intake, smoking cessation.
  - **Step 2—medications: Begin with a thiazide diuretic** unless there is an indication for another class (see Table 3-4). Consider starting two drugs initially if systolic BP is > 160.
  - Control other cardiovascular risk factors, such as diabetes, smoking, and high cholesterol.

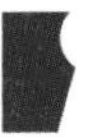

KEY FACT

The goal BP in patients with diabetes or chronic kidney disease is < 130/80.

Complications

Long-standing hypertension contributes to renal failure, heart failure (both systolic and diastolic), CAD, peripheral vascular disease, and stroke.

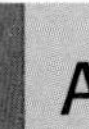

Aortic Dissection

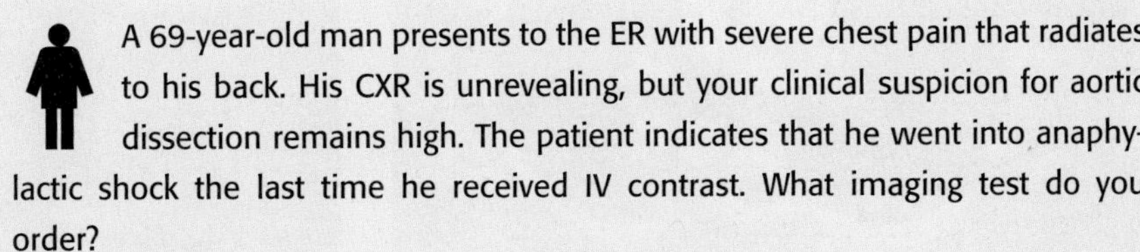

A 69-year-old man presents to the ER with severe chest pain that radiates to his back. His CXR is unrevealing, but your clinical suspicion for aortic dissection remains high. The patient indicates that he went into anaphylactic shock the last time he received IV contrast. What imaging test do you order?

Transesophageal echocardiography (TEE) in light of the contraindication to performing a CT scan with IV contrast in this patient.

Most common in patients with a history of long-standing hypertension, cocaine use, or aortic root disease such as Marfan's syndrome or Takayasu's arteritis.

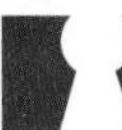

KEY FACT

Always think about dissection in patients with chest pain!

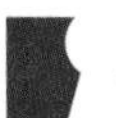

KEY FACT

Risk factors for aortic aneurysm include age > 60, smoking, hypertension, a family history of aortic aneurysm, and hypercholesterolemia. The risk of rupture is low for aneurysms < 4 cm.

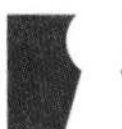

KEY FACT

Surgery is indicated for rapidly expanding aneurysms (> 0.5 cm per year) as well as for large aneurysms to avert the catastrophe of dissection.

Symptoms/Exam

- Presents with sudden onset of severe chest pain that sometimes radiates to the back. May also present with neurologic symptoms resulting from occlusion of vessels supplying the brain or spinal cord.
- On exam, look for aortic regurgitation, **asymmetric pulses and blood pressures,** and neurologic findings.

Differential

MI, pulmonary embolus, pneumothorax.

Diagnosis

- Requires a high index of suspicion.
- CXR has low sensitivity but may show a widened mediastinum or a hazy aortic knob (see Figure 3-3).
- **CT scan with IV contrast** is diagnostic and shows the extent of dissection.
- TEE is highly sensitive and specific.
- MRI may be used, but it is often time consuming and may not be optimal in the setting of an unstable patient.

Treatment

- **Initial medical stabilization:** Aggressive **HR and BP control,** first with β-blockers (typically IV esmolol) and then with IV nitroprusside if needed.
- **Ascending dissection—Stanford type A (involves the ascending aorta): Emergent surgical repair.**
- **Descending dissection—Stanford type B (distal to the left subclavian artery):** Medical management is indicated unless there is intractable pain, progressive dissection in patients with chest pain, or vascular occlusion of the aortic branches (see Figure 3-4).

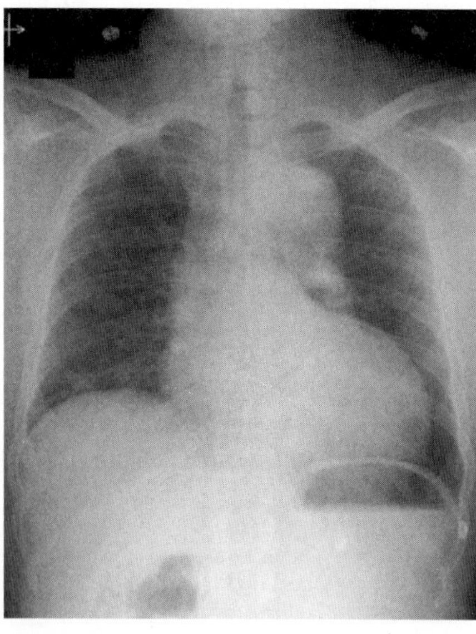

A

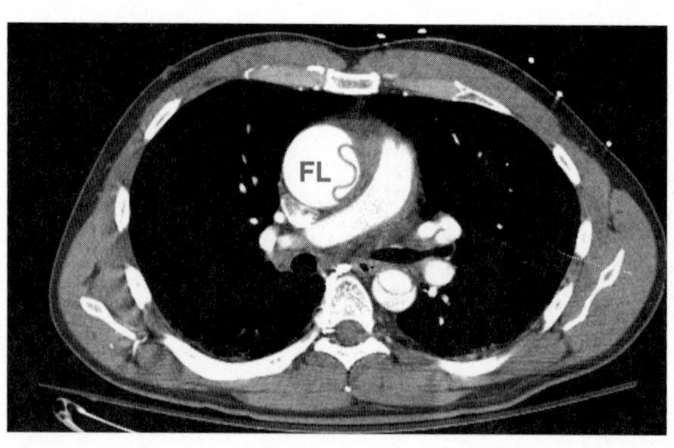

B

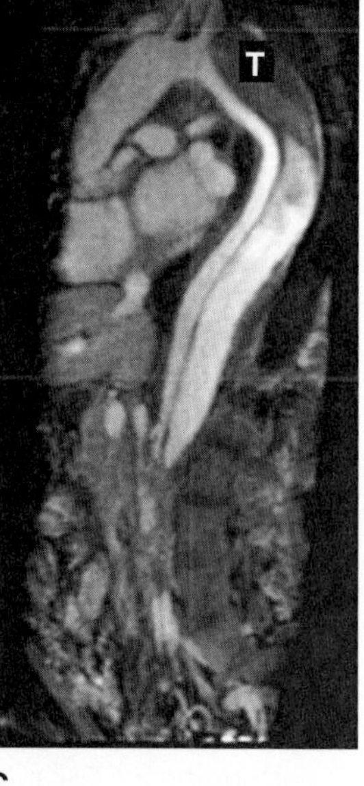

C

FIGURE 3-3. Aortic dissection. (A) Frontal CXR showing a widened mediastinum in a patient with an aortic dissection. (B) Transaxial contrast-enhanced CT showing a dissection involving the ascending and descending aorta (FL, false lumen). (C) Sagittal MRA image showing a dissection involving the descending aorta, with a thrombus (T) in the false lumen. (Images A and C reproduced with permission from USMLERx.com. Image B reproduced with permission from Doherty GM. *Current Diagnosis & Treatment: Surgery,* 13th ed. New York: McGraw-Hill, 2010, Fig. 19-17.)

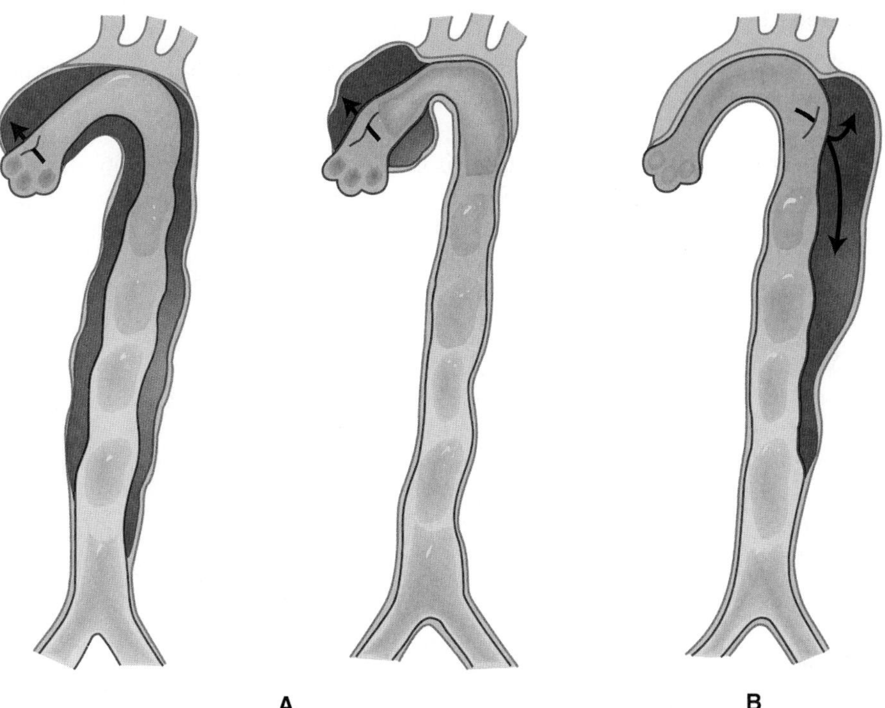

FIGURE 3-4. Ascending vs. descending aortic dissection. (**A**) Proximal or ascending (type A). (**B**) Distal or descending (type B). (Reproduced with permission from Doherty GM. *Current Diagnosis & Treatment: Surgery,* 13th ed. New York: McGraw-Hill, 2010, Fig. 19-16.)

Complications

Aortic rupture, acute aortic regurgitation, tamponade, neurologic impairment, limb or mesenteric ischemia, renal ischemia.

Peripheral Vascular Disease

Atherosclerotic disease of vessels other than the coronary arteries. Risk factors are similar to those for CAD and include **smoking,** diabetes, hypercholesterolemia, hypertension, and increasing age.

Symptoms

Presentation depends on the organ affected:

- **Mesenteric ischemia:** Postprandial abdominal pain and food avoidance.
- **Lower extremities:** Claudication, ulceration, rest pain.
- **Kidneys:** Usually asymptomatic, but may present with difficult-to-control hypertension.
- **CNS:** Stroke and TIA (see Chapter 13).

Exam

- **Mesenteric disease:** No specific findings. The patient may be thin because of weight loss from avoidance of food.
- **Lower extremity disease:** Exam reveals ulcers, diminished pulses, ↓ ankle-brachial indices, skin atrophy and loss of hair, and **bruits** over affected vessels (abdominal, femoral, popliteal).
- **Renal artery stenosis:** Listen for a **bruit during systole and diastole** (highly specific).

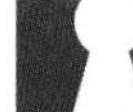

KEY FACT

Acute vessel occlusion from an embolus or an in situ thrombus presents with sudden pain (abdominal or extremity) and is an emergency.

DIFFERENTIAL

- **Abdominal pain:** Stable symptoms can mimic peptic ulcer disease or biliary colic. If the colon is predominantly involved, episodes of pain and bloody stool can look like infectious colitis.
- **Lower extremities: Spinal stenosis** can produce lower extremity discomfort similar to claudication. Claudication improves with standing still, but spinal stenosis classically improves with **sitting** (lumbar flexion improves spinal stenosis symptoms).

DIAGNOSIS

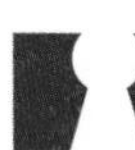

KEY FACT

Peripheral vascular disease is a predictor of CAD.

- **Mesenteric disease:** A diagnosis of exclusion. Angiography reveals lesions.
- **Lower extremity disease:** Diagnosed via the **ankle-brachial index** (compares BP in the lower and upper extremities) and Doppler ultrasound. Angiography or MRA is used in preparation for revascularization but is generally not used for diagnosis.
- **Renal artery stenosis:** CT angiography, MRA, conventional angiography, or ultrasound with Doppler flow (technically difficult).

TREATMENT

- Control risk factors, especially smoking.
- **Mesenteric disease:** Treat with surgical revascularization or angioplasty.
- **Lower extremity disease:** Treat with exercise to improve functional capacity, surgical revascularization, and sometimes angioplasty. Cilostazol is moderately useful (improves pain-free walking distance 50%), whereas pentoxifylline is of marginal benefit.
- **Renal artery stenosis:** Surgery or angioplasty may be of benefit.

Hypercholesterolemia

A 73-year-old man with a history of diabetes mellitus comes to your office for the results of his recent blood work. His fasting lipid panel is significant for an LDL of 130 mg/dL. In addition to educating him on diet and lifestyle changes, what medication would you start?

A statin.

One of the principal factors contributing to atherosclerotic vascular disease. An ↑ LDL and a low concentration of HDL are the 1° contributors. Hypercholesterolemia can be idiopathic, genetic, or 2° to other diseases, such as diabetes, nephrotic syndrome, and hypothyroidism.

SYMPTOMS

Asymptomatic unless the patient develops ischemia (eg, angina, stroke, claudication) or unless severe hypertriglyceridemia leads to pancreatitis.

EXAM

- Look for evidence of atherosclerosis—eg, carotid, subclavian, and other bruits; diminished pulses; or ischemic foot ulcers.
- Look for **xanthomas** (lipid depositions) over the tendons, above the upper eyelid, and on the palms.

Diagnosis

- Diagnosis is based on a lipid panel. A full fasting lipid panel consists of total cholesterol, HDL, LDL, and triglycerides.
  - Because triglycerides rise following a meal, only total cholesterol and HDL can be measured after a meal. Triglycerides and LDL can be measured only when fasting.
  - LDL is not measured directly; it is **calculated** on the basis of total cholesterol, HDL, and triglycerides. **High triglycerides** (> 400 mg/dL) make LDL calculation unreliable.
- Look for other contributing conditions. **Check glucose and TSH;** check body weight, and consider nephrotic syndrome.
- In patients with a family history of early heart disease, consider novel risk factors such as homocysteine, Lp(a), and C-reactive protein. These are treated with folic acid supplementation, niacin, and statins, respectively.

Treatment

Treatment is aimed at preventing pancreatitis when triglycerides are very high as well as preventing atherosclerotic disease (see Table 3-5).

- **Triglycerides:** If > 500 mg/dL, recommend dietary modification (↓ total fat and ↓ saturated fat) and aerobic exercise, and begin medication (fibrate or nicotinic acid). At lower levels, treatment can begin with diet and exercise, and medication can be added as needed. **Treat diabetes** if present.
- **LDL:** In patients with **diabetes or CAD, the goal LDL is < 70 mg/dL.** The mainstay of treatment is diet, exercise, and a statin. LDL control is the 1° cholesterol-related goal in patients with CAD or diabetes.
- **HDL:** Can be modestly ↑ with fibrate or nicotinic acid.

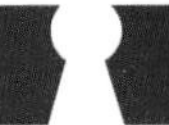
KEY FACT

LDL control is the number-one cholesterol-related goal in patients with CAD or diabetes!

TABLE 3-5. Mechanisms and Side Effects of Cholesterol-Lowering Medications

Medication	Primary Effect	Side Effects	Comments
HMG-CoA reductase inhibitors ("statins")	↓ LDL	Hepatitis, myositis.	A potent LDL-lowering medication.
Cholesterol absorption inhibitors (ezetimibe)	↓ LDL	Generally well tolerated; side effects are the same as those of placebo.	Introduced in 2003; its role in therapy is being defined.
Fibrates (gemfibrozil)	↓ triglycerides, slightly ↑ HDL	Potentiates myositis with statins.	–
Bile acid–binding resins	↓ LDL	Bloating and cramping.	Most patients cannot tolerate GI side effects.
Nicotinic acid (niacin)	↓ LDL, ↑ HDL	Hepatitis, flushing.	Aspirin before doses ↓ flushing.

Infective Endocarditis

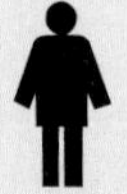

A 26-year-old IV drug user is admitted to the hospital with fevers and chills. Despite broad antibiotic therapy, blood cultures remain persistently ⊕. You suspect infective endocarditis and order a transthoracic echocardiogram (TTE), which is normal. What is your next step?

Order a TEE.

Inflammation of the heart valves. Can be infectious or noninfectious. Infectious endocarditis is commonly seen in IV drug abusers and in those with valvular lesions or prosthetic heart valves.

Symptoms

- **Acute endocarditis:** Presents with fever, rigors, heart failure from valve destruction, and symptoms related to systemic emboli (neurologic impairment, back pain, pulmonary symptoms).
- **Subacute bacterial endocarditis:** Characterized by weeks to months of fever, malaise, and weight loss. Also presents with symptoms of systemic emboli.
- **Noninfectious endocarditis:** Generally asymptomatic. Can cause heart failure by destroying valves.

Exam

- Look for a new **murmur.**
- Findings associated with emboli include focal neurologic deficits and tenderness to percussion over the spine.
- With infectious endocarditis, look at the fingers and toes for deep-seated, painful nodules (**Osler's nodes,** or "Ouchler's nodes") and small skin infarctions (**Janeway lesions**). Retinal exudates are called **Roth's spots.**

Differential

The differential diagnosis of endocarditis is outlined below and in Table 3-6.

- **Differential of a vegetation found on echocardiography:** Infectious endocarditis, nonbacterial thrombotic endocarditis (NBTE, also known as

TABLE 3-6. Causes of Endocarditis

Acute	Subacute	Culture Negative	NBTE (Marantic Endocarditis)	Verrucous (Libman-Sacks)
Most commonly *S aureus*	Viridans streptococci *Enterococcus* *Staphylococcus epidermidis* Gram-negative rods *Candida*	HACEK organisms[a] *Coxiella burnetii* Noncandidal fungi	Thrombus formation on the valve is seen in many cancers	Seen in lupus; vegetation is composed of fibrin, platelets, immune complexes, and inflammatory cells

[a] **HACEK** organisms: ***H**aemophilus aphrophilus* and ***H** parainfluenzae, **A**ctinobacillus actinomycetemcomitans, **C**ardiobacterium hominis, **E**ikenella corrodens, **K**ingella kingae.*

marantic endocarditis), verrucous endocarditis (Libman-Sacks endocarditis), valve degeneration.
- **Differential of bacteremia:** Infectious endocarditis, infected hardware (eg, from a central line), abscess, osteomyelitis.

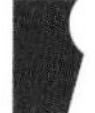

KEY FACT

Streptococcus bovis bacterial endocarditis should raise suspicions for occult GI malignancy. These patients need a colonoscopy.

Diagnosis

- The discovery of noninfectious endocarditis is usually an incidental finding on echocardiography. It may be found during the workup of systemic emboli.
- Infectious endocarditis is diagnosed by a combination of lab and clinical data. If suspicious, obtain **three sets of blood cultures** and an echocardiogram. If the TTE is ⊖, proceed to **TEE** (more sensitive). ⊕ blood cultures and echocardiogram findings diagnose endocarditis. The Duke criteria are often used for diagnosis.

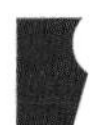

KEY FACT

Any patient with *S aureus* bacteremia should be evaluated for endocarditis with echocardiography.

Treatment

- Treat with **prolonged antibiotic therapy,** generally for 4–6 weeks. Begin empiric therapy with gentamicin and antistaphylococcal penicillin (**oxacillin or nafcillin).** If there is a risk of methicillin-resistant S *aureus,* use vancomycin instead of oxacillin/nafcillin.
- **Valve replacement** is appropriate for fungal endocarditis, **heart failure** from valve destruction, valve ring abscess, or systemic emboli despite adequate antibiotic therapy.
- Following treatment for infectious endocarditis, patients should receive endocarditis prophylaxis.
- For **NBTE,** treat the underlying disorder (often malignancy). Heparin is useful in the short term.
- For **verrucous endocarditis,** no treatment is required. Patients should receive endocarditis prophylaxis (see below).

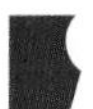

KEY FACT

Surgery is indicated in the setting of hemodynamic instability, valvular destruction, perivalvular extension, and persistently positive blood cultures and should not be delayed while the acute infection is cleared with antibiotics.

Prevention

- Administer endocarditis prophylaxis only to patients whose cardiac conditions are associated with the **highest risk of an adverse outcome from endocarditis.** These include the following:
  - **Congenital cardiac disease:**
    - Patients with unrepaired cyanotic disease, including those with palliative shunts and devices.
    - Patients with congenital cardiac defects that have been completely repaired through use of prosthetic material/devices, whether surgically or percutaneously, during the first six months after the repair procedure (endothelialization occurs after six months).
    - Patients with repaired congenital cardiac disease who have residual defects at or adjacent to the site of a patch device that may inhibit endothelialization.
  - **Other:** Patients with prosthetic heart valves, those with previous infective endocarditis, and cardiac transplant patients with cardiac valvulopathy.
- **Guidelines for antibiotic prophylaxis:**
  - **Dental procedures:** Prophylaxis is appropriate for all dental procedures that involve the manipulation of gingival tissue or the periapical region of teeth, or for procedures involving perforation of the oral mucosa (but **not** for routine anesthetic infections through noninfected tissue, dental radiographs, bleeding from trauma, adjustment of orthodontic devices, or shedding of deciduous teeth).

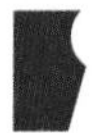

KEY FACT

Don't forget—infective endocarditis requires prolonged antibiotic therapy for 4–6 weeks.

    - **Respiratory tract procedures:** Prophylaxis is indicated for any of the above-mentioned cardiac patients who are undergoing an invasive procedure of the respiratory tract that involves incision or biopsy of the respiratory mucosa (but **not** for bronchoscopy if no biopsy is performed).
    - **Skin procedures:** Prophylaxis is appropriate for any of the above-mentioned cardiac patients who are undergoing procedures involving infected skin, skin structures, or musculoskeletal tissue.
    - **GI and GU procedures:** Prophylaxis is not recommended but may be considered in special scenarios involving the above-mentioned cardiac patients.
- **Prophylactic regimens:** Amoxicillin (or clindamycin/azithromycin for those with penicillin allergy) 30–60 minutes before the procedure.

COMPLICATIONS

Spinal osteomyelitis, valve destruction and heart failure, septic emboli, stroke.

CHAPTER 4

EMERGENCY MEDICINE

Trauma

The acute management of a trauma victim follows a linear algorithm that should be performed in the same order every time: **AcBCDE,** 1° survey, 2° survey. Stabilize the patient at each step before moving on.

ABCs AND THE 1° SURVEY

Trauma treatment should proceed as follows:

- **Ac:** Airway maintenance with **C**ervical spine control.
  - Check the patency of the airway first, and then give supplemental O_2 via nasal cannula, face mask, airway adjunct (nasopharyngeal or oropharyngeal airway), or bag-valve mask (Ambu-Bag) as appropriate.
  - **Indications for intubation** include impending airway compromise, a Glasgow Coma Scale (GCS) score of ≤ 8, ↓ mental status, apnea, and severe closed-head injuries.
  - A surgical airway (**cricothyroidotomy**) should be performed in the setting of significant maxillofacial trauma.
- **B:** **B**reathing with ventilation.
  - Quickly evaluate for **causes of impending cardiopulmonary death**—eg, tension pneumothorax, cardiac tamponade, open pneumothorax, massive hemothorax, or airway obstruction.
- **C:** **C**irculation with hemorrhage control.
  - **Resuscitation:** Think short and fat IV lines—eg, two large-bore (16- or 18-gauge) antecubital lines.
  - A good rule of thumb is to give three times as much isotonic fluid (NS or LR) as the estimated blood lost.
- **D:** **D**isability—determined by a brief neurologic examination:
  - **AVPU system: A** = **A**lert; **V** = responds to **V**ocal stimuli; **P** = responds to **P**ainful stimuli; **U** = **U**nresponsive.
  - **GCS:** Based on the **best** response of E + V + M (see Figure 4-1).
  - **Focused neurologic exam:** Examine for unequal pupils, depressed skull fracture, focal weakness, and posturing.
- **E:** **E**xposure/**E**nvironmental control: Completely undress the patient to assess for injury, but avoid hypothermia.

KEY FACT

Trauma nurses will help you with their own trauma mnemonic: **O-MI** (**O**xygen, cardiac **M**onitor, **I**V access).

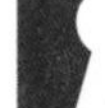

KEY FACT

The maximum score on the GCS is 15; the lowest is 3.

Eye Opening (E)	Verbal Response (V)	Motor Response (M)
4 Spontaneous	**5** Oriented	**6** Obeys commands
3 Responds to voice	**4** Confused speech	**5** Localizes pain
2 Responds to pain	**3** Inappropriate speech	**4** Withdraws to pain
1 No response	**2** Incomprehensible	**3** Abnormal flexion
	1 No response	**2** Abnormal extension
		1 No response

FIGURE 4-1. Scoring of the Glasgow Coma Scale.

2° SURVEY

The 2° survey consists of total patient evaluation as outlined below. This is also the time to order appropriate lab tests and radiographs based on the mechanism of injury, past medical history, and the like.

- **Obtain an AMPLE history:** Inquire about **A**llergies, **M**edications, **P**ast medical history, **L**ast oral intake, and **E**vents/**E**nvironmental factors related to the injury. If the patient can speak, ask about other symptoms that may not be obvious on exam. Obtain as much information as possible about the circumstances of the trauma from EMTs/paramedics, witnesses, and the like.
- **Conduct a focused physical exam:**
  - **Head and skull:** Inspect for trauma, pupils, and loss of consciousness. Examine for hemorrhage around the mastoid **(Battle's sign)**, eyes (**"raccoon eyes"**), and tympanic membrane, all of which are indicative of a **basilar skull fracture.** Inspect the nose for CSF leakage and for an unstable airway due to facial fractures.
  - **Neck:** Look for trauma; palpate for midline tenderness, crepitus, and tracheal deformity.
  - **Chest:** Inspect for irregular or paradoxical breathing patterns resulting from multiple rib fractures—ie, flail chest. Listen for equal and bilateral breath sounds (if not found, or if there is crepitus on palpation of the chest, suspect **pneumothorax**). Listen for clear heart sounds (if muffled and accompanied by JVD, suspect **cardiac tamponade**). A new diastolic murmur after trauma suggests **aortic dissection.**
  - **Abdomen:** Inspect the anterior and posterior abdomen for signs of trauma. Palpate the pelvis for tenderness or instability.
  - **Perineum/rectum/vagina:** Assess for trauma, including urethral bleeding (suggests urethral tear). Check for prostate position, rectal tone, and rectal blood. In female patients, check for vaginal trauma and blood in the vaginal vault.
  - **Musculoskeletal system:** Look for evidence of trauma, including contusions, lacerations, and deformities. Inspect the extremities for tenderness, crepitus, abnormal range of motion, and sensation. An externally rotated, shortened leg suggests **hip fracture**.
- **Management:**
  - **Head and skull:** Maintain the airway; continue oxygenation and ventilation. Obtain a CT scan of the head and face if indicated; intubate if necessary.
  - **Neck:** Maintain in-line immobilization and protection with a hard cervical collar. Obtain radiographs if the C-spine cannot be cleared clinically. If indeterminate, consider CT of the cervical spine (see Figure 4-2).
  - **Chest:** Obtain a CXR and, if necessary, a CT scan. **Tube thoracostomy** for pneumothorax (needle thoracostomy for tension pneumothorax); **pericardiocentesis** for cardiac tamponade; and emergent surgical repair for aortic disruption (see Figure 4-3). Consider placing an NG tube.
  - **Abdomen:** Obtain a pelvic x-ray; arrange for a **FAST (focused abdominal sonography for trauma)** and/or abdominal CT if indicated. Transfer to an OR in the presence of a penetrating wound to the abdomen deeper than the fascia or with any significant bleeding or bowel injury. **Keep any impaled objects in place,** and do not remove them until the patient has been taken to the OR. Stable patients who are cleared of metal shrapnel may have a triple-contrast CT exam first (see Figures 4-4 and 4-5).

KEY FACT

A "trauma series" consists of AP chest, AP abdomen/pelvis, and AP/lateral/odontoid C-spine x-rays.

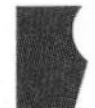

KEY FACT

Criteria for clinical clearance of the cervical spine: The patient is alert and not intoxicated; no posterior midline C-spine tenderness; no neurologic deficit; and no painful distracting injuries.

KEY FACT

The spleen is the most commonly injured solid organ in blunt abdominal trauma.

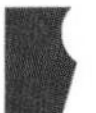

KEY FACT

Cushing's triad (widening pulse pressure, bradycardia, and irregular breathing) indicates ↑ ICP, as from a closed-head injury.

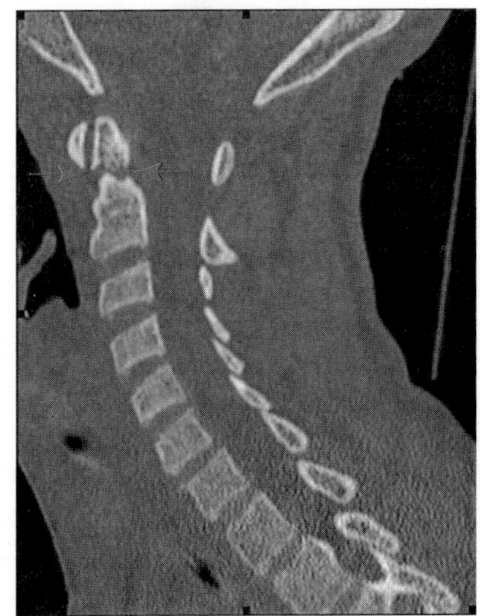

FIGURE 4-2. Cervical spine fracture. A sagittal reformation of a cervical spine CT shows a fracture through the base of the dens, a type 2 odontoid fracture (red arrows). (Reproduced with permission from USMLERx.com.)

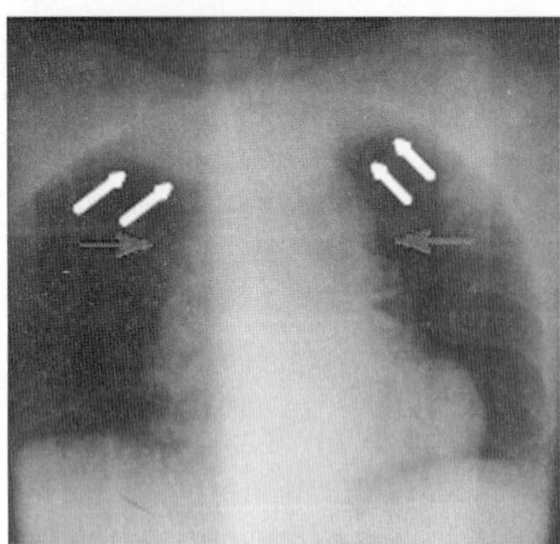

FIGURE 4-3. Aortic injury. A frontal CXR in a trauma patient shows widening of the superior mediastinum (red arrows) with bilateral "apical caps" (white arrows) corresponding to mediastinal bleeding extending into the extrapleural spaces above the lung apices. (Reproduced with permission from Brunicardi FC et al. *Schwartz's Principles of Surgery,* 9th ed. New York: McGraw-Hill, 2010, Fig. 7-23A.)

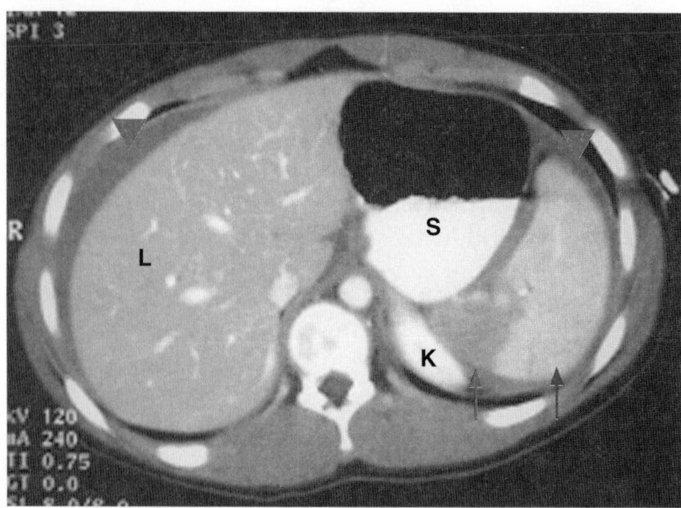

FIGURE 4-5. Abdominal trauma. A transaxial image from an abdominal CT in a trauma patient shows a splenic laceration (red arrow) that enhances less-than-normal splenic tissue (blue arrow) and hemoperitoneum (red arrowheads). L, liver; S, stomach; K, left kidney. (Reproduced with permission from Stone CK, Humphries RL. *Current Diagnosis & Treatment: Emergency Medicine,* 6th ed. New York: McGraw-Hill, 2008, Fig. 23-2.)

KEY FACT

Beck's triad (JVD, muffled heart tones, and hypotension) indicates cardiac tamponade. Sometimes pulsus paradoxus is also noted. Pericardiocentesis brings back unclotted blood.

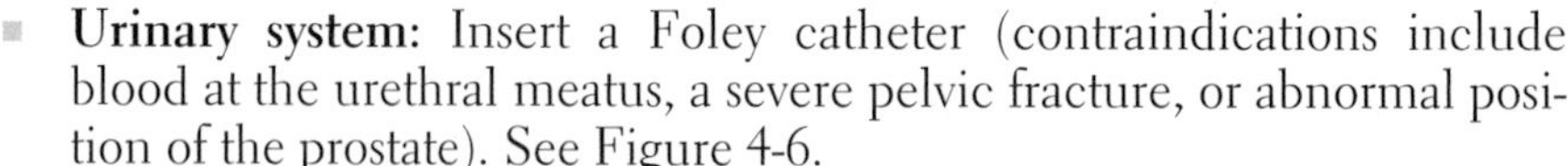

- **Urinary system:** Insert a Foley catheter (contraindications include blood at the urethral meatus, a severe pelvic fracture, or abnormal position of the prostate). See Figure 4-6.
- **Musculoskeletal system:** Wound irrigation and tissue debridement. Obtain an arteriogram if vascular injury is suspected. Obtain radiographs as needed. Maintain immobilization of the patient's thoracic and lumbar spine; apply a splint as indicated. Open fractures and suspected compartment syndromes require urgent orthopedic consultation. Administer tetanus immunization and antibiotics as required.

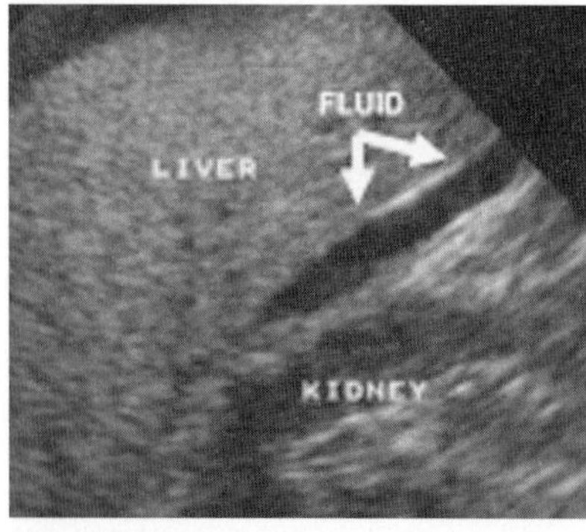

FIGURE 4-4. Positive FAST. Longitudinal image from a trauma FAST ultrasound shows hemoperitoneum (labeled "fluid") in the hepatorenal space. (Reproduced with permission from Brunicardi FC et al. *Schwartz's Principles of Surgery,* 9th ed. New York: McGraw-Hill, 2010, Fig. 7-28A.)

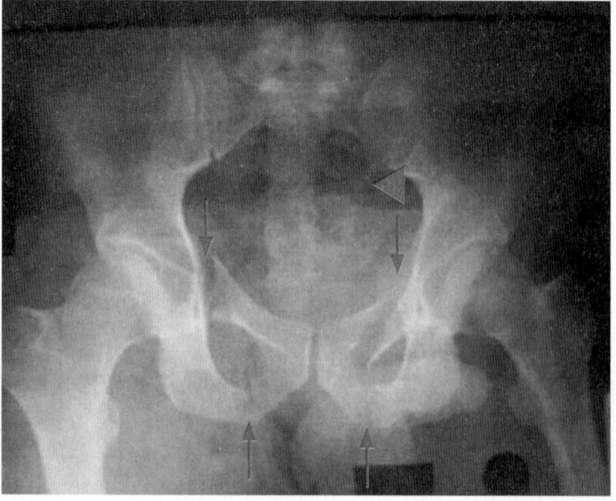

FIGURE 4-6. Pelvic fractures. Frontal pelvic radiograph in a trauma patient shows bilateral superior and inferior pubic ramus fractures (red arrows) and a left sacral fracture (red arrowhead). (Reproduced with permission from Brunicardi FC et al. *Schwartz's Principles of Surgery,* 9th ed. New York: McGraw-Hill, 2010, Fig. 7-30A.)

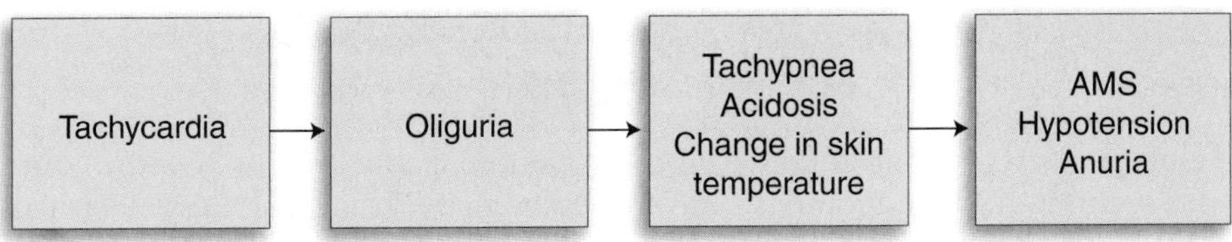

FIGURE 4-7. Symptoms of shock over time.

Shock

Described in the broadest strokes, **shock** is a physiologic **oxygen supply/demand mismatch.** ↓ tissue perfusion leads to cell hypoxia and eventual tissue death. Rapid clinical assessment of circulatory status includes pulse, skin color, and level of consciousness. The evolution of the symptoms of shock is shown in Figure 4-7.

Classically, shock has been divided into four types—**hypovolemic, cardiogenic, distributive,** and **obstructive**—based on physiologic response. Distributive shock, the penultimate, is further subdivided into septic, anaphylactic, and neurogenic shock. These types are all reviewed in Table 4-1.

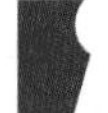

KEY FACT

With increasing blood loss, a patient's mental status progresses from anxiety to agitation to confusion and then to lethargy/unconsciousness.

TABLE 4-1. Hemodynamic Characteristics of Shock

Type of Shock	Major Causes	Cardiac Output	PCWP (≈ LA Pressure)	SVR (Vasoconstriction)	SVO_2	Treatment
Hypovolemic	Trauma, blood loss, inadequate fluid repletion, third spacing, burns.	↓	↓[a]	↑	↓	Crystalloid/blood.
Cardiogenic	MI, CHF, arrhythmia, structural heart disease (eg, severe mitral regurgitation, VSD).	↓[a]	↑	↑	↓	Treat the cause and give pressors (dopamine; norepinephrine or dobutamine if necessary).
Distributive	**Septic:** Bacteremia (especially gram ⊖). **Anaphylactic:** Bee stings; food/medication allergies. **Neurogenic:** Trauma to the spinal cord (leading to loss of autonomic/motor reflexes).	↑	Normal	↓[a]	↑	For **septic shock,** obtain cultures; then give antibiotics, fluid, and pressors (norepinephrine, dopamine). For **anaphylactic shock,** give diphenhydramine (epinephrine if severe).
Obstructive	Cardiac tamponade, tension pneumothorax, pulmonary embolism (PE).	↓	↑/↓[b]	↑	↓	For tamponade, needle pericardiocentesis. For PE, thrombolytics.

[a] Driving force.

[b] ↑ PCWP for tamponade; ↓ PCWP for PE.

KEY FACT

After a premature ventricular contraction (PVC), the sinus rhythm resumes as if the PVC never occurred. After a premature atrial contraction (PAC), however, the sinus rhythm resets as if the PAC were a normal beat.

KEY FACT

"Geminy" refers to the sequence of normal beats with PVCs; bigeminy is a pattern of one normal beat followed by a PVC; and trigeminy is that with two normal beats followed by a PVC.

Common Dysrhythmias

Tables 4-2 and 4-3 illustrate a variety of important dysrhythmias. **Narrow-complex arrhythmias** (eg, reentry supraventricular tachycardia, pulseless electrical activity [PEA]) are more likely to have noncardiac causes (eg, hypovolemia, poor vascular tone), whereas **wide-complex arrhythmias** (eg, V-tach, VF) are more likely to have cardiac causes (or electrolyte imbalances and toxins).

TABLE 4-2. Common Bradyarrhythmias

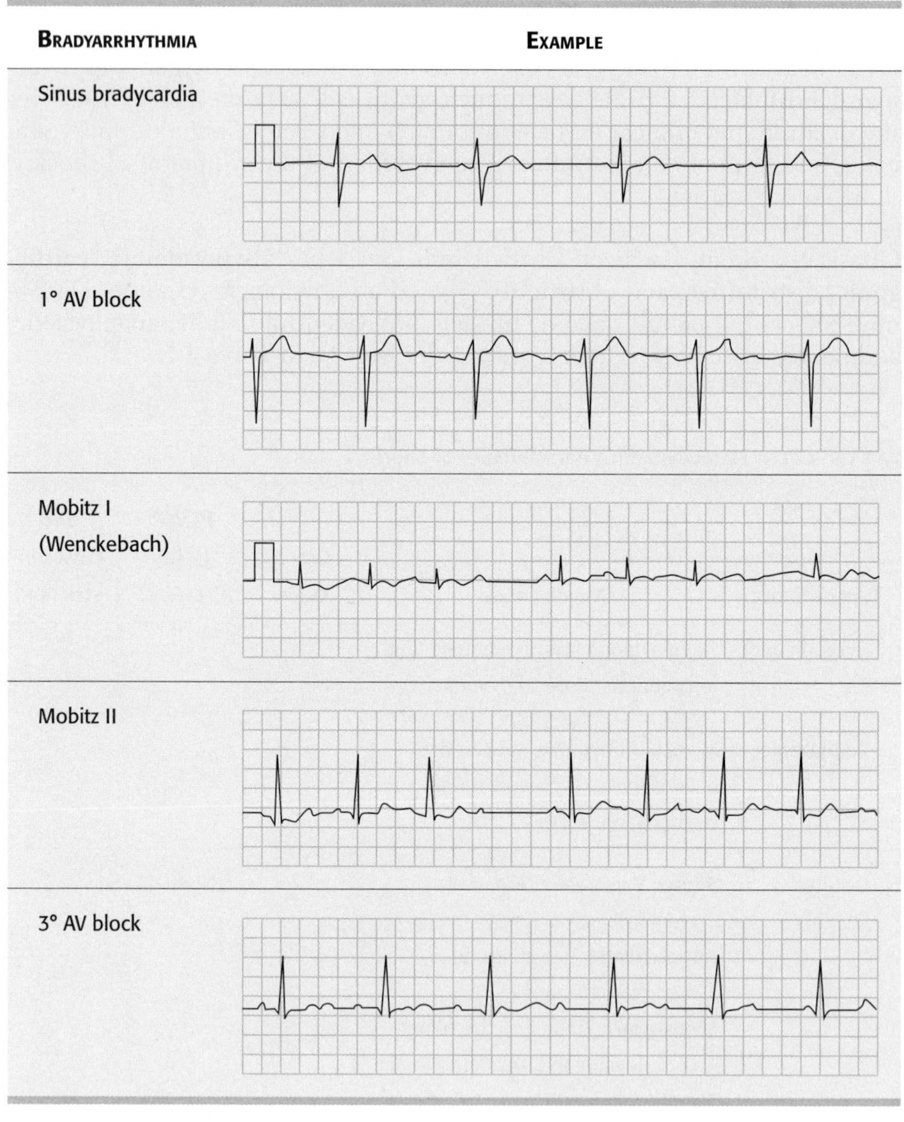

BRADYARRHYTHMIA	EXAMPLE
Sinus bradycardia	
1° AV block	
Mobitz I (Wenckebach)	
Mobitz II	
3° AV block	

TABLE 4-3. Common Tachyarrhythmias

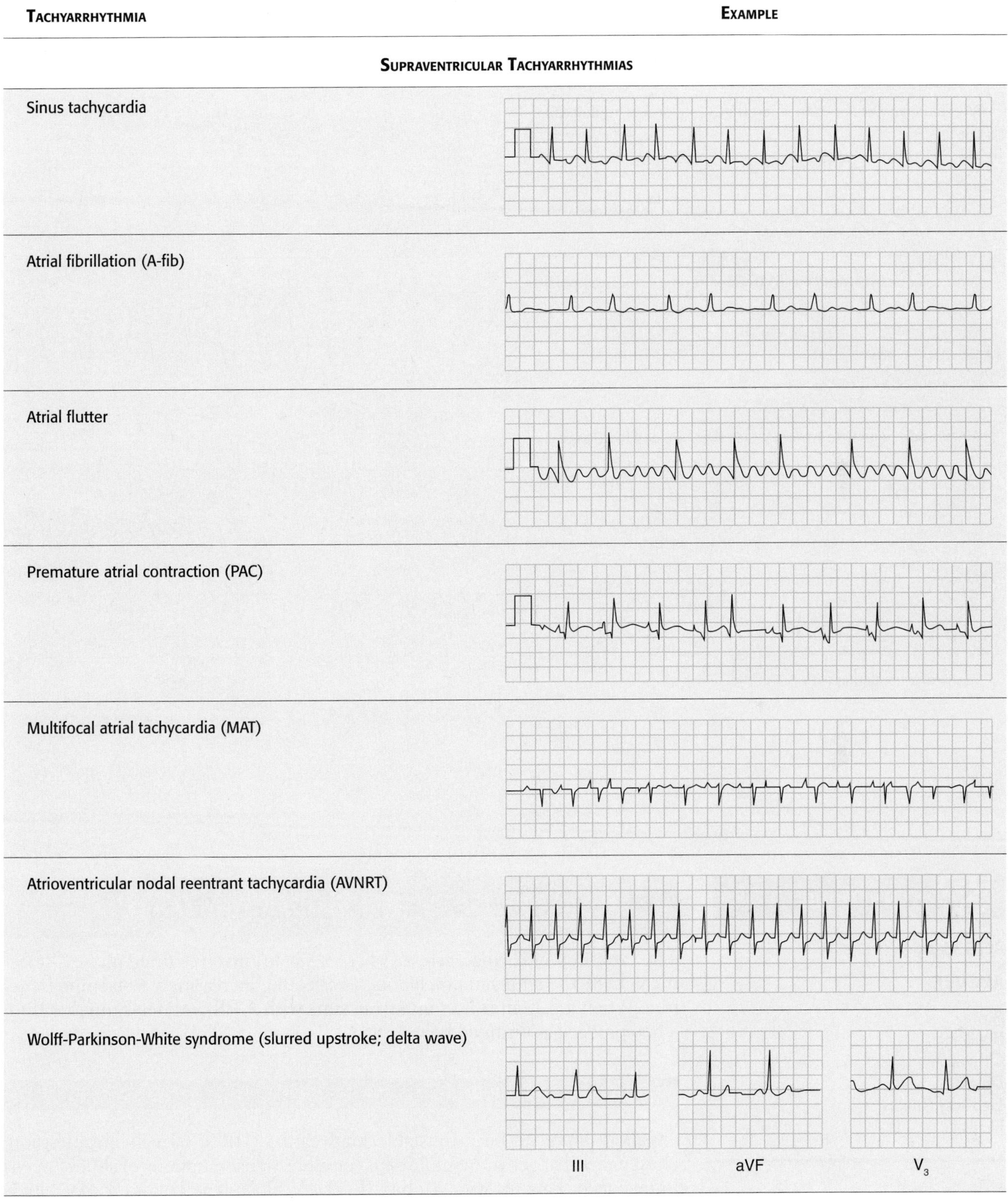

TACHYARRHYTHMIA	EXAMPLE
SUPRAVENTRICULAR TACHYARRHYTHMIAS	
Sinus tachycardia	
Atrial fibrillation (A-fib)	
Atrial flutter	
Premature atrial contraction (PAC)	
Multifocal atrial tachycardia (MAT)	
Atrioventricular nodal reentrant tachycardia (AVNRT)	
Wolff-Parkinson-White syndrome (slurred upstroke; delta wave)	III aVF V_3

(continues)

TABLE 4-3. Common Tachyarrhythmias *(continued)*

TACHYARRHYTHMIA	EXAMPLE
VENTRICULAR TACHYARRHYTHMIAS	
Premature ventricular contraction (PVC) (unifocal vs. multifocal)	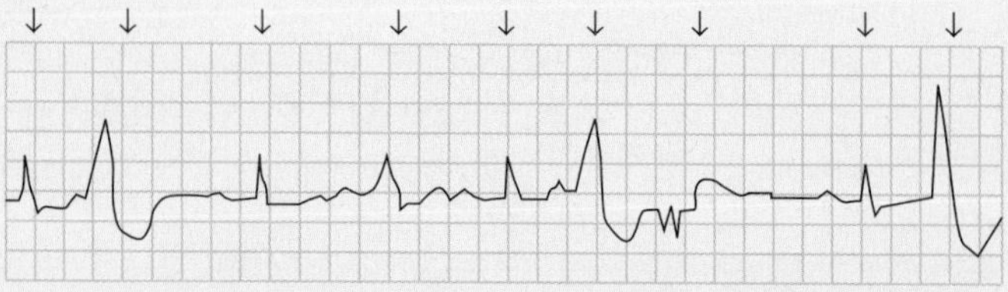
Ventricular tachycardia (V-tach) (monomorphic vs. polymorphic)	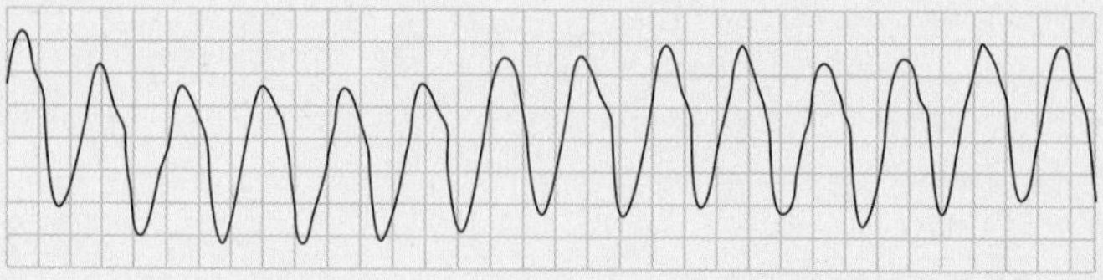
Torsades de pointes (a type of V-tach that can lead to VF as well)	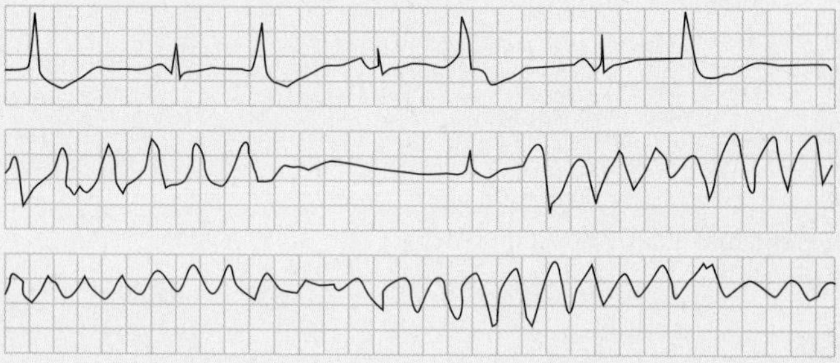
Ventricular fibrillation (VF)	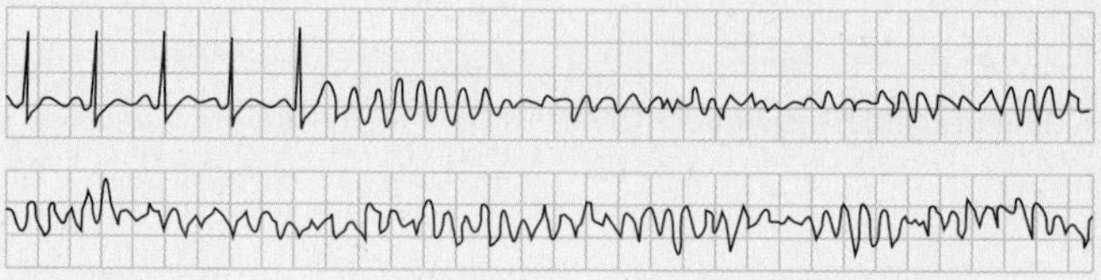

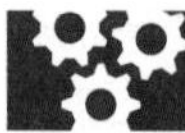

MNEMONIC

ACLS steps—

ABCDEF

Airway
Breathing
Circulation
Drugs
Electricity (shock)
Fluids

Advanced Cardiac Life Support (ACLS)

The evolution of **cardiac arrest** (VF → asystole) involves three phases—electrical, hemodynamic, and metabolic—reflecting increasingly worsening ischemia. When a patient suffers an arrest, **start with CPR** and determine rhythm. Then proceed as outlined below.

UNSTABLE BRADYCARDIA

A patient found to be in unstable bradycardia (HR < 60 with hypotension, chest pain, changes in mental status, or other signs/symptoms of shock) needs to be paced. Patients with Mobitz II (2° AV block type II) and 3° AV block, even if they are asymptomatic, also merit **transcutaneous pacing.** While preparing for pacing, give **atropine** 0.5 mg IV q 3–5 min × 3. Dopamine 2–10 μg/kg/min or epinephrine 2–10 μg/min may also be used, particularly if transcutaneous pacing is ineffective. Transvenous pacing and/or pressor drips may also be needed.

PULSELESS ARREST

In the setting of pulseless arrest, perform a 1° survey to determine which of four rhythms is involved: VF, pulseless V-tach, asystole, or PEA.

- **VF or pulseless V-tach:**
  - Attempt **unsynchronized cardioversion** (shock) prior to performing the 2° survey.
  - Next, give a **vasopressor: epinephrine** 1 mg IV q 3–5 min × 3 or **vasopressin** 40 units IV (replaces only the first or second dose of epinephrine).
  - Give another shock and then an **antiarrhythmic agent: amiodarone** 300 mg IV (150 mg for subsequent doses) q 3–5 min or **lidocaine** 1.0–1.5 mg/kg IV (0.50–0.75 mg/kg for subsequent doses) q 5–10 min.
  - Give another shock and return to the vasopressor step. Continue in this "vasopressor-shock-antiarrhythmic-shock" loop until the patient regains a pulse or resuscitation efforts are stopped.
  - If torsades de pointes develops, give magnesium 1–2 g IV.
- **Asystole or PEA:**
  - Proceed to the 2° survey (asystole and PEA are not shockable rhythms) and then give vasopressors only.
  - If bradycardia develops, give atropine 1 mg IV q 3–5 min × 3.
- Regardless of type, attempt to identify and treat the underlying cause(s) of cardiac arrest.

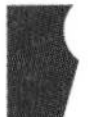

KEY FACT

When possible, pretreat the patient with sedation (eg, midazolam) before pacing. It won't reduce the pain, but it should keep the patient from remembering it.

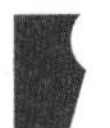

KEY FACT

For VF and pulseless V-tach, the defibrillator is set to 360 J if monophasic or 250 J if biphasic for unsynchronized cardioversion.

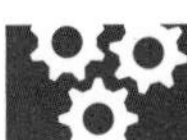

MNEMONIC

Potential underlying causes of pulseless electrical activity–

The 5 H's and 5 T's

Hypovolemia
Hypoxia
H+ (acidosis)
Hyper-/**H**ypokalemia
Hypothermia
Toxins/**T**ablets (drug overdose)
Cardiac **T**amponade
Tension pneumothorax
Coronary **T**hrombosis (ACS)
Pulmonary **T**hrombosis (PE)

TACHYCARDIA

- If signs/symptoms of **unstable tachycardia** develop (eg, shortness of breath, chest pain, hypotension, ischemic ECG changes), perform immediate **synchronized cardioversion** (at 100, 200, 300, and then 360 J).
- If **stable tachycardia** develops, quickly perform 1° and 2° surveys, and then determine if it is narrow complex (QRS < 0.12 sec) or wide complex.
  - **Narrow complex and regular:** First attempt **vagal stimulation,** and then try **adenosine** 6 mg IV followed by 12 mg q 2 min × 2. If the rhythm persists, give **metoprolol** 5 mg IV q 5 min × 3 or **diltiazem** 15–20 mg IV over 2 minutes (if no CHF).
  - **Narrow complex and irregular:** Give **metoprolol** or **diltiazem** as described above.
  - **Wide complex and regular:** Give **amiodarone** 150 mg IV over 10 minutes or **procainamide** 17 mg/kg at 50 mg/min (if no CHF). If the rhythm persists, proceed with **synchronized cardioversion.**
  - **Wide complex and irregular:** Further evaluate the rhythm.
    - **Torsades de pointes:** Give **magnesium** 1–2 g IV over 5–60 minutes with overdrive pacing.
    - **Wolff-Parkinson-White syndrome:** Follow the treatment pathway for regular wide-complex tachycardia (ie, amiodarone or procainamide, then synchronized cardioversion).
    - If neither of these rhythms exists, follow the treatment pathway for persistent regular narrow-complex tachycardia (ie, metoprolol or diltiazem).

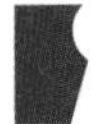

KEY FACT

Expert consultation is recommended for wide-complex tachycardia, irregular narrow-complex tachycardia, and persistent regular narrow-complex tachycardia.

Toxicology

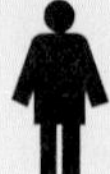

A 14-year-old boy is hospitalized for acute cholinergic toxicity after having been exposed to pesticides in a local orchard. Without treatment, what neuromuscular effects might he have experienced?

Muscle fasciculations, weakness, and paralysis.

In dealing with a patient who has been exposed to a toxin, begin by determining which toxin was involved and the **means** by which the patient was exposed—eg, through ingestion (most common), inhalation, injection, or absorption. Also determine the **time** and **extent** of the exposure, and ascertain if any **other substances** were involved. Ask about **symptoms** and **determine if the exposure was intentional.**

SYMPTOMS/EXAM/DIAGNOSIS

Vital signs may yield clues to the type of ingestion:

- **Hyperthermia:** Amphetamines, anticholinergics, ASA, cocaine, neuroleptics, nicotine, PCP, SSRIs, thyroid medication.
- **Hypothermia:** Alcohol, barbiturates, carbon monoxide, sedative-hypnotics.
- **Tachycardia:** Amphetamines, anticholinergics, cocaine, PCP, thyroid medication, TCAs.
- **Bradycardia:** β-blockers, calcium channel blockers (CCBs), cholinergics, clonidine, digitalis, opiates, parasympathomimetics.
- **Tachypnea:** Organophosphates (eg, pesticides), salicylates.
- **Respiratory depression:** Barbiturates, benzodiazepines, opiates.
- **Hypertension:** Amphetamines, anticholinergics, cocaine, PCP.
- **Hypotension:** Alcohol, β-blockers, CCBs, digitalis, opiates, organophosphates, sedative-hypnotics, TCAs.

Other diagnostic clues derived from physical findings include the following:

- **Breath odor:**
  - **Violets:** Turpentine.
  - **Pear:** Chloral hydrate.
  - **Bitter almonds:** Cyanide.
  - **Garlic:** Arsenic, DMSO, organophosphates.
  - **Mothballs:** Camphor, naphthalene.
- **Pupils:**
  - **Constricted (miosis): "COPS"** (**C**lonidine, **O**piates, **P**ontine bleed, **S**edative-hypnotics).
  - **Dilated (mydriasis):** Amphetamines, anticholinergics, cocaine.
- **Pulmonary edema:** Cocaine, ethylene glycol, opiates, organophosphates, salicylates, toxic inhalations (chlorine, nitric oxide, phosgene).
- **Bowel sounds:**
  - **Increased:** Sympathomimetics, opiate withdrawal.
  - **Decreased:** Anticholinergics, opiate toxicity.
- **Skin findings:**
  - **Needle tracks:** Opiates.
  - **Diaphoresis:** Organophosphates, salicylates, sympathomimetics.
  - **Jaundice:** Acetaminophen (after liver failure), mushroom poisoning.
  - **Alopecia:** Arsenic, chemotherapeutic agents, thallium.
  - **Cyanosis:** Drugs causing methemoglobinemia (eg, aniline dyes, "caine" anesthetics, chlorates, dapsone, nitrates/nitrites, sulfonamides).

KEY FACT

Meperidine is an exception to the opioid toxidrome and does not cause miosis.

TABLE 4-4. Classic Toxidromes

TOXIDROME	SYMPTOMS/SIGNS	EXAMPLES
Cholinergic	**DUMBBELS: D**iarrhea, **U**rination, **M**iosis, **B**radycardia, **B**ronchospasm, **E**mesis, **L**acrimation, **S**alivation.	Muscarine-containing mushrooms, organophosphates, pilocarpine, pyridostigmine.
Anticholinergic	"Hot as a hare, red as a beet, dry as a bone, mad as a hatter, blind as a bat": fever, skin flushing, dry mucous membranes, psychosis, mydriasis. Also tachycardia and urinary retention.	Antihistamines, antipsychotics, atropine, Jimson weed, scopolamine, TCAs.
Opioid	Triad of coma, respiratory depression, and miosis. Also bradycardia, hypothermia, and diminished bowel sounds.	Heroin, morphine, oxycodone.
Sedative-hypnotic	CNS depression, respiratory depression, and coma.	Alcohol, barbiturates, benzodiazepines.
Hallucinogenic	Disorientation, panic, seizures, hypertension, tachycardia, tachypnea.	Amphetamines, cocaine, PCP.
Extrapyramidal	Parkinsonian symptoms: tremor, torticollis, trismus, rigidity, oculogyric crisis, opisthotonos, dysphonia, and dysphagia.	Haloperidol, metoclopramide, phenothiazines.

Table 4-4 lists symptoms and signs associated with common toxin-induced syndromes ("toxidromes").

TREATMENT

Treatment options are as follows:

- **Elimination:**
  - **Activated charcoal:** Constitutes first-line treatment. Administer in a dose of 1 g/kg. Avoid multiple doses of cathartics (eg, sorbitol), especially in young children.
  - **Whole bowel irrigation** (eg, polyethylene glycol with electrolytes to wash toxins from the GI tract): Useful for ingestions of lithium, iron, heavy metals, sustained-released drugs, and "body packers" (eg, cocaine).
- **Removal of unabsorbed toxin:**
  - **Emesis:** Induced vomiting through use of ipecac. (No longer within the standard of care.)
  - **Gastric lavage:**
    - **Indications:** The ingestion is known or suspected to be serious; the ingestion was recent (< 30–60 minutes before presentation); the patient is awake and cooperative or is intubated; the patient can be placed in the left lateral decubitus position.

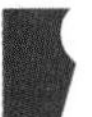

KEY FACT

The anticholinergic and sympathomimetic toxidromes are similar, but the latter is associated with hyperactive bowel sounds and diaphoresis.

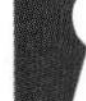

KEY FACT

With a paucity of objective data to support their theoretical benefits, emesis and gastric lavage have fallen out of favor. Gastric lavage is rarely performed in practice today, and emesis not at all.

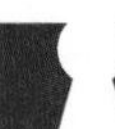

KEY FACT

For patients presenting with altered mental status of unknown etiology, start out by giving them a **ThONG: Th**iamine, **O**xygen, **N**aloxone, and **G**lucose.

- **Contraindications:** Altered mental status, ↓ or absent gag reflex, caustic agents (to prevent reinjury of the esophagus if the patient vomits), esophageal trauma (eg, Mallory-Weiss tears), agents that are easily aspirated, nontoxic ingestion.
- **Removal of absorbed toxin:**
  - **Alkalization methods:** Involve mixing D_5W with 2–3 amps of $NaHCO_3$.
    - Alkalinization of blood improves clearance of TCAs.

TABLE 4-5. Specific Antidotes and Treatments

Toxin	Antidote/Treatment
Acetaminophen	*N*-acetylcysteine
Anticholinesterases (eg, organophosphates)	Atropine, pralidoxime
Anticholinergics (antimuscarinics—eg, atropine; antinicotinics)	Physostigmine (crosses the blood-brain barrier)
Benzodiazepines	Flumazenil
β-blockers	Glucagon
Carbon monoxide	O_2
Cyanide	Amyl nitrite pearls, sodium nitrite, sodium thiosulfate, hydroxocobalamin
Digoxin	Anti-digitalis Fab; magnesium, lidocaine (for torsades)
Ethylene glycol (antifreeze), methanol	Fomepizole, ethanol drip, dialysis; calcium gluconate for ethylene glycol
Heparin	Protamine sulfate
Iron	Deferoxamine
Isoniazid (INH)	Pyridoxine (vitamin B_6)
Lead[a]	Chelator agents: penicillamine and succimer for lower levels; EDTA and dimercaprol (British anti-Lewisite, aka BAL) for higher levels
Nitrites (eg, methemoglobin)	Methylene blue
Opioids	Naloxone
Phenothiazines	Diphenhydramine, benztropine
Salicylates	Sodium bicarbonate, dialysis
TCAs	Sodium bicarbonate (for QRS prolongation); benzodiazepines (for seizures)
tPA, streptokinase	Aminocaproic acid
Warfarin	Vitamin K, fresh frozen plasma (FFP)

[a] Arsenic, copper, gold, and mercury are also treated with similar combinations of chelator agents.

- Alkalinization of urine to a pH > 8 ionizes weak acids into ionized molecules, thereby increasing the excretion of salicylates, phenobarbital, and chlorpropamide.
- **Charcoal hemoperfusion:** ↑ absorption of toxic substances in the blood by filtering blood from a shunt through a column of activated charcoal. Particularly useful for aminophylline, barbiturates, carbamazepine, and digoxin.
- **Hemodialysis:** Filters small, ionized molecules such as salicylates, theophylline, methanol, lithium, barbiturates, and ethylene glycol.

Substance-specific antidotes are outlined in Table 4-5. Drug withdrawal treatments are delineated in Table 4-6. Additional information on drug intoxication and withdrawal can be found in Chapter 17.

MNEMONIC

Indications for emergent hemodialysis–

AEIOU

Metabolic **A**cidosis that cannot be corrected with $NaHCO_3$
Severe **E**lectrolyte imbalances (eg, hyperkalemia)
Toxic **I**ngestions (eg, lithium or aspirin)
Fluid **O**verload that is resistant to treatment with diuretics
Uremia (eg, uremic encephalopathy, uremic serositis)

TABLE 4-6. Drug Withdrawal Syndromes and Treatment

DRUG	WITHDRAWAL SYMPTOMS	TREATMENT
Alcohol	**6–12 hours:** Tremor. **Within 48 hours:** Tachycardia, hypertension, agitation, seizures. **Within 2–7 days:** Hallucinations, **DTs** (autonomic instability, including tachycardia, hypertension, and delirium). Mortality is 15–20%.	**Benzodiazepines;** haloperidol for hallucinations. Thiamine (B_1), folate, B_{12}, and multivitamin replacement–ie, **banana bag** (does not affect withdrawal but may prevent Wernicke's encephalopathy). Give thiamine before glucose.
Barbiturates	Anxiety, seizures, delirium, tremor, cardiac and respiratory depression.	Benzodiazepines.
Benzodiazepines	Rebound anxiety, seizures, tremor. May lead to **DTs.**	Benzodiazepine taper.
Cocaine, amphetamines	Depression, hyperphagia, hypersomnolence.	Supportive treatment. Avoid β-blockers (may lead to uninhibited α-cardiac stimulation with cocaine use–ie, hypertension).
Opioids	Anxiety, insomnia, **flulike symptoms,** sweating, piloerection, fever, rhinorrhea, nausea, stomach cramps, diarrhea, mydriasis.	Symptom management. Clonidine and/or buprenorphine for moderate withdrawal; methadone for severe symptoms. Naltrexone can be used when the patient has been drug free for 7–10 days.

Sexual Assault

In working with a victim of sexual assault, begin by diagnosing and treating the victim's **physical and emotional injuries.** It is also critical to collect legal evidence as well as to document that evidence carefully and completely. Information sought should include the following:

- **Where and when** did the assault occur?
- What happened **during the assault?** Determine the **number** of assailants; the use of force, weapons, objects, or restraints; which **orifices** were penetrated; and whether alcohol and/or drugs were involved.
- What happened **after the assault?** Are there any specific symptoms or pains? Did the patient bathe, defecate, urinate, brush teeth, or change clothes? Has the patient had **sexual intercourse in the last 72 hours?**
- Determine the **risk of pregnancy.** Last menstrual period? Any birth control?

Diagnosis

- Conduct a general trauma and pelvic exam.
- Collect **physical evidence** (eg, debris, fingernail scrapings, dried secretions from the skin, pubic hairs).
- Medically indicated tests include a pregnancy test; cultures for gonorrhea and chlamydia; serology for syphilis; and HBV, HCV, and HIV testing.

Treatment

- Treat traumatic injuries.
- **Infection prevention:**
  - Where appropriate, treat gonorrhea, chlamydia, trichomoniasis, and bacterial vaginosis.
  - Institute HBV and HIV prophylaxis.
- **Pregnancy prevention:**
  - Administer two Ovral (ethinyl estradiol and norgestrel) tablets PO immediately and again 12 hours later.
  - Offer counseling.

Animal and Insect Bites

KEY FACT

Tearing dog bites cause considerably more physical trauma, but puncture-like cat bites are more likely to become infected.

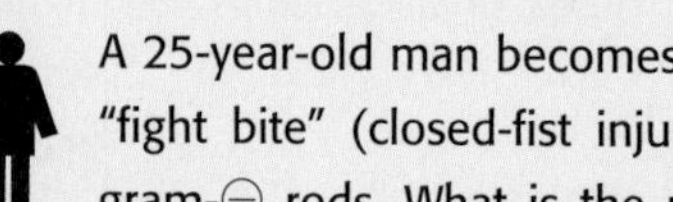

A 25-year-old man becomes involved in a barroom brawl and sustains a "fight bite" (closed-fist injury) to his hand. The wound culture grows gram-⊖ rods. What is the most likely pathogen in this case, and how should it be treated?

Eikenella corrodens; treat with amoxicillin/clavulanate.

KEY FACT

Scorpion stings are treated with antivenom and a midazolam drip to control agitation and involuntary muscle movements. Monitor for hypertension, arrhythmias, and pancreatitis.

- The rabies treatment protocol for animal bites is as follows:
  - If the bite is from a domestic animal that can be captured/secured and its behavior observed as normal for 10 days, no treatment is necessary.
  - If the bite is from a domestic animal that exhibits abnormal behavior or becomes ill, the animal should be sacrificed and its head/brain tested for rabies via a direct immunofluorescent antibody study. If that study is ⊖, no treatment is necessary. If it is ⊕, immediate treatment is indicated.
  - If the animal is wild, immediate treatment is indicated.

TABLE 4-7. Bite Types, Infecting Organisms, and Treatment

Bite Type	Likely Organisms/Toxins	Treatment
Dog	α-hemolytic streptococci, *S aureus, Pasteurella multocida,* and anaerobes.	**Amoxicillin/clavulanate** or a first-generation cephalosporin +/– tetanus and rabies prophylaxis.
Cat	***P multocida*** (high rate of infection), anaerobes.	**Amoxicillin/clavulanate** +/– tetanus prophylaxis.
Human	Polymicrobial. Viridans streptococci are most frequently implicated.	Second- or third-generation cephalosporins, dicloxacillin + penicillin, **amoxicillin/clavulanate** or clarithromycin +/– tetanus prophylaxis, HBV vaccine, HBIG, and postexposure HIV prophylaxis.
Rodent	*Streptobacillus moniliformis, P multocida, Leptospira* spp.	**Penicillin VK** or doxycycline.
Bat	Rabies and other viruses.	Vaccination against rabies.
Snake	*Pseudomonas aeruginosa, Proteus* spp, *Bacteroides fragilis, Clostridium* spp, venom.	Antivenom as appropriate. Venomous snakes (eg, coral snake, pit viper, rattlesnake) may not require antibiotics; ampicillin/sulbactam (or, alternatively, a fluoroquinolone or clindamycin + TMP-SMX) are given to combat the snake's oral flora. Monitor for rhabdomyolysis, neurologic impairment, and serum sickness.
Spider	Venom (can cause tissue necrosis and/or rigid paralysis, depending on species).	Antivenom as appropriate; otherwise supportive care (analgesics, antihistamines, wound irrigation/debridement). Tetanus prophylaxis. Dapsone may be used to prevent further tissue necrosis.

- Treatment options for rabies include the following:
  - **Active immunization** with human diploid cell vaccine (HDCV).
  - **Passive immunization** with **human rabies immune globulin** (HRIG).
- Regardless of treatment, be sure to reevaluate the wound 24–48 hours after injury.
- Table 4-7 summarizes bite types (including human), associated infecting organisms, and appropriate treatment.

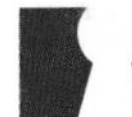

KEY FACT

For monkey bites, add postexposure prophylactic valacyclovir or acyclovir x 14 days.

Tetanus

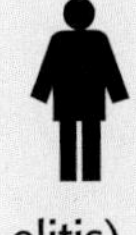

A 42-year-old carpenter presents to the ER after a rusty nail pierces his work boot. What are the most likely pathogens involved?

Clostridium tetani (tetanus) and *Pseudomonas aeruginosa* (osteomyelitis).

Presents with trismus (ie, lockjaw), glottal spasm, and convulsive spasms. High-risk patients include the elderly (due to inadequate immunization), IV drug users, and ulcer patients.

TABLE 4-8. Tetanus Prophylaxis Schedule

	Non-Tetanus-Prone Wounds	Tetanus-Prone Wounds[a]	
History of Adsorbed Tetanus Toxoid (doses)	**Td**	**Td**	**TIG**
Unknown or < 3 doses	√	√	√
Three doses:			
Last dose > 5 years		√	
Last dose > 10 years	√	√	

[a] Tetanus-prone wounds are those that are present > 6 hours; are nonlinear; are > 1 cm deep; and show signs of infection, devitalized tissue, and contamination.

Treatment

- Benzodiazepines to control muscle spasms; neuromuscular blockade if needed to control the airway.
- **Metronidazole** is the antibiotic of choice.
- Administer tetanus immune globulin (TIG) and/or adsorbed tetanus and diphtheria toxoid (Td) vaccine as indicated in Table 4-8.

Environmental Emergencies

COLD EMERGENCIES

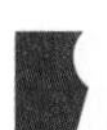

KEY FACT

Do not rewarm frostbite until refreezing can be prevented.

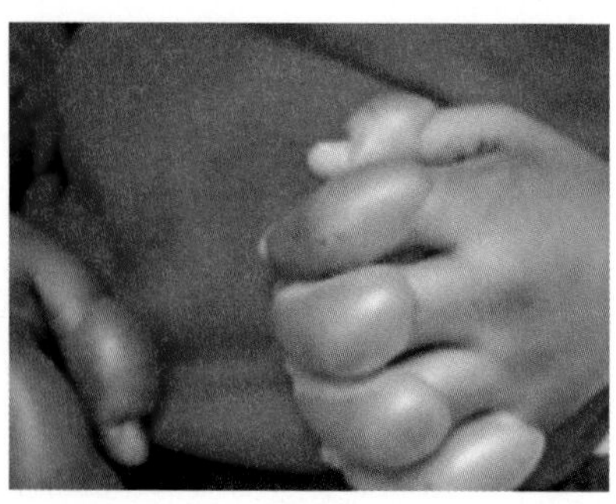

FIGURE 4-8. Frostbite injury in a child. (Courtesy of Mark Sochor, MD.)

Frostbite

- Cold injury with pallor and loss of cold sensation. Results from exposure to cold air or direct contact with cold materials. Nonviable structures demarcate and slough off. Subtypes are as follows:
  - **Superficial:** Injury to cutaneous and subcutaneous tissue. Skin is soft under a frozen surface. Large, clear, fluid-filled vesicles develop within two days (indicating a good prognosis); sloughing leaves new skin that is pink and hypersensitive (see Figure 4-8).
  - **Deep:** Injury to the above tissues plus deep structures (muscle, bone). Skin is hard under a frozen surface.
- **Tx:** Rapidly rewarm once refreezing can be prevented. Circulating water at 40°C (104°F); wound care; tetanus prophylaxis.

Hypothermia

A 20-year-old woman is pulled from the water unconscious five minutes after her sailboat capsizes. Despite the problems associated with hypothermia, victims of cold-water submersion injuries usually have a better outcome. Why is this?

Activation of the diving reflex (reflex bradycardia and breath holding), which reduces metabolic demands (and the effects of hypoxemia), shunts blood to the vital organs, and limits aspiration of water.

- Defined as a core body temperature of < 35°C (< 95°F).
- Causes include environmental exposure, **alcohol ingestion,** drugs (barbiturates, benzodiazepines, narcotics), hypoglycemia, CNS or hypothalamic dysfunction (via loss of stimulus of shivering response and adrenal activity), hypothyroidism, skin disorders, and sepsis.
- **Dx:** Look for arrhythmias and/or **Osborn/J waves** (positive deflection in the QRS complex) on ECG (see Figure 4-9).
- **Tx:**
  - ABCs, CPR, and stabilization.
  - **Rewarming:**
    - **Passive external:** Blankets.
    - **Active external:** Warmed blankets; hot-water bottles.
    - **Active internal:** Warm humidified O_2; heated IV fluids; gastric, colonic, bladder, or peritoneal lavage; extracorporeal rewarming.
  - Do not pronounce patients until they have been rewarmed to 35°C (95°F); full recovery is not uncommon.
  - Associated with a risk of dysrhythmias, especially VF at core temperatures of < 30°C (86°F). **Bretylium** is generally the drug of choice.

KEY FACT

The "J" in J waves refers not only to the approximate shape of these waves but also to the initials of the man who first described them: John J. Osborn.

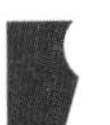

KEY FACT

"No one is dead until they're warm and dead."

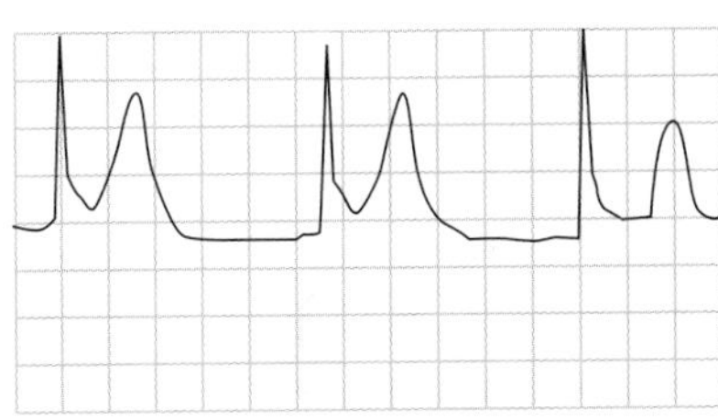

FIGURE 4-9. Sinus bradycardia, Osborn wave. J-point elevation with ST-segment elevation and a prolonged QT interval (0.56 sec) is seen in a patient with hypothermia.

HEAT EMERGENCIES

Heat Exhaustion

- Extreme fatigue with **profuse sweating.** Also presents with nausea/vomiting and a dull headache.
- **Sx/Exam:** Body temperature is **normal** or slightly elevated. Patients are tachypneic, tachycardic, and hypotensive.
- **Tx:** Treat with IV NS and a cool environment.

Heat Stroke

A 35-year-old migrant worker with no past medical history has a syncopal episode while harvesting tobacco. His exam reveals diminished mentation, tachypnea, and rales. His blood work reveals hypovolemic hyponatremia, hypoglycemia, leukocytosis, and elevated LFTs. What single diagnosis can account for all of these abnormalities?

Exertional heat stroke.

- Elevation of body temperature above normal due to temperature dysregulation (> 40°C [104°F]). **Constitutes a true emergency.** Monitor for convulsions and cardiovascular collapse.
- **Sx/Exam:** Presents with ↑ **body temperature** and altered mental status. Patients have hot, dry skin, often with no sweating. Ataxia may be seen.
- **Tx:** Treat with **aggressive cooling.** Remove from the heat source and undress. Use an atomized tepid water spray; apply ice packs to the groin/axillae. (Some facilities use cooled IV fluids run through a central line.) Treat neuroleptic malignant syndrome and drug fever with **dantrolene.** Treat seizures with **diazepam.**

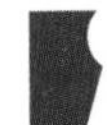

KEY FACT

Heat stroke presents with altered mental status and ↑ temperature, often with no sweating.

Burns

In dealing with burn patients, begin by determining if the victim was in an enclosed or an open space. Are there any toxic products of combustion? Any respiratory symptoms? Consider **carbon monoxide poisoning** (symptoms are nonspecific).

Exam

- Gauge the body surface area (BSA) involved. Observe the **rule of 9's: 9% BSA** for the head and each arm; **18% BSA** for the back torso, the front torso, and each leg. In **children,** the rule is 9% BSA for each arm; 18% BSA for the head, back torso, and front torso; and 14% BSA for each leg.
- Determine the **depth of the burn** (see Table 4-9 and Figure 4-10).

Treatment

- **Prehospital treatment:**
  - Administer IV fluids and high-flow O_2.
  - Remove the patient's clothes and cover with clean sheets or dressings.
  - Administer pain medications.
- **In-hospital treatment:**
  - **ABCs: Early airway control** is critical. Intubate if:
    - The patient is unconscious or obtunded.
    - The patient is in respiratory distress with facial burns, soot in the airway, singed nasal hairs, and carbonaceous sputum.
  - **Fluid resuscitation:** Appropriate for patients with > 20% BSA second-degree burns.
    - Give 4 cc/kg per % total BSA (**Parkland formula**) over 24 hours—the first half over the first 8 hours and the second half over the next 16 hours.
    - Maintain a urine output of 1 cc/kg/hr.
    - Tetanus prophylaxis; pain control.
- **Disposition:**
  - **Minor burns:** Discharge with pain medications.
  - **Moderate burns** (partial-thickness 15–25% or full-thickness < 10% BSA): Admit to the hospital.

TABLE 4-9. Burn Classification

Severity of Burn	Tissue Involvement	Findings
First degree	Epidermis only.	Red and painful.
Second degree (superficial)	Epidermis and superficial dermis.	Red, wet, and painful with **blisters.**
Second degree (deep)	Epidermis and deep dermis.	White, dry, and tender.
Third degree	Epidermis and **entire dermis.**	Charred/leathery, pearly white, and **nontender.**
Fourth degree	Below the dermis to bone, muscle, and fascia.	

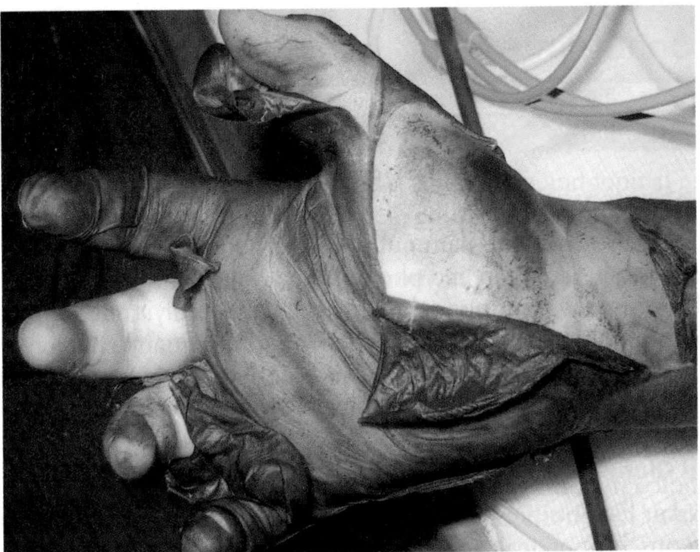

FIGURE 4-10. Fourth-degree burns involving underlying bone and/or muscle. (Reproduced with permission from Wolff K et al. *Fitzpatrick's Dermatology in General Medicine,* 7th ed. New York: McGraw-Hill, 2008, Fig. 94-1D.)

- **Major burns** (partial-thickness > 25% BSA or full-thickness > 10% BSA; burns to the face, hands, joints, feet, or perineum; electrical or circumferential burns): Refer to a burn center.

Electrical Injuries

Electrical current flows most easily through tissues of low resistance, such as nerves, blood vessels, mucous membranes, and muscles. The current pathway determines which organs are affected.

Symptoms/Exam

Symptoms vary according to the nature of the current.

- **Alternating current (household and commercial):**
  - Associated with explosive exit wounds (see Figure 4-11).
  - Effects are worse with AC than with DC current at the same voltage.
  - VF is common.
- **Direct current (industrial, batteries, lightning):**
  - Causes discrete exit wounds.
  - Asystole is common.

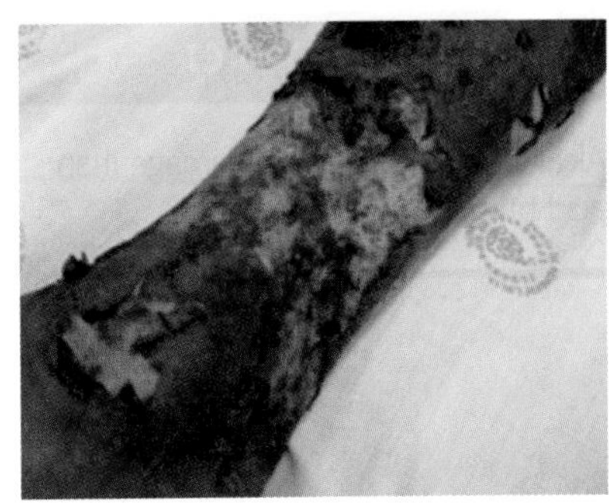

FIGURE 4-11. Circumferential electrical burn of the right lower extremity. (Courtesy of Benjamin Silverberg, MD.)

Treatment

- ABCs; IV fluids for severe burns.
- Administer pain medications and treat burns.
- Treat **myoglobinuria** by administering IV fluids to maintain a urine output of 1.5–2.0 cc/kg/hr.
- Tetanus prophylaxis.
- Asymptomatic low-voltage (< 1000-V) burn victims can be discharged.

NOTES

CHAPTER 5

ENDOCRINOLOGY

Diabetes Mellitus (DM)

TYPE 1 DIABETES MELLITUS

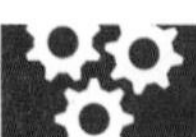

MNEMONIC

The 3 P's of DM type 1:

Polyuria
Polydipsia
Polyphagia

Destruction of pancreatic beta cells leads to insulin deficiency (see Table 5-1). Generally immune mediated.

SYMPTOMS/EXAM

Presents with the classic symptoms of **P**olyuria (including nocturia), **P**olydipsia, and **P**olyphagia (the **3 P's**). Patients may also have rapid or unexplained weight loss, blurry vision, or recurrent infections (eg, candidiasis).

DIFFERENTIAL

Pancreatic disease (eg, chronic pancreatitis), glucagonoma, Cushing's disease, iatrogenic factors (eg, corticosteroids), gestational diabetes, diabetes insipidus.

DIAGNOSIS

At least one of the following is required to make the diagnosis:

- A random plasma glucose concentration of ≥ 200 mg/dL with classic symptoms of diabetes.
- A fasting plasma glucose level of ≥ 126 mg/dL on two separate occasions.

TABLE 5-1. Type 1 vs. Type 2 DM

	TYPE 1 (INSULIN-DEPENDENT DM)	TYPE 2 (NON-INSULIN-DEPENDENT DM)
Pathophysiology	Failure of the pancreas to secrete insulin as a result of autoimmune destruction of beta cells.	Insulin resistance and inadequate insulin secretion by the pancreas to compensate.
Incidence	15%.	85%.
Age (exceptions are common)	< 30 years of age.	> 40 years of age.
Association with obesity	No.	Yes.
"Classic symptoms"	Common.	Sometimes.
Diabetic ketoacidosis	Common.	Rare.
Genetic predisposition	Weak, polygenic.	Strong, polygenic.
Association with HLA system	Yes (HLA-DR3 and -DR4).	No.
Serum C-peptide	↓; can be normal during the "honeymoon period."	↓ late in the disease.

- A two-hour postprandial glucose level of ≥ 200 mg/dL after a 75-g oral glucose tolerance test on two separate occasions.
- A hemoglobin A_{1c} (HbA_{1c}) level > 6.5% has recently been added to the diagnostic criteria by the American Diabetes Association.

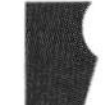

KEY FACT

The **"honeymoon period"** is a remission phase that is seen in type 1 diabetics days after the initiation of insulin therapy. During this phase, which may last several months, patients often have ↓ insulin requirements.

TREATMENT

- Type 1 diabetics should be started on insulin (see Table 5-2). Both basal and bolus insulin are required. Oral hypoglycemic agents are not effective.
- Most patients with type 1 diabetes are on a multiple-daily-injection (MDI) regimen consisting of premeal short-acting insulin (eg, lispro or aspart) and bedtime glargine or twice-daily NPH. Others are on insulin pumps consisting of short-acting insulin.
- Long-term management should include the following:
  - Check an **HbA_{1c} level** every three months. Maintain an HbA_{1c} < 7.
  - Maintain a low-fat, reduced-carbohydrate diet, and refer patients to a dietitian.
  - Manage **CAD risk factors** (hypertension, smoking, obesity, hyperlipidemia).
  - Obtain a baseline ECG if the patient has heart disease or is > 35 years of age.
  - Check eyes annually for retinopathy or cataracts. An ophthalmologic exam is also indicated if the patient is planning a pregnancy.
  - Screen newly diagnosed type 1 diabetics for **thyroid disease.**
  - Order an annual BUN/creatinine and UA for **microalbuminuria** to screen for diabetic nephropathy.
  - Check the **feet** annually for neuropathy, ulcers, and peripheral vascular disease. Patients should inspect their feet daily and wear comfortable shoes.
  - Administer an annual flu shot and keep pneumococcal vaccinations up to date.

TABLE 5-2. Types of Insulin[a]

INSULIN	ONSET	PEAK EFFECT	DURATION
Regular	30–60 minutes	2–4 hours	5–8 hours
Humalog (lispro)	5–10 minutes	0.5–1.5 hours	6–8 hours
NovoLog (aspart)	10–20 minutes	1–3 hours	3–5 hours
Apidra (glulisine)	5–15 minutes	1.0–1.5 hours	1.0–2.5 hours
NPH	2–4 hours	6–10 hours	18–28 hours
Levemir (detemir)	2 hours	No discernible peak	20 hours
Lantus (glargine)	1–4 hours	No discernible peak	20–24 hours

[a] Combination preparations mix longer-acting and shorter-acting types of insulin together to provide immediate and extended coverage in the same injection, eg, 70 NPH/30 regular = 70% NPH + 30% regular.

(Reproduced with permission from Le T et al. *First Aid for the USMLE Step 2 CK,* 7th ed. New York: McGraw-Hill, 2007: 114.)

TYPE 2 DIABETES MELLITUS

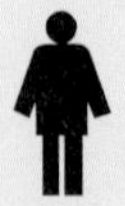

A 45-year-old obese man presents with polyuria and weight loss. What level of serum glucose is diagnostic of diabetes mellitus (DM)?

A serum glucose level of ≥ 200 mg/dL is diagnostic of DM in a symptomatic patient.

Patients with type 2 DM have two defects: insufficient insulin secretion and ↑ insulin resistance (see Table 5-1).

Symptoms/Exam

The 3 P's (see type 1 DM), recurrent blurred vision, paresthesias, and fatigue are common to both forms of diabetes. Because of the insidious onset of hyperglycemia, however, patients with type 2 DM may be asymptomatic at the time of diagnosis.

Differential

Similar to that of type 1 DM.

Diagnosis

Similar to that of type 1 DM.

Treatment

- Diet and exercise are critical. Type 2 diabetics should be started on an oral antidiabetic medication (see Table 5-3).
- Typical stepwise pharmacologic management includes metformin, a "glitazone," and a sulfonylurea (eg, glyburide).
- If the patient continues to have inadequate control on three oral antidiabetic drugs, glyburide should be replaced with NPH or glargine insulin at bedtime.
- For those who require more intense therapy, a split/mixed regimen of regular or short-acting and NPH or glargine insulin may be used.
  - **Prebreakfast glucose level:** Reflects predinner NPH dose.
  - **Prelunch glucose level:** Reflects prebreakfast regular insulin dose.
  - **Predinner glucose level:** Reflects prebreakfast NPH dose.
  - **Bedtime glucose level:** Reflects predinner regular insulin dose.
- Long-term management includes **monitoring blood glucose** (see Table 5-4) and checking a fasting glucose level once a day. Otherwise, management is similar to that of type 1.

KEY FACT

Step 3 loves to ask about lifestyle changes in diseases like diabetes!

TABLE 5-3. Oral Antidiabetic Medications

Medication	Examples	Mechanism of Action	Side Effects	Contraindications
Sulfonylureas	**First generation:** Chlorpropamide **Second generation:** Glipizide, glyburide	↑ insulin secretion.	Hypoglycemia.	Renal/liver disease.
Meglitinides	Repaglinide	↑ insulin secretion.	Hypoglycemia.	Renal/liver disease.
Biguanides	Metformin	Inhibit hepatic gluconeogenesis; ↑ glucose utilization; ↓ insulin resistance.	Lactic acidosis, diarrhea, GI discomfort, metallic taste, weight loss.	Renal insufficiency, any form of acidosis, liver disease, severe hypoxia.
α-glucosidase inhibitors	Acarbose	↓ glucose absorption.	↑ flatulence, GI discomfort, elevated LFTs.	Renal/liver disease.
Thiazolinediones ("glitazones")	Rosiglitazone, pioglitazone	↓ insulin resistance; ↑ glucose utilization.	Hepatocellular injury, anemia, pedal edema, CHF.	Liver disease, CHF (class III/IV), LFTs > 2 times normal.
Glucagon-like peptide-1 (GLP-1) agonists	Exenatide	↑ postprandial glucose utilization.	Nausea, vomiting, weight loss, hypoglycemia.	Renal disease.
Dipeptidyl peptidase (DPP-4) inhibitors	Sitagliptin, vildagliptin	Same as that of GLP-1 agonists.	Same as those of GLP-1 agonists.	Same as that of GLP-1 agonists.

TABLE 5-4. Target Glucose Levels in Diabetics

	Normal Glucose Level (mg/dL)	Target Glucose Level with Drug Treatment (mg/dL)	Adjust Dosage of Drug When Glucose Level Is:
Preprandial glucose	< 110	80–120	< 80 or > 140
Bedtime glucose	< 120	100–140	< 100 or > 160

COMPLICATIONS OF DIABETES MELLITUS

Diabetic Ketoacidosis (DKA)

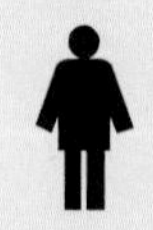

An eight-year-old boy presents with a two-day history of a productive cough and a fever of 38.4°C (101.1°F). Labs reveal leukocytosis, a blood glucose level of 341 mg/dL, a serum bicarbonate level of 13 mEq/L, and a UA positive for 2+ ketones. CXR reveals lobar pneumonia. Which serum ketone is likely elevated?

β-hydroxybutyrate.

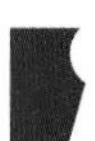

KEY FACT

Symptoms and signs of DKA:

- "Fruity" breath
- Kussmaul hyperpnea
- Dehydration
- Abdominal pain
- ↑ anion gap
- Hyperkalemia
- Hyperglycemia
- Ketones in blood/urine

DKA may be the initial manifestation of **type 1 DM** and is usually precipitated by a stressor (eg, infection, surgery). ↑ catabolism due to lack of insulin action plus ↑ counterregulatory hormones lead to life-threatening metabolic acidosis. Hyperkalemia is due to ↓ insulin and hyperosmolality, **not** to H^+-K^+ shifts.

Symptoms/Exam

Symptoms and signs of DKA include a "fruity" breath odor, Kussmaul hyperpnea (an abnormal ↑ in the depth and rate of breathing), dehydration, abdominal pain, an ↑ anion gap, hyperkalemia, hyperglycemia, and ketones in the blood and urine.

Diagnosis

- Order a CBC, electrolytes, BUN/creatinine, glucose, ABGs, serum ketones, a CXR, a blood culture, a UA and urine culture, and an ECG.
- Labs reveal hyperglycemia (blood glucose > 250 mg/dL), acidosis with a blood pH < 7.3, serum bicarbonate < 15 mEq/L, and ↑ serum/urine ketones.

Treatment

- Admission to the ICU/floor may be necessary depending on the patient's clinical status.
- Fluid resuscitate (3–4 L in eight hours) with NS and IV insulin.
- Sodium, potassium, phosphate, and glucose must be monitored and repleted every two hours (change NS fluids to D_5NS when glucose levels are < 250 mg/L).
- Change IV insulin to an SQ insulin sliding scale once the anion gap normalizes.
- Continue IV insulin for at least 30 minutes following the administration of the first dose of SQ insulin.

KEY FACT

In DKA, improvement is monitored via anion gap, not blood glucose levels.

Hyperglycemic Hyperosmolar Nonketotic State (HHNK)

Typically occurs in **type 2 DM.** Can be precipitated by dehydration, infection, or medications (eg, β-blockers, steroids, thiazides).

Symptoms/Exam

Patients are acutely ill and dehydrated with altered mental status.

Diagnosis

Diagnostic criteria for HHNK are as follows:

- Serum glucose > 600 mg/dL (hyperglycemia).
- Serum pH > 7.3.
- Serum bicarbonate > 15 mEq/L.
- Anion gap < 14 mEq/L (normal).
- Serum osmolality > 310 mOsm/kg.

Treatment

- Fluid resuscitate with 4–6 L NS within the first eight hours.
- Identify the precipitating cause and treat.
- Monitor and replete sodium, potassium, phosphate, and glucose every two hours. Give IV insulin only if glucose levels remain elevated after sufficient fluid resuscitation.

Other Complications

Both type 1 and type 2 diabetics are at ↑ risk for macro- and microvascular disease and infections. The three most common microvascular complications are as follows:

- **Retinopathy:**
  - Correlates with the duration of DM and the degree of glycemic control.
  - **Sx/Exam:** Classified as nonproliferative or proliferative.
    - **Nonproliferative diabetic retinopathy:** Characterized by retinal vascular microaneurysms, blot hemorrhages, and cotton-wool spots. Macular edema may be seen.
    - **Proliferative diabetic retinopathy:** Neovascularization in response to retinal hypoxia is the hallmark.
  - **Tx:** Prevention, regular eye exams, and laser therapy are the mainstays of therapy.
- **Nephropathy:**
  - **Sx/Exam:** Usually asymptomatic, but can present with bilateral lower extremity edema (from nephrotic syndrome).
  - **Dx:**
    - Kimmelstiel-Wilson lesions (nodular glomerulosclerosis) may be seen on kidney biopsy.
    - Look for **coexisting retinopathy.**
  - **Tx:**
    - Patients with microalbuminuria or proteinuria should be started on an ACEI to keep their BP < 130/80.
    - End-stage nephropathy requires chronic hemodialysis or transplantation.
- **Neuropathy:**
  - **Sx/Exam:** Can present as polyneuropathy, mononeuropathy, and/or autonomic neuropathy. Patients are also at ↑ risk for the development of diabetic foot ulcers.
  - **Tx:**
    - Strict glycemic control improves nerve conduction.
    - TCAs, carbamazepine, and gabapentin are used to treat sensory dysfunction.

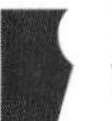

KEY FACT

The risk of microvascular complications in DM is ↓ by tight glycemic control.

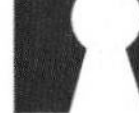

KEY FACT

Diabetics have ↑ susceptibility to the following:

- Pseudomonal otitis externa
- Mucormycosis facial infection
- Pyelonephritis
- Emphysematous cholangitis

Thyroid Disorders

FUNCTIONAL THYROID DISORDERS

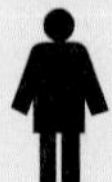

A 30-year-old woman presents with weight loss and heat intolerance and is found to be tachycardic. Labs reveal a suppressed TSH and an elevated T_4 level. What is the most common cause of hyperthyroidism?

Graves' disease.

Classified as hyperthyroidism or hypothyroidism.

Symptoms/Exam

Table 5-5 lists distinguishing features of hypo- and hyperthyroidism.

Diagnosis

- Order a TSH and a free T_4 to distinguish hyperthyroidism from hypothyroidism.
  - **Hyperthyroid patients (↓ TSH):** Order a radioactive iodine uptake scan as well as thyroid-stimulating immunoglobulin assays.
  - **Hypothyroid patients (↑ TSH):** Order an anti–thyroid peroxidase (anti-TPO) antibody assay.
- Figure 5-1 and Table 5-6 outline the workup, differential, and treatment of functional thyroid disease.

TABLE 5-5. Clinical Presentation of Functional Thyroid Disease

	Hypothyroidism	Hyperthyroidism
General	Fatigue, lethargy.	Hyperactivity, nervousness, fatigue.
Temperature	Cold intolerance.	Heat intolerance.
GI	Constipation leading to ileus; weight gain despite a poor appetite.	Diarrhea; weight loss despite good appetite.
Cardiac	Bradycardia, pericardial effusion, hyperlipidemia.	Tachycardia, atrial fibrillation, CHF; systolic hypertension, ↑ pulse pressure.
Neurologic	Delayed DTRs.	Fine resting tremor; apathetic hyperthyroidism (elderly).
Menstruation	Heavy.	Irregular.
Dermatologic	Dry, coarse skin; thinning hair; thin, brittle nails; myxedema.	Warm, sweaty skin; fine, oily hair; nail separation from matrix.
Other	Arthralgias/myalgias.	**Osteoporosis.**

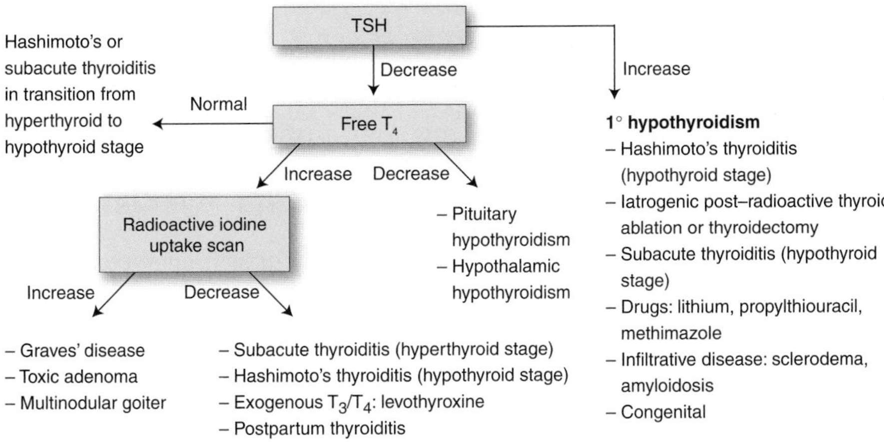

FIGURE 5-1. Workup of functional thyroid disease.

TREATMENT

- Symptomatic hyperthyroidism:
  - Treat with **propranolol,** hydration, rest, and adequate nutrition. Cooling measures are required for severe hyperthermia.
  - Mild cases of hyperthyroidism can then be treated with **propylthiouracil** or **methimazole, which block thyroid hormone synthesis.** More severe cases require radioactive ^{131}I thyroid ablation.
  - **Thyroidectomy** is indicated for large goiters, pregnant patients, or obstruction of the trachea. Patients who have undergone radioactive ablation or thyroidectomy become hypothyroid and are treated with levothyroxine.

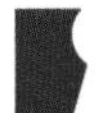

KEY FACT

Methimazole should **not** be given during pregnancy because it can cause aplasia cutis in the fetus.

TABLE 5-6. Differential and Treatment of Functional Thyroid Disease

	Graves' Disease	Subacute Thyroiditis	Hashimoto's Thyroiditis
Etiology/ pathophysiology	Antibody directed at TSH receptor. More prevalent in females.	Viral (possibly mumps or coxsackievirus).	Autoimmune disorder.
Symptoms/ exam	Hyperthyroidism; diffuse, painless goiter. Proptosis, lid lag, diplopia, conjunctival injection. Pretibial myxedema.	Hyperthyroidism leading to hypothyroidism. Tender thyroid. Malaise, upper respiratory tract symptoms, fever early on.	Hypothyroidism. Painless thyroid enlargement.
Diagnosis	↑ radioactive uptake scan, ⊕ thyroid-stimulating immunoglobulin.	↓ radioactive uptake scan, high ESR.	⊕ anti-TPO antibody.
Disease-specific treatment	Propylthiouracil, methimazole, thyroid ablation with ^{131}I. Ophthalmopathy may require surgical decompression, steroids, or orbital radiation.	NSAIDs for pain control; steroids for severe pain. Self-limited.	Levothyroxine.

- **Thyroid storm** is a form of severe hyperthyroidism that is characterized by high fever, dehydration, tachycardia, coma, and high-output cardiac failure.
- **Hypothyroidism:**
  - Treat with **levothyroxine.** Patients with myxedema coma require IV levothyroxine and IV hydrocortisone.
  - Mechanical ventilation and warming blankets are required for hypoventilation and hypothermia, respectively.
  - **Myxedema coma** is a form of severe hypothyroidism characterized by altered mental status and hypothermia.

THYROID NODULES

A 55-year-old woman on no medications presents with abdominal pain, nausea, and fatigue. Routine lab evaluations reveal an elevated serum calcium level. What is the next step in the diagnostic workup?

Laboratory screening with a CBC and a chemistry panel that includes PO_4, 24-hour urine calcium, PTH, 25-OH vitamin D, and SPEP.

The basic workup of a solitary thyroid nodule is outlined in Figure 5-2.

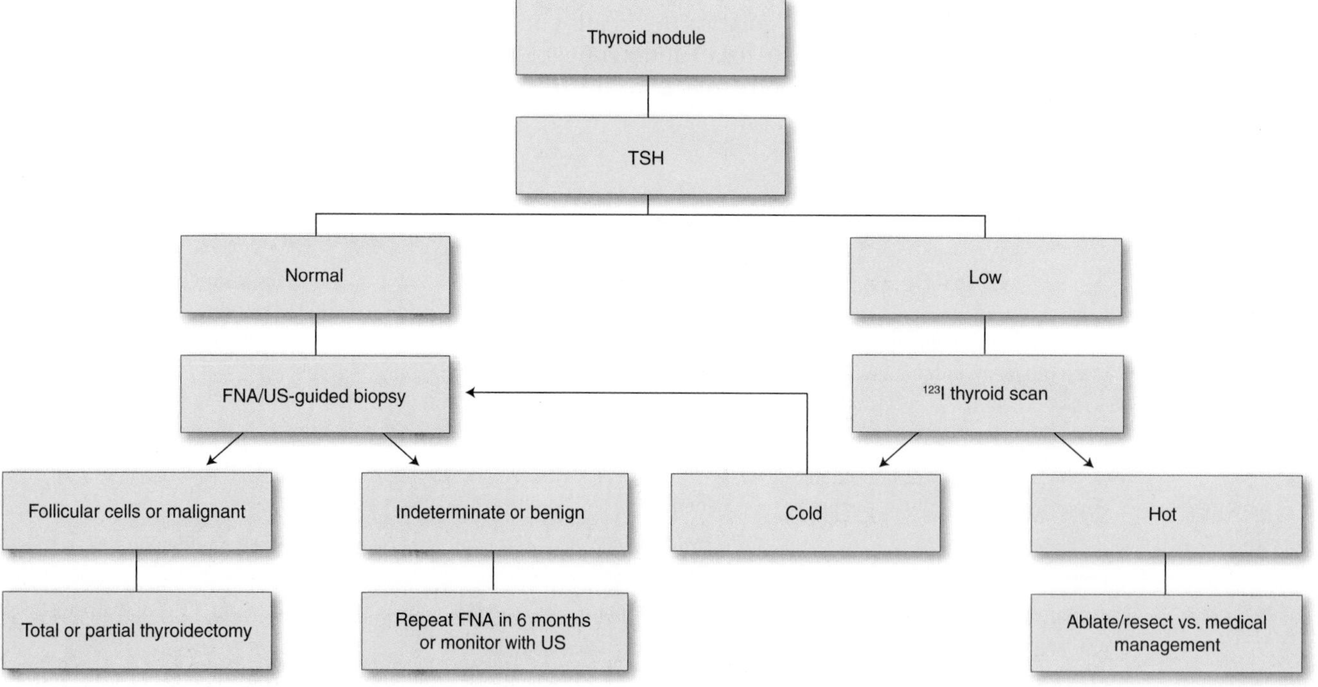

FIGURE 5-2. Workup of a thyroid nodule.

Hypercalcemia

Most cases of 1° hyperparathyroidism are caused by a parathyroid adenoma. Initial treatment is focused on correcting the underlying hypercalcemia. Table 5-7 lists the clinical characteristics of 1° hyperparathyroidism and other causes of hypercalcemia.

TABLE 5-7. Clinical Characteristics of Hypercalcemia

	1° Hyperparathyroidism	Other
Etiology	Adenoma. Multiglandular disease.	Malignancy that produces PTH-related peptide, multiple myeloma, sarcoidosis, vitamin D excess, vitamin A excess, thiazide diuretics, lithium, bone metastasis.
Symptoms/exam	Fatigue, constipation, polyuria, polydipsia, bone pain, nausea.	Presentation is the same as that of 1° disease.
Diagnosis	↑ calcium and PTH; low PO_4.	↑ calcium; low PTH; sometimes ↑ PO_4.
Treatment	Parathyroidectomy. Hydrate with IV fluids; give furosemide after volume deficit is corrected; bisphosphonates for severe hypercalcemia.	Sarcoidosis, multiple myeloma: steroids. Low-calcium diet. Hydrate with IV fluids; give furosemide after volume deficit is corrected; bisphosphonates for severe hypercalcemia.
Complications	Nephrolithiasis, nephrocalcinosis, osteopenia, osteoporosis, pancreatitis, cardiac valve calcifications.	Same as those for 1° disease.

Osteoporosis

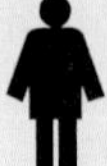

A 68-year-old woman presents to her primary care physician for a routine checkup. The physician orders a DEXA scan of the spine and hip. What T-score value denotes osteoporosis?

T-score ≤ –2.5.

A common metabolic bone disease characterized by ↓ bone strength and abnormal bone density. More common among inactive, **postmenopausal Caucasian women.**

SYMPTOMS/EXAM

Commonly asymptomatic. Patients may present with **hip fractures, vertebral compression fractures** (resulting in loss of height and progressive thoracic kyphosis), and/or distal radius fractures following minimal trauma.

DIFFERENTIAL

Osteomalacia (inadequate bone mineralization), hyperparathyroidism, multiple myeloma, metastatic carcinoma (pathologic fracture).

DIAGNOSIS

- All patients > 65 years of age, as well as patients 40–60 years of age with at least one risk factor for osteoporotic fractures after menopause, should be screened with a DEXA scan of the spine and hip.
- Take the lowest **T-score** between the hip and the spine:
  - **T-score –1 to –2.5:** Osteopenia.
  - **T-score ≤ –2.5:** Osteoporosis.
- Rule out 2° causes, including smoking, alcoholism, renal failure, hyperthyroidism, multiple myeloma, 1° hyperparathyroidism, vitamin D deficiency, hypercortisolism, heparin use, and chronic steroid use.

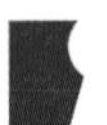

KEY FACT

Avoid HRT in osteoporotic patients in view of the risk of cardiovascular mortality and breast cancer.

TREATMENT

- Treat when a T-score is < –2 or when a T-score is < –1.5 in a patient with risk factors for osteoporotic fractures.
- Drugs of choice, in order of efficacy, include **bisphosphonates** (alendronate, risedronate, etidronate, ibandronate), teriparatide, selective estrogen receptor modulators (SERMs) such as raloxifene, and intranasal calcitonin.
- Eliminate or treat 2° causes, and add weight-bearing exercises and calcium/vitamin D supplementation.
- A DEXA scan should be repeated 1–2 years after the initiation of drug therapy. If the T-score is found to have worsened, combination therapy (eg, a SERM and a bisphosphonate) or a change in therapy should be initiated, with consideration given to ruling out 2° causes.

Cushing's Syndrome (Hypercortisolism)

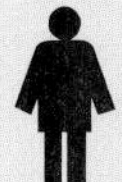

A 30-year-old woman with a history of SLE who is on chronic steroids presents with ↑ truncal obesity, a "buffalo hump," and moon facies. What is the first step in diagnosis?

A 24-hour urine collection should reveal an elevated cortisol level, which is diagnostic for Cushing's syndrome.

Cushing's disease is Cushing's syndrome caused by hypersecretion of ACTH from a pituitary adenoma. The etiologies of hypercortisolism include adrenal (adenoma, carcinoma), pituitary (adenoma), ectopic (lung cancer), and exogenous (corticosteroid administration).

Symptoms/Exam

- Look for truncal obesity with moon facies and a "**buffalo hump.**"
- Psychiatric disturbances, hypertension, hyperglycemia, impotence, oligomenorrhea, growth retardation, hirsutism (excessive hair growth, acne), easy bruisability, and purple striae can also be seen.
- Table 5-8 lists the laboratory characteristics of Cushing's syndrome according to etiology.

Differential

Chronic alcoholism, depression, DM, chronic steroid use, adrenogenital syndrome, acute stress, obesity.

Diagnosis

- ↑ 24-hour urine cortisol is diagnostic for Cushing's syndrome.
- Check A.M. serum ACTH.
  - **A.M. serum ACTH < 5 pg/mL:** Obtain an adrenal CT scan or an MRI to look for an adrenal adenoma or carcinoma (unilateral) or adrenal hyperplasia (bilateral).

TABLE 5-8. Laboratory Characteristics of Endogenous Cushing's Syndrome

	ACTH Dependent	ACTH Independent
Plasma cortisol	↑	↑
Urinary cortisol	↑	↑
ACTH	↑	↓
Source	Pituitary (suppressible) Ectopic (nonsuppressible)	Adenoma (↓ DHEA) Carcinoma (↑ DHEA)

- **A.M. serum ACTH > 5 pg/mL:** Administer a high-dose dexamethasone suppression test.
  - **Suppressed cortisol response:** Cushing's disease (eg, ACTH-secreting pituitary adenoma). Confirm with a pituitary MRI.
  - **Nonsuppressed cortisol response:** Ectopic ACTH-producing tumor such as carcinoid tumors and small cell lung cancer. Can be seen on octreotide scan and/or MRI/CT of the chest. If ⊖, do a pituitary MRI.
- DHEA is most elevated in adrenal carcinoma.

TREATMENT

- **Ectopic ACTH-secreting tumor:** Surgical resection of the tumor.
- **Adrenal carcinoma, adenoma, or hyperplasia:** Adrenalectomy.
- **ACTH-secreting pituitary adenoma:** Transsphenoidal resection or radiation treatment.
- **Exogenous steroids:** Minimize use.

Adrenal Insufficiency

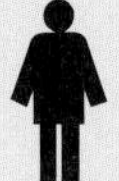

A 65-year-old man with a known recent diagnosis of melanoma presents with vague complaints of dizziness, weakness, fatigue, and weight loss. Basic lab testing reveals hyponatremia. What testing will help determine the diagnosis?

A.M. serum cortisol and A.M. serum ACTH.

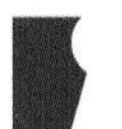

KEY FACT

Addison's **D**isease is due to **A**drenocortical **D**eficiency.

Adrenocortical hypofunction can stem from adrenal failure (1° adrenal insufficiency, also known as **Addison's disease**) or from ↓ ACTH production from the pituitary (2° adrenal insufficiency). Etiologies are as follows:

- **1° adrenal insufficiency:** Autoimmune disease (idiopathic), metastatic tumors, hemorrhagic infarction (from coagulopathy or septicemia), adrenalectomy, granulomatous disease (TB, sarcoid).
- **2° adrenal insufficiency:** Withdrawal of exogenous steroids; hypothalamic or pituitary pathology (tumor, infarct, trauma, infection, iatrogenic).

SYMPTOMS/EXAM

- Symptoms include weakness, anorexia, weight loss, nausea, vomiting, postural hypotension, diarrhea, abdominal pain, and myalgias/arthralgias.
- Infection, surgery, or other stressors can trigger an **addisonian crisis** with symptomatic adrenal insufficiency, confusion, and vasodilatory shock.

KEY FACT

Hyperpigmentation, dehydration, hyperkalemia, and salt craving are specific to 1° adrenal insufficiency.

DIAGNOSIS

- An A.M. serum cortisol < 5 μg/dL or a serum cortisol < 20 μg/dL after an ACTH stimulation test or an ↑ of < 9 μg/dL in serum cortisol after the same test is diagnostic.

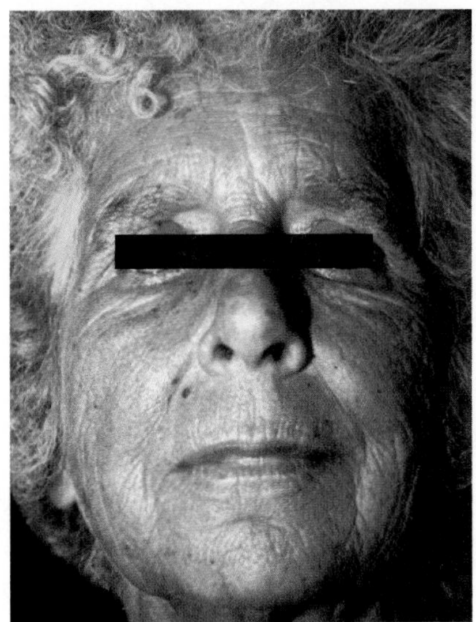

A

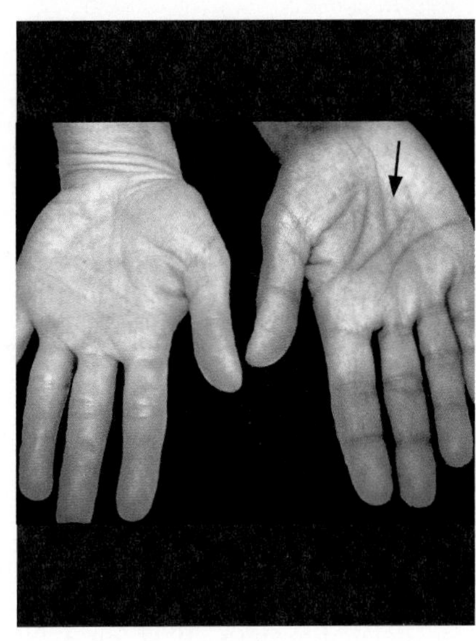

B

FIGURE 5-3. Addison's disease. (**A**) Note the characteristic hyperpigmentation in sun-exposed areas. (**B**) Contrast the hyperpigmented palmar creases (arrow) with the normal hand of a different patient. (Reproduced with permission from Wolff K et al. *Fitzpatrick's Dermatology in General Medicine,* 7th ed. New York: McGraw-Hill, 2008, Fig. 152-16.)

- Nonspecific findings include hyponatremia, hyperkalemia, hyperpigmentation (see Figure 5-3), and eosinophilia.
- Check A.M. serum ACTH to distinguish 1° from 2° adrenal insufficiency (see Table 5-9).

Treatment

- Treat with glucocorticoids, and add mineralocorticoids in the setting of 1° adrenal insufficiency.
- **Hydrocortisone** is the drug of choice. Add **fludrocortisone** for orthostatic hypotension, hyponatremia, or hyperkalemia. Glucocorticoid doses should be ↑ in times of illness, trauma, or surgery.
- Patients in **adrenal crisis** need immediate fluid resuscitation and IV hydrocortisone.

TABLE 5-9. 1° vs. 2° Adrenal Insufficiency

	Addison's Disease	2° Adrenal Insufficiency
ACTH	↑	↓
Cortisol after ACTH challenge	↓	↑

(Reproduced with permission from Le T et al. *First Aid for the USMLE Step 2 CK,* 4th ed. New York: McGraw-Hill, 2004: 121.)

Prolactinoma

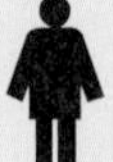

A 60-year-old man with a history of erectile dysfunction presents with headaches and associated temporal field visual loss. Lab testing reveals elevated prolactin levels. What is the imaging test of choice?

MRI to assess the pituitary for possible prolactinoma.

The most common functional pituitary tumor.

Symptoms/Exam

Women typically present with galactorrhea and amenorrhea. Men may develop impotence and, later in the disease (and often when the adenoma is larger), symptoms related to mass effect (eg, CN III palsy, diplopia, temporal field visual loss, headache).

Diagnosis

↑ prolactin levels; ↓ LH and FSH. Order an MRI to confirm the tumor (see Figure 5-4).

Treatment

Treat medically with a dopamine agonist such as bromocriptine or cabergoline. If medical therapy is not tolerated or if the tumor is large, transsphenoidal surgery followed by irradiation is indicated.

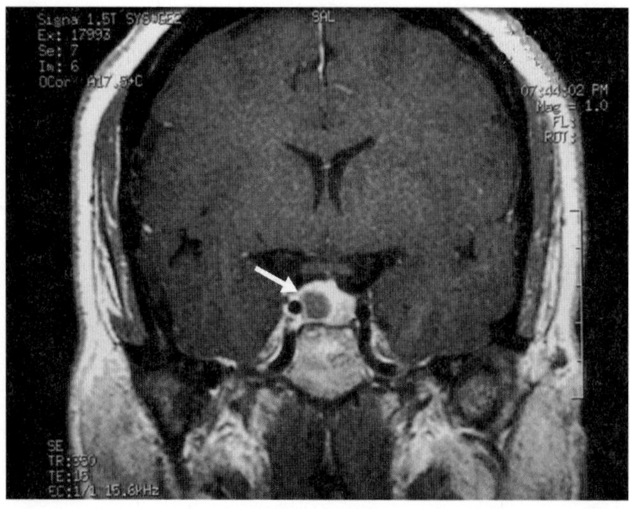

A

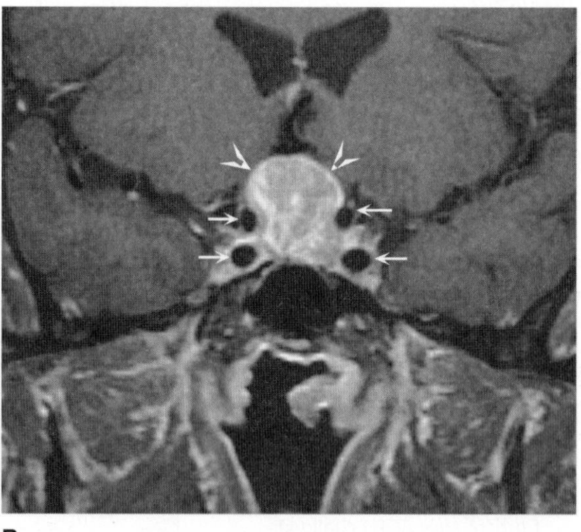

B

FIGURE 5-4. Pituitary adenomas. Coronal gadolinium-enhanced MR images demonstrating (**A**) a microadenoma (arrow), which enhances less than the adjacent pituitary tissue, and (**B**) a pituitary macroadenoma (arrowheads) extending superiorly from the sella turcica to the suprasellar region. Arrows denote the internal carotid arteries. (Image A reproduced with permission from Schorge JO et al. *Williams Gynecology.* New York: McGraw-Hill, 2008, Fig. 15-8A. Image B reproduced with permission from Fauci AS et al. *Harrison's Principles of Internal Medicine,* 17th ed. New York: McGraw-Hill, 2008, Fig. 333-4.)

Multiple Endocrine Neoplasia (MEN)

A group of familial, autosomal dominant syndromes (see Table 5-10).

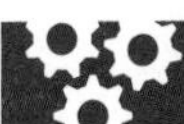

MNEMONIC

The 3 P's of primary MEN:

Parathyroid hyperplasia
Pancreatic islet cell tumor
Pituitary adenoma

PHEOCHROMOCYTOMA

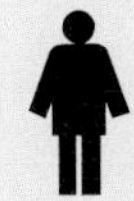

A 40-year-old woman with a history of difficult-to-control hypertension presents with a headache. A review of systems reveals associated palpitations and diaphoresis. On exam, she is found to have a BP of 200/100. What lab test will yield the suspected diagnosis?

Urine or plasma free metanephrines and normetanephrines.

- A clinical syndrome that typically presents as hypertension along with the triad of headache, palpitations, and sweating.
- **Dx:** The diagnosis is confirmed with lab testing for urine or plasma free metanephrines and normetanephrines along with a CT/MRI.
- **Tx:** Treat preoperatively with α-blockade (phenoxybenzamine) followed by surgical resection.

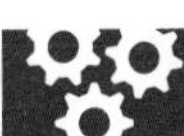

MNEMONIC

MEN 2A and 2B—two common characteristics:

Thyroid medullary cancer
Pheochromocytoma

TABLE 5-10. Characteristics of MEN Syndromes

SYNDROME	TYPE	CHARACTERISTICS
Wermer's syndrome	1	**P**arathyroid hyperplasia **P**ancreatic islet cell tumor **P**ituitary adenoma
Sipple's syndrome	2A	Parathyroid hyperplasia **T**hyroid medullary cancer **P**heochromocytoma
	2B	**T**hyroid medullary cancer **P**heochromocytoma Mucocutaneous neuromas Ganglioneuromatosis of the colon Marfan-like habitus

NOTES

CHAPTER 6

ETHICS AND STATISTICS

Basic Principles

Be familiar with the following principles:

- **Autonomy:** The right to make decisions for oneself according to one's own system of morals and beliefs.
- **Paternalism:** Providing for patients' needs without their input.
- **Beneficence:** Action intended to bring about a good outcome.
- **Nonmaleficence:** Action not intended to bring about harm.
- **Truth telling:** Revealing all pertinent information to patients.
- **Proportionality:** Ensuring that a medical treatment or plan is commensurate with the illness and with the goals of treatment.
- **Distributive justice:** Allocation of resources in a manner that is fair and just, though not necessarily equal.

Autonomy

A 22-year-old man who is a Jehovah's Witness presents with GI bleeding. The patient clearly states that he does not want a blood transfusion. His hematocrit falls from 40 to 22, and his blood pressure is decreasing as well. The physicians urge the patient to accept lifesaving treatments, but the patient refuses. When his blood pressure reaches a critical level, one of the physicians initiates plans to transfuse the patient. The rest of the team vetoes the plan. Which two principles of ethics are involved, and which principle trumps the other?

This is a conflict between beneficence and autonomy. The physician aims to bring a good outcome for the patient, but the patient is making a decision in accordance with his belief system. The principle of autonomy trumps beneficence in this situation.

INFORMED CONSENT

Involves discussing diagnoses and prognoses with patients as well as any proposed treatment, its risks and benefits, and its alternatives. Only with such information can a patient reach an informed decision. **Do not conceal a diagnosis from a patient;** doing so violates the principle of truth telling. However, respect your patients' wishes if they tell you to share only certain things with them.

RIGHTS OF MINORS

The treatment of patients < 18 years of age requires parental consent unless:

- They are emancipated (ie, financially independent, married, raising children, living on their own, or serving in the armed forces).
- They are requesting contraception or treatment of pregnancy, STDs, or psychiatric illness. Note that many states require parental consent or notice for termination of pregnancy in a minor.

Most questions on the Step 3 test regarding parental consent will deal with situations such as those cited above. In general, this means that for the Step 3 test, the governing principle should be to let minors make their own decisions.

Competency

COMPETENCY VS. CAPACITY

It is a mistake to use the terms **competency** and **capacity** interchangeably. Competency is a **legal** determination made only by a court, whereas capacity is a **clinical** assessment. Each involves the assessment of a patient's ability to think and act rationally (not necessarily wisely). Incompetence is permanent (eg, severe dementia), and incompetent patients are generally assigned a surrogate by the court. Incapacity may be temporary (eg, delirium), and careful decision making is important when considering therapeutic interventions for patients with questionable capacity.

DETENTION AND USE OF RESTRAINTS

Psychiatric patients may be held against their will only if they are a danger to themselves or to others (in accordance with the principle of beneficence). The use of restraints can be considered if a patient is at risk of doing harm to self or others, but such use must be evaluated on at least a daily basis.

DURABLE POWER OF ATTORNEY (DPoA) FOR HEALTH CARE

DPoA has two related meanings. First, it can refer to a document signed by the patient assigning a surrogate decision maker in the event that he or she becomes incapacitated. Second, it can refer to the person to whom that authority has been granted.

SURROGATE/PROXY

Defined as an alternate decision maker, designated by the patient (DPoA), by law, or by convention. If no person has been formally designated to represent the patient, surrogacy falls to relatives in accordance with a hierarchy that may vary from state to state (typically, a spouse is at the top of this hierarchy).

Confidentiality

IMPORTANCE OF CONFIDENTIALITY (AND HIPAA)

Maintaining the confidentiality of patient information is critical. Violations are unethical, can result in legal troubles, and may irreparably harm the patient-physician relationship. The Health Insurance Portability and Accountability Act (HIPAA) outlines rules and guidelines for preserving patient privacy.

WHEN TO VIOLATE CONFIDENTIALITY

If a physician learns about a threat to an individual's life or well-being (ie, a danger to self or to others), violating confidentiality is mandatory. In a similar manner, information about child abuse or elder abuse must be reported.

REPORTABLE CONDITIONS

Most contagious, rare, and incurable infections, as well as other threats to public health, are reportable. The list of reportable infections varies by state but often includes HIV/AIDS, syphilis, gonorrhea, chlamydia, TB, mumps, measles, rubella, smallpox, and suspected bioterrorist events. Such reporting is mandatory and does not constitute a violation of confidentiality.

ASKING FOLLOW-UP QUESTIONS

Follow-up questions should be used to clarify unclear issues regarding questions such as which family members can be included in discussions of care, who is the primary surrogate, and what patients want to know about their own conditions.

End-of-Life Care

Patients in the end stages of a terminal illness have the right to obtain medical treatment that is intended to preserve human dignity in dying. The best means of reaching an agreement with the patient and his or her family regarding end-of-life care is to continue to talk about the patient's condition and to resolve decision-making conflicts. Ultimately, this is the same task that an ethics consultant would attempt to perform for the physician and the patient.

There is a growing body of literature addressing the importance of cultural issues in end-of-life care. In the United States, emphasis is placed on patient autonomy, full disclosure of medical information, and the primacy of objective over subjective medical findings. However, members of other cultures may lend more credibility to family-based decisions, particular methods of diagnosis communication, and the importance of subjective aspects of illness. It is important to elicit and respect these frameworks and interactional dynamics in end-of-life care.

ADVANCE DIRECTIVES

Defined as oral or written statements regarding what a patient would want in the event that intensive resuscitative intervention becomes necessary to sustain life. These instructions can be detailed—which is obviously preferable—or they can be broad. Oral statements are ethically binding but are not legally binding in all states. Remember that an informed, competent adult can refuse treatment even if it means that doing so would lead to death. Such instructions must be honored.

DO NOT RESUSCITATE (DNR) ORDERS/CODE STATUS

The express wishes of a patient (eg, "I do not want to be intubated") supersede the wishes of family members or surrogates. Physicians should inquire about and follow DNR orders during each hospitalization. If code status has not been addressed and the matter becomes relevant, defer to the surrogate.

PAIN IN TERMINALLY ILL PATIENTS

Terminally ill patients are often inadequately treated for pain. Prescribe as much narcotic medication as is needed to relieve patients' pain and suffering. Do not worry about addiction in this setting. Two-thirds of patients in their last three days of life stated that they felt moderate to severe pain.

THE PRINCIPLE OF "DOUBLE EFFECT"

Actions can have more than one consequence, some intended, others not. Unintended medical consequences are acceptable if the intended consequences are legitimate and the harm proportionately smaller than the benefit. For example, a dying patient can be given high doses of analgesics even if it may unintentionally shorten life.

PERSISTENT VEGETATIVE STATE (PVS)

Defined as a state in which the brain stem is intact and the patient has sleep-wake cycles, but there is no awareness, voluntary activity, or ability to interact with the environment. Reflexes may be normal or abnormal. Some patients survive this way for five years or more, with the aggregate annual cost reaching into the billions of dollars.

KEY FACT

The Elisabeth Kübler-Ross psychological stages at the end of life are denial, anger, bargaining, depression, and acceptance.

QUALITY OF LIFE

Defined as a subjective evaluation of a patient's current physical, emotional, and social well-being. This must be evaluated from the perspective of the patient.

EUTHANASIA

Euthanasia is assisting an informed, competent, terminally ill patient to end life, usually through the administration of a lethal dose of medication. Euthanasia is different from physician-assisted suicide, in which the physician prescribes a medication that the patient administers to himself or herself to end life. Neither of these is the same as withdrawal of care. Currently, euthanasia is illegal in all states, and physician-assisted suicide is legal only in Oregon.

PALLIATION AND HOSPICE

These related concepts involve the provision of end-of-life care within (palliation) or outside (hospice) a traditional medical system. Each is an attempt to manage psychosocial and physical well-being in a manner that preserves dignity and maximizes comfort. Both involve interdisciplinary collaboration (MD, RN, chaplain, social worker, aide), focusing on patient-defined goals of care.

WITHDRAWAL OF TREATMENT

Withdrawal of treatment is the removal of life-sustaining treatment and is legally and ethically no different from never starting treatment. The decision to withdraw treatment may come from the patient, an advance directive, a DPoA, or, absent any of these, the closest relative and/or a physician. It is easiest when all parties are in agreement, although this is not required. When there is conflict, the patient's wishes take precedence. In futile cases or those involving extreme suffering, a physician may withdraw or withhold treatment; if the family disagrees, the physician should seek input from an ethics committee or a court's approval.

Biostatistics

Not everyone with a given disease will test positive for that disease, and not everyone with a positive test result has the disease.

SENSITIVITY AND SPECIFICITY

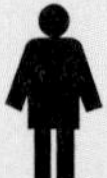

You have a test that has a sensitivity of 0.95 and a specificity of 0.95. How helpful is this test in your diagnostic reasoning for the following scenarios?

1. Disease prevalence of 1%
2. Disease prevalence of 10%
3. Disease prevalence of 50%
4. Disease prevalence of 90%

1. Not helpful. Most of the positives will be false positives, so further evaluation will be necessary.
2. Somewhat helpful. A negative test reduces the probability of disease below a threshold for further testing, while a positive test helps stratify a high-risk population that requires further testing.
3. Very helpful. Both positive and negative results make significant changes in disease probability and can confirm or disprove a diagnosis. This is the situation in which a laboratory test is most helpful.
4. Not helpful. The positive result adds nothing to your clinical suspicion, and a negative test is likely to be a false negative.

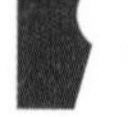

KEY FACT

Sense (sensitivity) who does have a disease. **Specify (specificity)** who does not.

Sensitivity is the probability that a person with a disease will have a positive result on a given test. High sensitivity is useful in a screening test, as the goal is to identify everyone with a given disease. **Specificity** is the probability that a person without a disease will have a negative result on a test. High specificity is desirable for a confirmatory test.

Ideally, a test will be highly sensitive and specific, but this is rare. A test that is highly sensitive but not specific will yield many false positives, whereas one that is highly specific but not sensitive will yield many false negatives.

TABLE 6-1. Determination of PPV and NPV

	DISEASE PRESENT	NO DISEASE	
Positive test	a	b	PPV = a/(a + b)
Negative test	c	d	NPV = d/(c + d)
	Sensitivity = a/(a + c)	Specificity = d/(b + d)	

PREDICTIVE VALUES

Positive predictive value (PPV) is the probability that a person with a positive test result has the disease (true positives/all positives; see Table 6-1). If a disease has a greater prevalence, then the PPV is higher. **Negative predictive value (NPV)** is the probability that a person with a negative test result is disease free (see Table 6-1). A test has a higher NPV value when a disease has a lower prevalence. It is important to note that PPV and NPV can be determined only if the incidence in the sample is representative of the population. For example, if the data for Table 6-1 are derived from a case-control study, then the PPV and NPV cannot be calculated. Generally, one needs a cohort study design to get PPV or NPV.

INCIDENCE

Defined as the number of **new** cases of a given disease per year; for example, four cases of X per year.

PREVALENCE

Defined as the total number of **existing** cases of a given disease in the entire population; for example, 20 people have X (right now).

ABSOLUTE RISK

The **probability** of an event in a given time period; for example, 0.1% chance of developing X in 10 years.

RELATIVE RISK (RR)

Used to evaluate the results of cohort (prospective) studies. The RR compares the incidence of a disease in a group exposed to a particular risk factor with the incidence in those not exposed to the risk factor (see Table 6-2). An RR

TABLE 6-2. Determination of RR and OR

	DISEASE DEVELOPS	NO DISEASE	
Exposure	a	b	RR = [a/(a + b)]/[c/(c + d)]
No exposure	c	d	OR = ad/bc

< 1 means that the event is less likely in the exposed group; conversely, an RR > 1 signifies that the event is more likely in that group.

ODDS RATIO (OR)

Used in case-control (retrospective) studies. The OR compares the rate of exposure among those with and without a disease (see Table 6-2). It is considered less accurate than RR, but in rare diseases the OR approximates the RR.

ABSOLUTE RISK REDUCTION (ARR) OR ATTRIBUTABLE RISK

Measures the risk accounted for by exposure to a given factor, taking into account the background of the disease. Useful in randomized controlled trials. Numerically, ARR = the absolute risk (rate of adverse events) in the placebo group minus the absolute risk in treated patients.

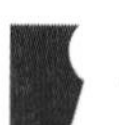

KEY FACT

ARR and RRR give very different values and should not be confused. ARR is a much better measure of benefit; because it is a ratio, RRR can look deceptively large. Watch out for drug advertising that touts RRR.

RELATIVE RISK REDUCTION (RRR)

Also used in randomized controlled trials, this is the ratio between two risks. Numerically, RRR = [the event rate in control patients minus the event rate in experimental patients] ÷ the event rate in control patients.

RRR can be deceptive and is clinically far less important than ARR. Consider a costly intervention that reduces the risk of an adverse event from 0.01% to 0.004%. ARR is 0.01 – 0.004 = 0.006%, but RRR is (0.01 – 0.004)/0.01 = 0.6, or 60%! Would you order this intervention?

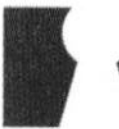

KEY FACT

If a 95% CI includes 1.0, the results are not significant. So if an RR is 1.9 but the 95% CI is 0.8–3.0, the RR is not significant.

NUMBER NEEDED TO TREAT (NNT)

The number of patients who would need to be treated to prevent one event. NNT = 1/ARR. In the example above, the NNT is 167.

STATISTICAL SIGNIFICANCE/*p*-VALUE

The *p*-value expresses the likelihood that an observed outcome was due to random chance. A *p*-value < 0.05 is generally accepted as indicating that an outcome is statistically significant.

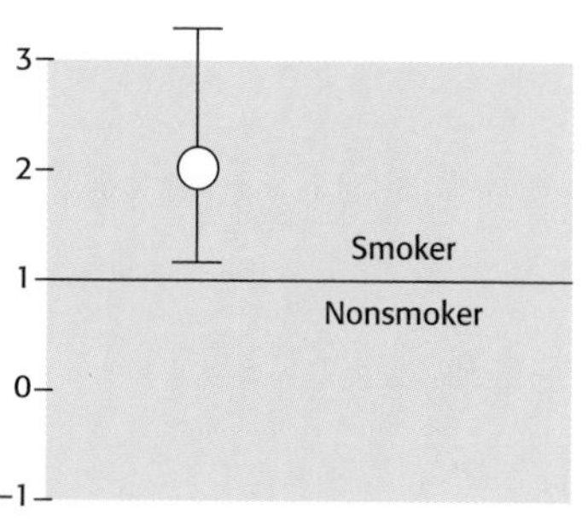

FIGURE 6-1. Relative risk of cancer.

CONFIDENCE INTERVAL (CI)

Like the *p*-value, the CI expresses the certainty that the observation is real or is a product of random chance. Used with ORs and RR, the 95% CI says that the observed risk or odds have a 95% chance of being within the interval. Thus, in Figure 6-1, the relative risk of cancer with smoking is 2.0 with a 95% CI of 1.3–3.5—meaning that the **observed** RR of cancer was 2.0, and that there is a 95% certainty that the **actual** RR of cancer from smoking falls somewhere between 1.3 and 3.5.

Study Design

Statistical analyses are used as a means of assessing relationships between events and outcomes. They do not prove irrefutably that a relationship exists but point to the likelihood. The validity of the results depends on the strength of the design.

SURVEYS

These are self-reporting of symptoms, exposures, feelings, and other subjective data. Such data may be analyzed with descriptive statistics or qualitative methodologies.

PROSPECTIVE AND RETROSPECTIVE STUDIES

Prospective studies assess future outcomes relating to present or future events; this enables the study designer to control for biases and to modify inputs/exposures. Retrospective studies relate to outcomes from past events. They may be less reliable than prospective studies.

COHORT STUDY

In a **cohort study** (see Figure 6-2), a population is observed over time, grouped on the basis of exposure to a particular factor, and watched for a specific outcome. Such studies are not good for rare conditions. Studies can be prospective or retrospective. Use RR to interpret results. Examples include the Nurses' Health Study and the Framingham Heart Study.

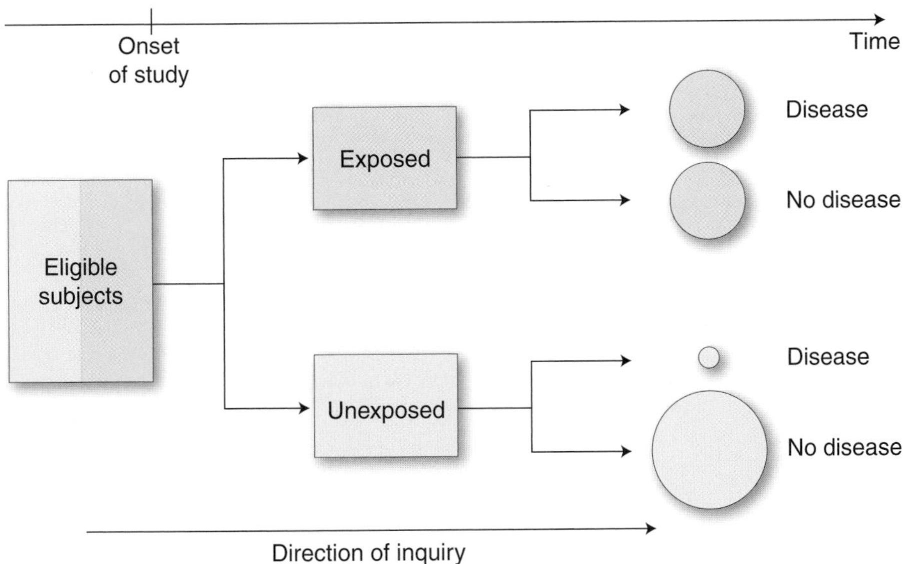

FIGURE 6-2. Schematic diagram of a cohort study. Shaded areas in the diagram represent exposed persons; unshaded areas represent unexposed persons. (Reproduced with permission from Greenberg RS et al. *Medical Epidemiology,* 4th ed. New York: McGraw-Hill, 2005, Fig. 8-2.)

CASE-CONTROL STUDY

A **case-control study** (see Figure 6-3) is a retrospective study involving a group of people with a given disease and an otherwise similar group of people without the disease who are compared for exposure to risk factors. Good for rare diseases. Use OR to interpret results.

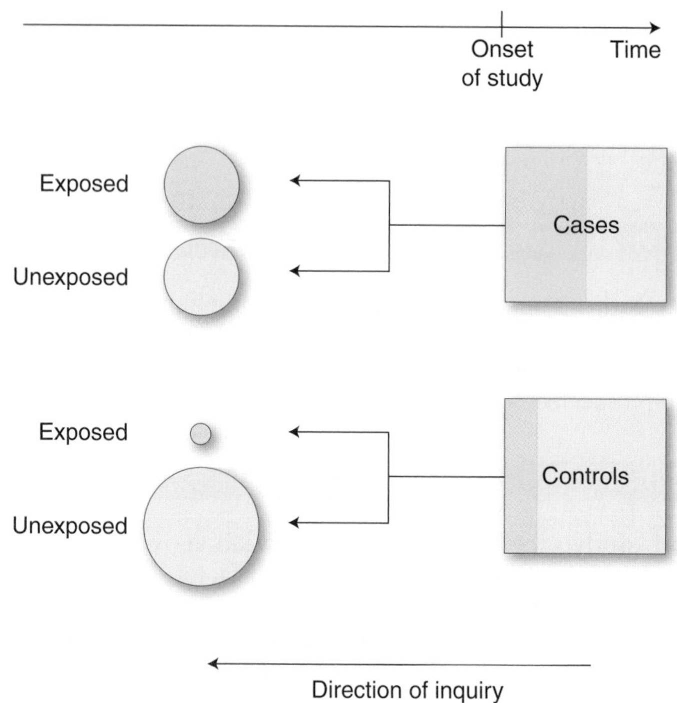

FIGURE 6-3. Schematic diagram of a case-control study. Shaded areas represent subjects who were exposed to the risk factor of interest. (Reproduced with permission from Greenberg RS et al. *Medical Epidemiology,* 4th ed. New York: McGraw-Hill, 2005, Fig. 9-1.)

RANDOMIZED CONTROLLED TRIAL (RCT)

A prospective study that randomly assigns participants to a treatment group or to a placebo group (see Figure 6-4). The placebo group and the treatment group are then compared to determine if the treatment made a difference. The double-blind RCT is the gold standard of experimental design.

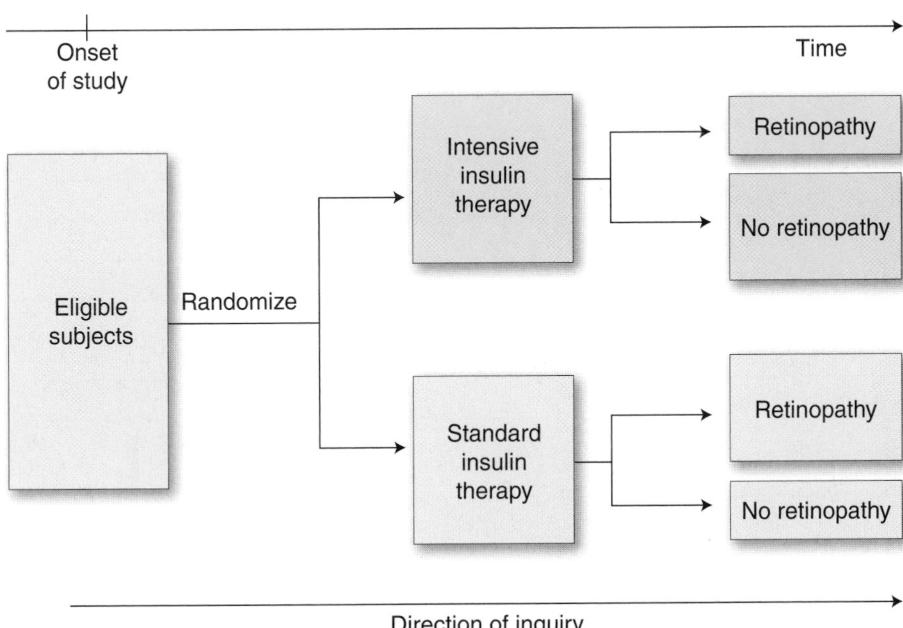

FIGURE 6-4. Schematic diagram of a randomized controlled clinical trial. The study above compares standard therapy with intensive insulin therapy for the treatment of diabetes mellitus. Shaded areas correspond to patients randomized to intensive insulin therapy. (Reproduced with permission from Greenberg RS et al. *Medical Epidemiology,* 4th ed. New York: McGraw-Hill, 2005, Fig. 7-2.)

NOTES

CHAPTER 7

GASTROENTEROLOGY

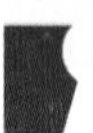

KEY FACT

Warning signs of more serious disease than PUD include age > 45, weight loss, anemia, and heme-⊕ stools.

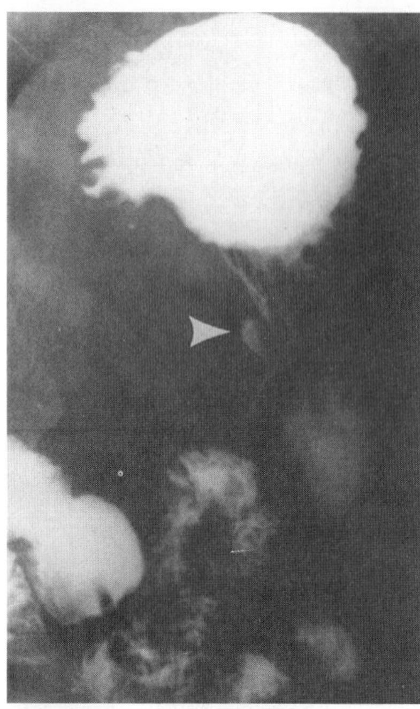

FIGURE 7-4. Gastric ulcer on barium upper GI. A benign gastric ulcer can be seen as pooling of contrast (arrowhead) extending beyond the adjacent gastric wall. (Reproduced with permission from Chen MY et al. *Basic Radiology.* New York: McGraw-Hill, 2004, Fig. 10-21.)

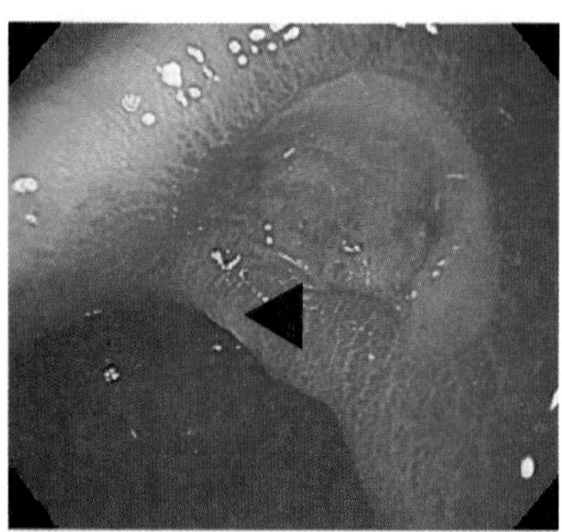

FIGURE 7-5. Benign gastric ulcer on endoscopy. (Reproduced with permission from Fauci AS et al. *Harrison's Principles of Internal Medicine,* 17th ed. New York: McGraw-Hill, 2008, Fig. 285-2A.)

Peptic Ulcer Disease (PUD)

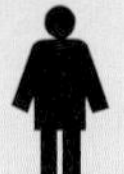

A 56-year-old woman was recently diagnosed with osteoarthritis. Two months later she started having abdominal pain that is aggravated by the consumption of food. What is the likely diagnosis?

Gastric ulcer 2° to the use of NSAIDs for joint pain.

The most common sites of PUD are the **stomach** and **duodenum.** ***H pylori*** infection and **NSAID/ASA use** are the major causes; Zollinger-Ellison syndrome, HSV infection, CMV, and cocaine use are less common etiologies.

SYMPTOMS/EXAM

- Presents with **epigastric** abdominal pain that patients describe as a "**gnawing**" or "**aching**" sensation that comes in waves. May also present with dyspepsia and upper GI bleed. Perforation and/or penetration into adjacent structures (eg, the pancreas, vascular structures such as the SMA, and the bile ducts) can lead to hemodynamic instability and associated symptoms (ie, pancreatitis).
- Symptoms can often be further distinguished by disease site:
  - **Duodenal ulcers:** Pain is relieved by food and comes on **postprandially.**
  - **Gastric ulcers:** Pain worsens with food **(pain with eating).**
- **Red flags:** With diarrhea, weight loss, and excessive gastric acid (elevated basal acid output), think of more uncommon causes (Zollinger-Ellison syndrome, systemic mastocytosis, hyperparathyroidism, extensive small bowel resection, gastric cancer).

DIAGNOSIS

- **Detect the ulcer:** Perform **endoscopy** with rapid urease testing for *H pylori;* biopsy any gastric ulcers to rule out malignancy (see Figures 7-4 and 7-5).
- **Look for *H pylori* infection** by the following means:
  - **Urease testing** of the biopsy sample.
  - **Serum antibody:** Easy to obtain, but a ⊕ antibody may not necessarily indicate active infection. Antibody remains ⊕ even after treatment.
  - **Urea breath test:** Good for detecting active infection, but patients must be off PPIs for two weeks and off antibiotics and bismuth for four weeks.
  - **Fecal antigen test:** Can also be used to test for *H pylori,* but as above, patients must be off antibiotics, PPIs, and bismuth.

TREATMENT

- **Discontinue ASA/NSAIDs;** promote smoking cessation and encourage weight loss.
- Give PPIs to control symptoms, ↓ acid secretion, and heal the ulcer (4 weeks for duodenal ulcers; 8–12 weeks for gastric ulcers).
- For *H pylori* infection, initiate multidrug therapy. Two of the following three drugs may be used—**amoxicillin 1 g BID, clarithromycin 500 mg BID,** or **metronidazole 500 mg BID**—along with a PPI **(omeprazole, lansoprazole) for 10–14 days.**

- Indications for surgery include recurrent/refractory upper GI bleed, gastric outlet obstruction, recurrent/refractory ulcers, perforation, and Zollinger-Ellison syndrome.

Inflammatory Bowel Disease (IBD)

Describes two distinct chronic idiopathic inflammatory diseases: **Crohn's disease** and **ulcerative colitis.** IBD clusters in families and is more common among **Jewish persons** and four times more common in **Caucasians but can occur in anyone, including young children and older adults.**

CROHN'S DISEASE

A 30-year-old man comes to your office complaining of diarrhea and weight loss. He states that his diarrhea often has mucus, but he denies any blood in his stool. He also mentions having difficulty eating food because of ulcers in his mouth. What is the next step in management?

In light of his age and presenting symptoms, this patient needs a colonoscopy and an evaluation for possible Crohn's disease.

Transmural inflammation (skip lesions) anywhere from the mouth to the anus. Most often affects the **terminal ileum,** small bowel, and colon. Has a bimodal distribution with peaks in the 20s and 50s–70s.

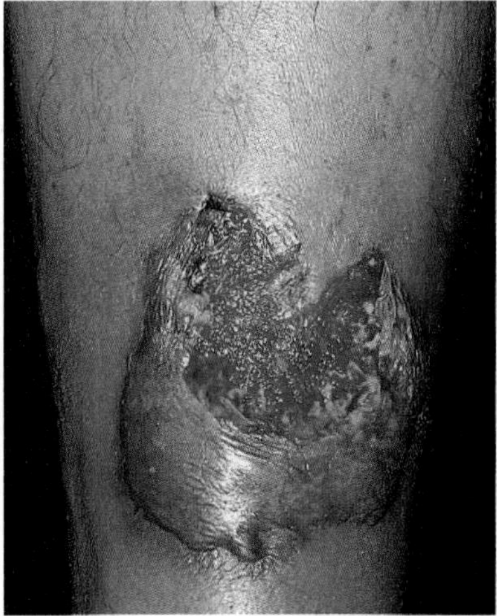

FIGURE 7-6. Pyoderma gangrenosum. (Reproduced with permission from Wolff K et al. *Fitzpatrick's Color Atlas & Synopsis of Clinical Dermatology*, 5th ed. New York: McGraw-Hill, 2005: 153.)

Symptoms/Exam

- Patients may be pale or thin with temporal wasting and often have RLQ tenderness/fullness; some present with perianal fistula.
- Symptoms include the following:
  - **GI: Colicky RLQ pain,** diarrhea (mucus-containing, nonbloody stools), weight loss, anorexia, low-grade fever, **perirectal abscess/fistula,** and, less often, GI blood loss, fecal incontinence, and oral ulcers.
  - **Other: Low-grade fever,** erythema nodosum, pyoderma gangrenosum (see Figure 7-6), iritis and episcleritis, gallstones, kidney stones, and peripheral arthritis.

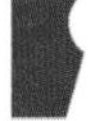

KEY FACT

Crohn's involves transmural inflammation, so the outer layers can make fistulas. Ulcerative colitis is **not** transmural and therefore is not associated with fistulas.

Diagnosis

- **Labs:** Obtain a CBC, iron, folate, B_{12}, ESR, LFTs, a stool WBC count, an RBC count, and a stool O&P.
  - Look for normocytic anemia of chronic disease or anemia due to iron, vitamin B_{12}, or folate deficiency.
  - ESR or C-reactive protein (CRP) may be ↑; ASCA is ⊕.
  - O&P is ⊖, but fecal leukocytes and occult blood may be ⊕.
  - LFTs should be normal or mildly elevated.
- **Imaging:**
  - **Skip lesions** are seen on colonoscopy; **cobblestoning** is seen on barium enema.
  - Biopsy may show noncaseating granulomas with mononuclear cell infiltrate (see Figure 7-7A and B).
  - Stricture formation, pseudodiverticula, abscesses, and fistulas (to the skin, bladder, vagina, or other bowel loops) may be seen on imaging (see Figure 7-8).

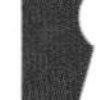

KEY FACT

Crohn's disease often affects the terminal ileum, so think of things that are absorbed in the terminal ileum.

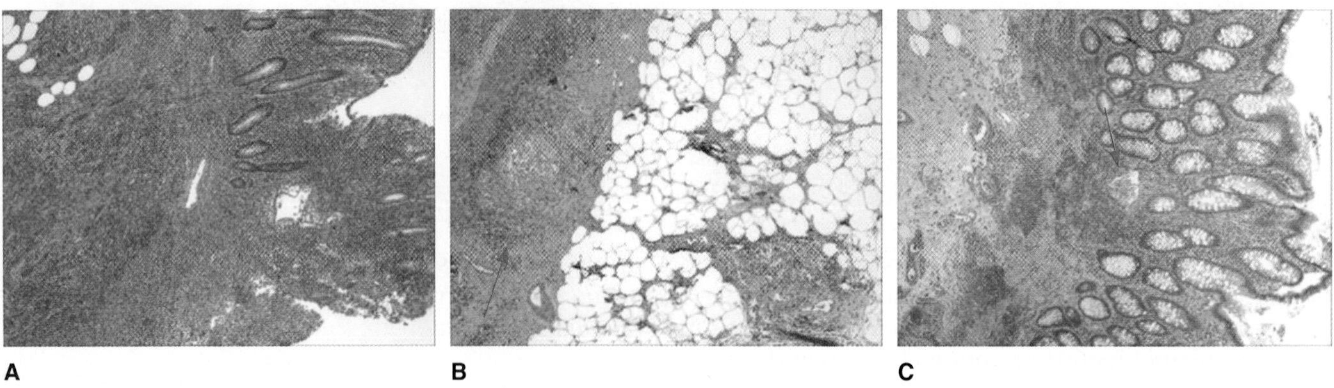

FIGURE 7-7. Inflammatory bowel disease. (**A**)–(**B**) **Crohn's disease.** Transmural inflammation with noncaseating granulomas (arrow) is seen deep in the serosal fat on pathology. (**C**) **Ulcerative colitis.** Inflammation is confined to the mucosa and submucosa, with a crypt abscess (arrow). (Reproduced with permission from USMLERx.com.)

Treatment

- **Mild cases: 5-ASA** compounds.
- **Moderate cases:** Oral corticosteroids +/– azathioprine, 6-mercaptopurine (6-MP), or methotrexate.
- **Refractory disease:** IV steroids +/– immunomodulators (anti-TNF). Imaging (CT, MRI, CT enterography) is important for ruling out perforation, megacolon, fistula, or abscess formation. In some cases, stricturoplasty +/– resection may be needed.
- **Follow-up:** Surveillance colonoscopy with multiple biopsies to look for dysplasia in patients with a large extent of colonic involvement 8–10 years after diagnosis and biannually or annually thereafter.

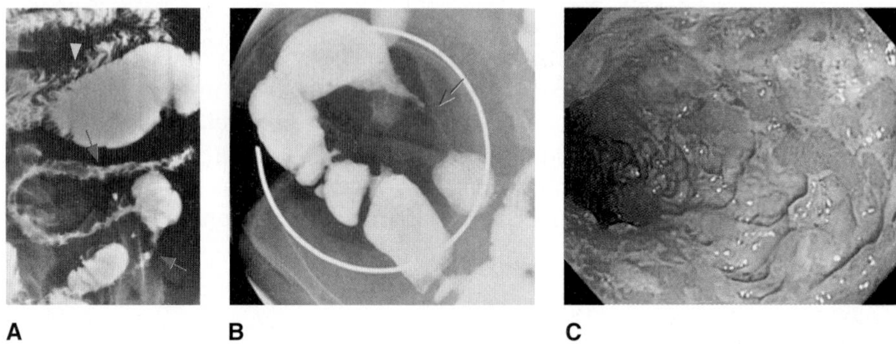

FIGURE 7-8. Crohn's disease. (**A**) Small bowel follow-through (SBFT) barium study shows skip areas of narrowed small bowel with nodular mucosa (arrows) and ulceration. Compare with normal bowel (arrowhead). (**B**) Spot compression image from SBFT shows "string sign" narrowing (arrow) due to stricture. (**C**) Deep ulcers in the colon of a patient with Crohn's disease, seen at colonoscopy. (Image A reproduced with permission from Chen MY et al. *Basic Radiology.* New York: McGraw-Hill, 2004, Fig. 10-30. Image B reproduced with permission from USMLERx.com. Image C reproduced with permission from Fauci AS et al. *Harrison's Principles of Internal Medicine,* 17th ed. New York: McGraw-Hill, 2008, Fig. 285-4B.)

ULCERATIVE COLITIS

Continuous colonic mucosal inflammation extending proximally for variable distances from the anal verge. Usually occurs in a bimodal distribution (ages 15–30 and 60–80). Can lead to **toxic megacolon.**

Symptoms/Exam

- Presents with **cramping** abdominal pain, **urgency, bloody diarrhea,** weight loss, and fatigue.
- Exam reveals low-grade fever, tachycardia, orthostatic hypotension, heme-⊕ stools, and mild tenderness in the lower abdomen.

Diagnosis

- **Labs:** Laboratory studies reveal **normocytic, normochromic anemia or iron-deficiency anemia;** low albumin; ⊕ **p-ANCA;** and ⊖ stool cultures.
- **Imaging:**
  - Colonoscopy shows **friable mucosa** with ulcerations and erosions along with inflammation that is continuous from the anus up.
  - Barium enema shows a **lead-pipe colon** and loss of haustra (characteristic of long-standing disease; see Figure 7-9).
  - Biopsy reveals crypt abscess and microulcerations but no granulomas (see Figure 7-7C).

Treatment

- **Mild cases: 5-ASA** compounds.
- **Moderate cases:** Oral corticosteroids +/– azathioprine, 6-MP, or methotrexate.
- **Refractory disease:** IV steroids +/– cyclosporine, +/– anti-TNF antibody. Serial imaging to rule out perforation or toxic megacolon. In some cases resection may be needed, especially if complications arise or if the patient fails medical therapy.
- **Follow-up: Surveillance colonoscopy with multiple biopsies** 8–10 years after diagnosis and biannually or annually thereafter.
- Some patients may elect to get a **prophylactic colectomy** given that the incidence of colon cancer is 0.5–1.0% per year after 10 years of disease. Total colectomy cures the disease.

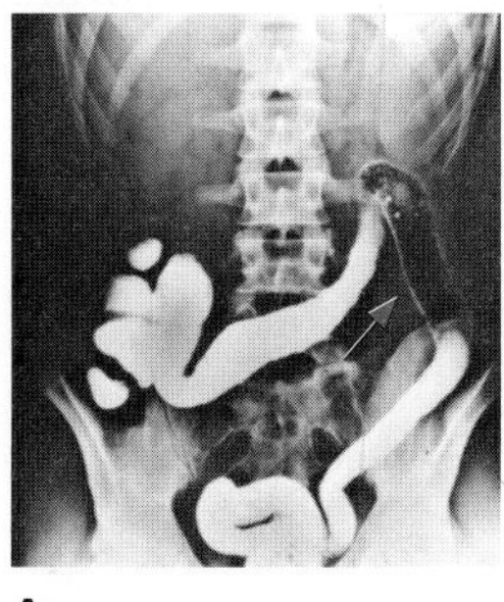

A

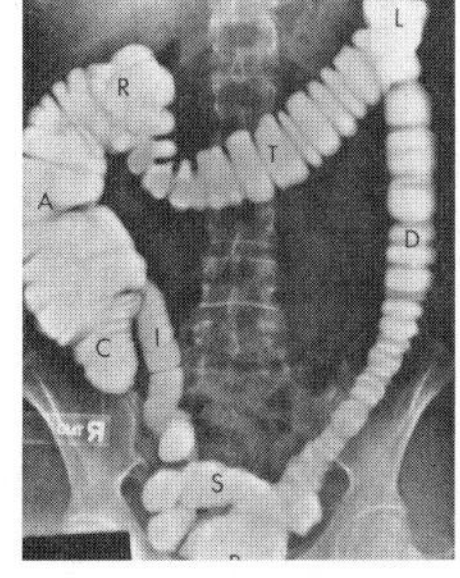

B

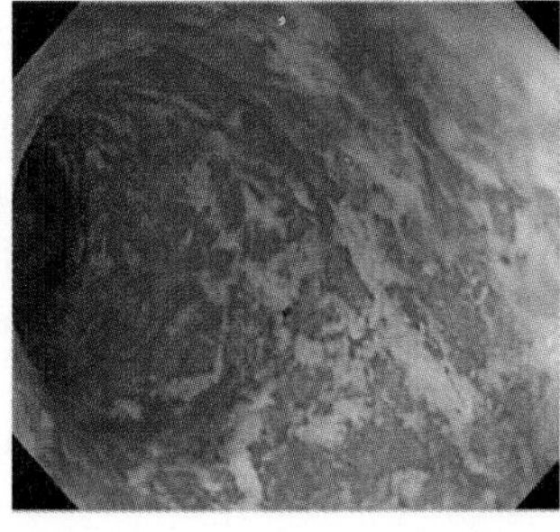

C

FIGURE 7-9. Ulcerative colitis. (**A**) Radiograph from a barium enema showing a featureless ("lead pipe") colon with small mucosal ulcerations (arrow). Compare with normal haustral markings in (**B**). (**C**) Diffuse mucosal ulcerations and exudates at colonoscopy in chronic ulcerative colitis. (Image A reproduced with permission from Doherty GM. *Current Diagnosis & Treatment: Surgery,* 13th ed. New York: McGraw-Hill, 2010, Fig. 30-17. Image B reproduced with permission from Chen MY et al. *Basic Radiology.* New York: McGraw-Hill, 2004, Fig. 10-10A. Image C reproduced with permission from Fauci AS et al. *Harrison's Principles of Internal Medicine,* 17th ed. New York: McGraw-Hill, 2008, Fig. 285-4A.)

Irritable Bowel Syndrome (IBS)

A 30-year-old woman comes to your clinic complaining of vague, crampy abdominal pain that is mitigated with defecation. The patient is concerned that her illness may be serious and that her children may be taken away from her, as she recently divorced and is now a single mother. What is the likely diagnosis?

Irritable bowel syndrome. The patient has pain associated with defecation, and her background points to recent stressors and a possible anxiety disorder.

A GI disorder characterized by abdominal pain and altered bowel function (diarrhea or constipation) with or without bloating. Possible etiologies include altered gut motor function, **autonomic nervous system abnormalities,** and **psychological factors.**

KEY FACT

Pain that is unrelated to defecation or that is induced with activity, menstruation, or urination is unlikely to be IBS.

Symptoms/Exam

- Characterized by **abdominal pain** with complete or incomplete relief with defecation; **intermittent diarrhea or constipation;** a feeling of incomplete rectal evacuation; urgency; passage of mucus; and bloating.
- Abdominal pain is poorly localized, migratory, and variable in nature.

Diagnosis

- A **diagnosis of exclusion** based primarily on the history and physical exam. Basic labs to exclude other causes should include CBC, BMP, calcium, TSH, and stool O&P.
- The **Rome III criteria** can be used to aid in diagnosis and consist of 12 weeks of the following within one year:
  - Improvement of pain with bowel movement.
  - Often associated with a change in frequency of bowel movements.
  - Onset associated with a change in the form/appearance of stool.

Treatment

- **High-fiber diet** (20–30 g/day), **exercise,** and adequate fluid intake.
- **TCAs** are often used even in the absence of depression, especially in the setting of chronic pain and diarrhea.
- Additional treatment options depend on symptom predominance.
  - **If constipation predominates:** Use bulking agents (psyllium), lactulose, PEG, or enemas.
  - **If diarrhea predominates:** Give loperamide, cholestyramine, or TCAs.
  - **If bloating predominates:** Simethicone, charcoal, or *Lactobacillus* may be used.
- **Postprandial symptoms:** Treat with anticholinergic agents, dicyclomine, or hyoscyamine.

Diarrhea

A 74-year-old woman is transported from a rehabilitation facility where she was being treated for osteomyelitis. She was sent to the hospital after having had many foul-smelling bowel movements over the past two days. What is the likely cause of her diarrhea, and what is the treatment of choice?

This patient was likely receiving long-term antibiotics for osteomyelitis, thereby putting her at risk for *Clostridium difficile* infection. She needs to be treated with metronidazole.

Described as watery consistency and/or ↑ frequency of bowel movements. Stool weight is > 200–300 g/day. Small bowel pathology will show voluminous watery diarrhea; large bowel pathology is associated with more frequent but smaller-volume output. Distinguish acute from chronic diarrhea as follows:

- **Acute diarrhea:** Defined as < 2 weeks in duration; usually infectious.
- **Chronic diarrhea:** Defined as lasting > 4–6 weeks.

Symptoms/Exam

- The most important goal is to assess the degree of fluid loss/dehydration and nutritional depletion. If bloating predominates, it is suggestive of malabsorption. If fever is present, think of infectious causes. If guaiac ⊕, consider inflammatory processes or enteroinvasive organisms.
- Etiologies can be further distinguished as follows:
  - **Infectious:** The **leading cause of acute diarrhea.** Characterized by vomiting, pain, fever, or chills. If stools are bloody, think of enteroinvasive organisms. To characterize, check stool leukocytes, Gram stain, culture, and stool O&P. Treat severe disease with ciprofloxacin or metronidazole for C *difficile*.
  - **Osmotic:** Associated with lactose intolerance and with the ingestion of magnesium, sorbitol, or mannitol; ↑ stool osmotic gap. Bloating and gas are prominent with malabsorption. Treat by stopping the offending agent.
  - **Secretory:** Caused by hormonal stimulation (gastrin, VIP) or by viruses or toxins. Stool osmotic gap is normal; no change in the diarrhea occurs with fasting. Treatment is mainly supportive. Viral syndromes are common and self-limited.
  - **Exudative:** Associated with mucosal inflammation, enteritis, TB, colon cancer, and IBD. Labs reveal ↑ ESR and CRP. Characterized by tenesmus, often small volume, and frequent diarrhea. Diagnose by colonoscopy, endoscopy with small bowel biopsies (celiac disease), and imaging studies. Treatment varies depending on the etiology.
  - **Rapid transit:** Associated with laxative abuse or, rarely, hyperthyroidism. Management involves checking TSH or stopping laxative use.
  - **Slow transit:** Small bowel bacterial overgrowth syndromes, structural abnormalities (small bowel diverticulum, fistulas), radiation damage, slow motility (DM, scleroderma). Treat the underlying cause; give a short course of antibiotics to ↓ bacterial growth.

Diagnosis

- **Evaluation of acute diarrhea:**
  - In the setting of high fever, bloody diarrhea, or a duration of > 4–5 days, obtain fecal leukocytes and bacterial cultures and test for C *difficile* toxin; obtain a stool O&P for immunocompromised patients.
  - If symptoms started within six hours of ingestion, think of a preformed toxin such as *Staphylococcus* or *Bacillus cereus*. If symptoms started after 12 hours, the etiology is more likely to be bacterial or viral, especially if symptoms are accompanied by vomiting.
- **Evaluation of chronic diarrhea:**
  - Consider malabsorption syndromes, lactose intolerance, previous bowel surgery, medications, systemic disease, and IBD.
  - Tests to consider include fecal leukocytes, occult blood, flexible sigmoidoscopy with biopsy, endoscopy with small bowel biopsies, small bowel imaging, or colonoscopy.
- **Calculate the osmotic gap:** 290 – 2 (stool Na + stool K). A normal gap is < 50.
  - **Normal gap:** If the stool is of normal weight, consider IBS and factitious causes. If weight is ↑, consider a secretory cause or laxative abuse.
  - **Increased gap:** Normal stool fat points to lactose intolerance or sorbitol, lactulose, or laxative abuse. ↑ stool fat is associated with small bowel malabsorption, pancreatic insufficiency, or bacterial overgrowth.

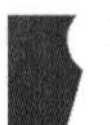

KEY FACT

Common bugs in acute diarrhea:

- **Bacterial:** *E coli, Shigella, Salmonella, Campylobacter jejuni, Vibrio parahaemolyticus, Yersinia.*
- **Viral:** Rotavirus, Norwalk virus.
- **Parasitic:** *Giardia, Cryptosporidium, Entamoeba histolytica.*

Treatment

Treat according to the etiology as indicated above. General treatment guidelines are as follows:

- If acute, give oral or IV fluids and electrolyte repletion. Loperamide may be given if the patient does not have bloody stools or high fevers, as this may precipitate toxic megacolon (especially with C *difficile* colitis).
- Avoid antimotility agents in the presence of a high fever, bloody diarrhea, severe abdominal pain, or systemic toxicity.
- If testing for C *difficile* toxin is ⊕, treat initially with oral metronidazole; if refractory to metronidazole, treat with oral vancomycin.

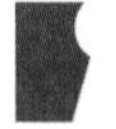

KEY FACT

If a patient is on antibiotics, think C *difficile.*

Celiac Sprue

Usually affects those of **northern European** ancestry. Can be **familial;** thought to be an **autoimmune disease** triggered by an environmental agent (wheat, rye, barley, and some oats). More prevalent than previously thought; associated with osteoporosis, an ↑ risk of GI malignancies (small bowel lymphoma), and **dermatitis herpetiformis.**

Symptoms/Exam

- Celiac sprue leads to **malabsorption** with **chronic diarrhea.** Patients complain of **steatorrhea** and **weight loss.**
- Can also present with nonspecific symptoms (nausea, abdominal pain, weight loss), iron-deficiency anemia, increased LFTs, or muscle wasting.

Diagnosis

- Histology reveals **flattening or loss of villi** and inflammation.
- Antibody assays are ⊕ for **antiendomysial antibody** or **anti–tissue transglutaminase antibodies** and are ⊖ only with IgA deficiency.
- A gluten-free diet improves symptoms and the histology of the small bowel.

Treatment

Institute a **gluten-free diet.** Gluten is found in most grains in the Western world (eg, wheat, barley, rye, some oats, additives, many prepared foods).

Upper GI Bleed

Bleeding in the section of the GI tract extending from the upper esophagus to the duodenum to the **ligament of Treitz.** Primarily due to **PUD, gastritis, varices,** or **Mallory-Weiss syndrome** (see Figure 7-10).

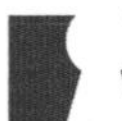

KEY FACT

Melena by definition points to an upper GI bleed. There is no other location in the GI tract that is acidic enough to result in melena.

Symptoms

- May present with **dizziness,** lightheadedness, weakness, and nausea.
- Patients may also report vomiting of blood or dark brown contents (**hematemesis**—vomiting of fresh blood, clots, or coffee-ground material) or passing of black stool (**melena**—dark, tarry stools composed of degraded blood from the upper GI tract).

Exam

- Associated with pallor, **abdominal pain,** tachycardia, and hypotension; rectal exam reveals blood.
- If patients show signs of **cirrhosis** (telangiectasia, spider angiomata, gynecomastia, testicular atrophy, palmar erythema, caput medusae), think varices.
- **Vital signs** reveal **tachycardia** at 10% volume loss, orthostatic **hypotension** at 20% blood loss, and **shock** at 30% loss.

Diagnosis

- Assess the severity of the bleed beginning with the **ABCs.**
- Check **hematocrit** (may be normal in acute blood loss), **platelet count, BUN/creatinine** (an ↑ ratio reflects volume depletion), PT/PTT, and LFTs.
- NG tube placement and lavage can help determine the activity and severity of the bleed (if clear, the bleed could be intermittent or from the duodenum).
- If perforation is suspected, obtain upright and abdominal x-rays.
- Endoscopy can be both diagnostic and therapeutic.

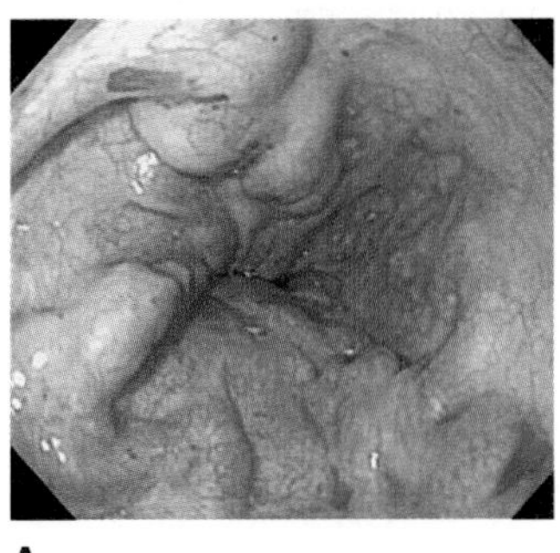

A

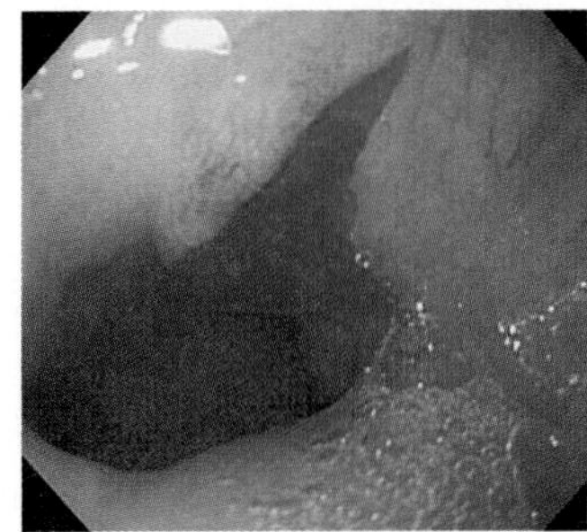

B

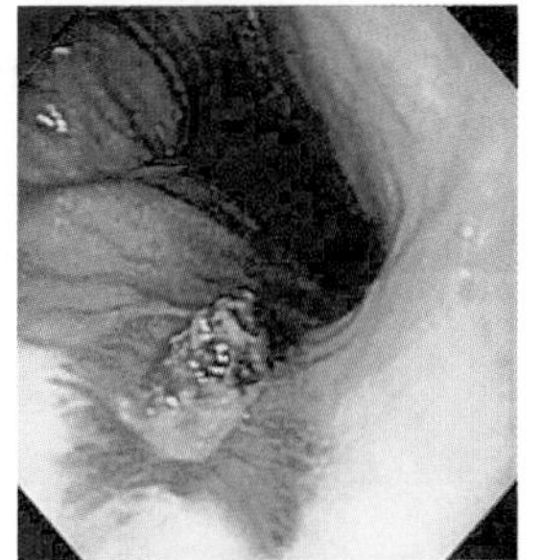

C

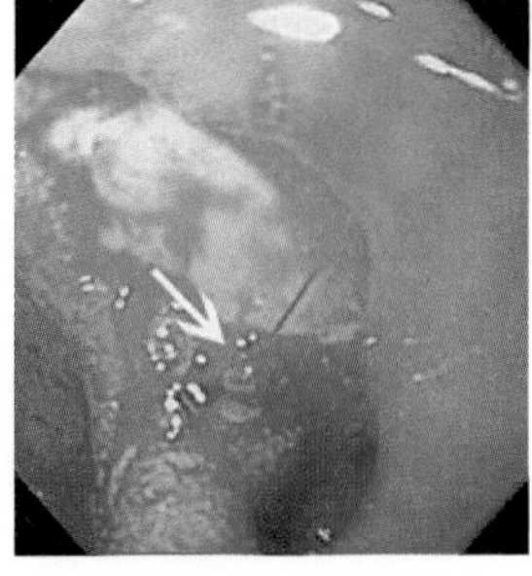

D

FIGURE 7-10. Causes of upper GI bleed at endoscopy. (**A**) Esophageal varices. (**B**) Mallory-Weiss tear. (**C**) Gastric ulcer with protuberant vessel. (**D**) Duodenal ulcer with active bleeding (arrow). (Reproduced with permission from Fauci AS et al. *Harrison's Principles of Internal Medicine,* 17th ed. New York: McGraw-Hill, 2008, Figs. 285-16, 285-18, and 285-15D and E.)

TREATMENT

- Start with the **ABCs.** Use at least **two large-bore** peripheral IV catheters. **Transfusion** and intravascular volume replacement are indicated.
- Consult GI and surgery if bleeding does not stop or if difficulty is encountered with resuscitation 2° to a brisk bleed.
- Treat **variceal bleeds** with **octreotide,** endoscopic **sclerotherapy,** or **band ligation.** If the bleed is severe, balloon tamponade is appropriate, followed by embolization, transjugular intrahepatic portosystemic shunt **(TIPS),** or a surgical shunt if endoscopic therapy fails.
- To prevent variceal bleeds, treat with **nonselective** β-blockers (eg, propranolol), obliterative endoscopic therapy, **shunting,** and, if the patient is an appropriate candidate, liver transplantation.
- For **PUD,** use **PPIs, endoscopic** epinephrine injection, thermal contact, and laser therapy. Begin *H pylori* eradication measures.
- **Mallory-Weiss tears** usually stop bleeding **spontaneously.**
- Treat **esophagitis/gastritis** with PPIs or H_2 antagonists. Avoid ASA and NSAIDs.

Lower GI Bleed

Bleeding that is distal to the ligament of Treitz.

SYMPTOMS/EXAM

- Presents with **hematochezia** (fresh blood or clot per rectum).
- Diarrhea, tenesmus, bright red blood per rectum, or maroon-colored stools are also seen.
- As with upper GI bleeds, check vital signs to assess the severity of the bleed. Obtain orthostatics; perform a rectal exam for hemorrhoids, fissures, or a mass.

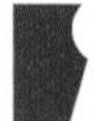

KEY FACT

A small number of GI bleeds (3.5%) are called obscure GI bleeds because they are associated with a ⊖ EGD and colonoscopy followed by a ⊖ small bowel pill camera.

DIFFERENTIAL

Hemorrhoids, diverticulosis, angiodysplasia, carcinoma, enteritis, IBD, polyps, Meckel's diverticulum.

DIAGNOSIS

- First **rule out an upper GI bleed.**
- Bleeding usually **stops spontaneously.** However, colonoscopy should be performed; in the majority of cases, the diagnosis can be made at the time of visualization.
- If the bleed continues, a bleeding scan (**^{99}Tc-tagged RBC scan**) can be done to detect bleeding if it is > 1.0 mL/min.
- If the bleed is refractory, **arteriography** or **exploratory laparotomy** may be done.

KEY FACT

Think diverticulosis with painless lower GI bleeding. Think diverticulitis in the presence of pain.

TREATMENT

- Although bleeding generally stops spontaneously, resuscitative efforts should be initiated, as with upper GI bleeds, until the source is found and the bleeding stops.
- With diverticular disease, bleeding usually stops spontaneously, but **epinephrine injection,** catheter-directed **vasopressin,** or **embolization** can be used. In some cases, surgery may be needed.

Pancreatitis

A 32-year-old man presents to the ER with sharp abdominal pain. He states that the pain radiates to his back and is constant in nature. He adds that the pain started after he attended a barbecue with friends, at which he drank 14 beers. What is your diagnosis, and how should this patient be managed?

The patient likely has alcoholic pancreatitis. Initial management should consist of bowel rest, IV hydration, and pain control.

Gallstones and **alcohol** account for 70–80% of acute cases. Other causes include **obstruction** (pancreatic or ampullary tumors), **metabolic** factors (severe hypertriglyceridemia, hypercalcemia), abdominal **trauma,** endoscopic retrograde cholangiopancreatography **(ERCP), infection** (mumps, CMV, clonorchiasis, ascariasis), and **drugs** (thiazides, azathioprine, pentamidine, sulfonamides).

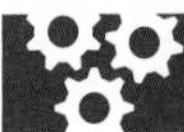

MNEMONIC

Causes of acute pancreatitis–

GET SMASH'D

Gallstones
Ethanol, **E**RCP
Trauma
Steroids
Mumps
Autoimmune
Scorpion bites
Hyperlipidemia
Drugs

Symptoms

- Acute pancreatitis often presents with abdominal pain, typically in the **midepigastric** region, that **radiates to the back,** may be relieved by sitting forward, and lasts hours to days.
- Nausea, vomiting, and fever also are seen.

Exam

- Exam reveals **midepigastric tenderness,** ↓ bowel sounds, guarding, jaundice, and fever.
- **Cullen's sign** (periumbilical ecchymoses) and **Grey Turner's sign** (flank ecchymoses) reflect hemorrhage and severe pancreatitis, although they are often seen long after symptoms manifest and the diagnosis has been made.

Diagnosis

- Typically, both **amylase and lipase** will be elevated; however, amylase may be normal, especially if the disease is due to hyperlipidemia. **Lipase** has the **greatest specificity and remains more significantly elevated than amylase in acute pancreatitis.**
- **Abdominal CT within 48–72 hours** is especially useful in detecting complications of pancreatitis, such as necrotic or hemorrhagic pancreatitis. In **chronic pancreatitis (especially alcohol induced), calcifications** may be seen (see Figure 7-11). However, CT scans are not required if the patient is improving.
- **Elevated ALT levels suggest gallstone pancreatitis.**
- If patients are female and > 60 years of age or if they abstain from alcohol or use it only moderately, gallstones are the more likely etiology.
- Ultrasound may allow visualization of gallstones or sludge in the gallbladder.
- In **chronic pancreatitis, a 72-hour fecal fat test** (100-g/day fat diet) is ⊕ if there are > 7 **g/day of fat in the stool.** The etiology of chronic pancreatitis includes alcohol, cystic fibrosis, a history of severe pancreatitis, and idiopathic causes (excluding gallstones).

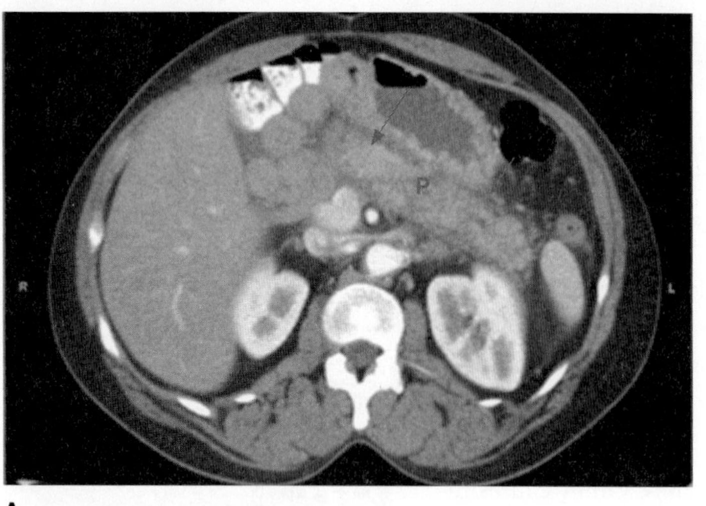

A

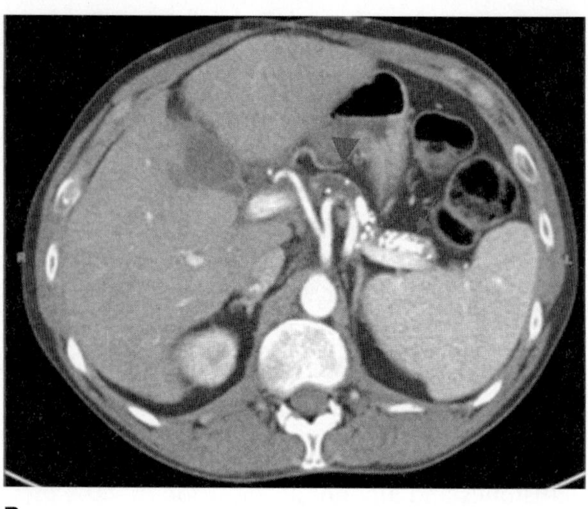

B

FIGURE 7-11. Pancreatitis. Transaxial contrast-enhanced CT images. **(A) Uncomplicated acute pancreatitis.** Peripancreatic fluid and fat stranding can be seen (arrows). P = pancreas. **(B) Chronic pancreatitis.** Note the dilated pancreatic duct (arrowhead) and pancreatic calcifications (arrow). (Reproduced with permission from USMLERx.com.)

TREATMENT

- Acute:
  - **Supportive** (NPO, IV fluids; pain management).
  - In the setting of **gallstone pancreatitis,** ERCP with sphincterotomy is appropriate if the common bile duct is obstructed or if there is evidence of cholangitis. If the gallstone has passed, perform a cholecystectomy once the patient is sufficiently stable for surgery.
  - **Prophylactic antibiotics** are used for severe pancreatitis and consist of imipenem monotherapy or a fluoroquinolone + metronidazole.
- Chronic:
  - Treat malabsorption with pancreatic enzyme and vitamin B_{12} replacement.
  - Treat glucose intolerance; encourage alcohol abstinence.
  - Management of chronic pain.

COMPLICATIONS

- **Acute: Pseudocyst,** peripancreatic effusions, **necrosis,** abscess, ARDS, hypotension, splenic vein thrombosis.
- **Chronic: Malabsorption,** osteoporosis, DM, **pancreatic cancer.**

Approach to Liver Function Tests

A 48-year-old woman with a past medical history of diabetes, obesity, and hyperlipidemia comes to your clinic for a routine physical and lab work. Routine labs show a normal bilirubin level but an AST and ALT of 58 and 72 U/L, respectively; alkaline phosphatase is within normal limits. What is the likely cause of her transaminitis?

Nonalcoholic fatty liver disease.

The algorithm in Figure 7-12 outlines a general approach toward the interpretation of LFTs.

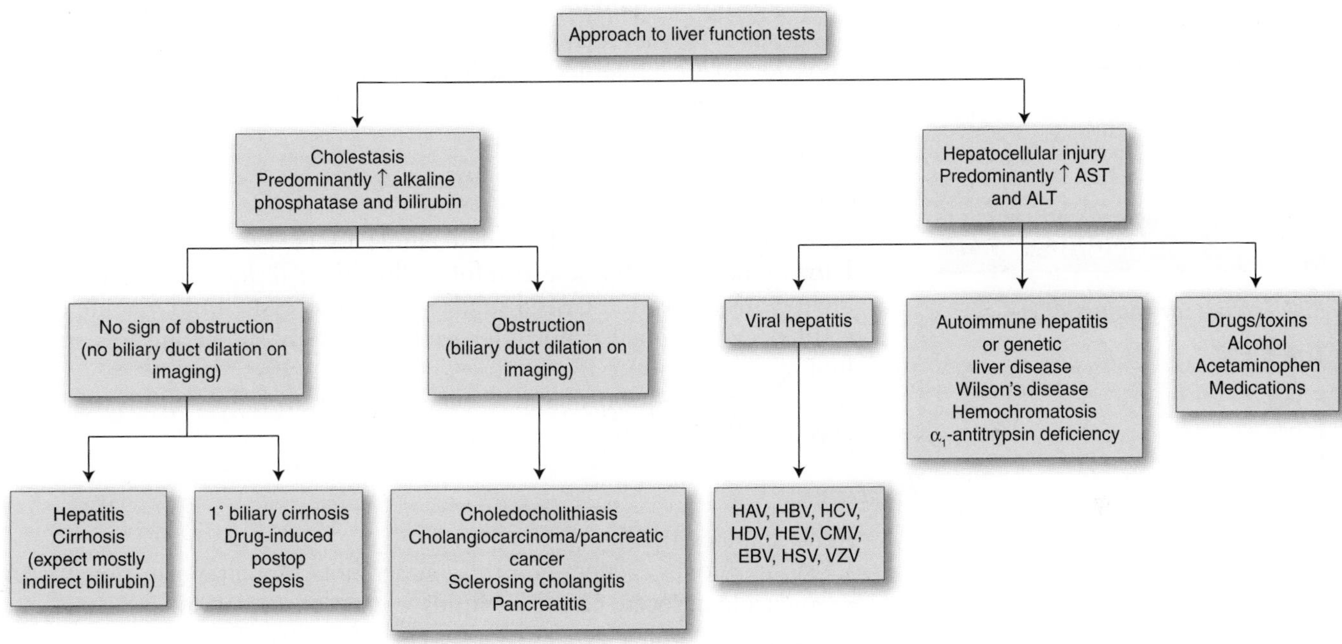

FIGURE 7-12. Abnormal liver tests.

Gallstone Disease

In the United States, gallstone disease is most likely due to **cholesterol stones.** In trauma patients, burn patients, or those on TPN, acute cholecystitis may occur in the absence of stones **(acalculous cholecystitis).**

SYMPTOMS/EXAM

- Most patients with gallstones are **asymptomatic** (80%).
- May also present as follows:
  - **Biliary colic:** Characterized by **episodic RUQ** or epigastric pain that may radiate to the right shoulder; usually **postprandial** and accompanied by vomiting. **Nocturnal** pain that awakens the patient is common. Associated with **fatty food** intolerance.
  - **Cholangitis:** Suggested by the presence of fever and persistent RUQ pain.
    - **Charcot's triad:** RUQ pain, jaundice, and fever/chills.
    - **Reynolds' pentad:** Charcot's triad plus shock and altered mental status may be seen in suppurative cholangitis.
- Look for RUQ tenderness and **Murphy's sign** (inspiratory arrest during deep palpation of the RUQ). Look for jaundice as a sign of common bile duct obstruction.

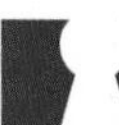

KEY FACT

Symptoms of cholangitis:
- RUQ pain
- Fever
- Jaundice

DIAGNOSIS

- Labs reveal **leukocytosis,** ↑ amylase, and ↑ LFTs.
- **Ultrasound** is 85–90% sensitive for gallbladder gallstones and cholecystitis (**echogenic focus that casts a shadow**; pericholecystic fluid = acute cholecystitis). A thickened gallbladder wall and biliary sludge are less specific findings (see Figure 7-13).
- If ultrasound is equivocal and suspicion for acute cholecystitis is high, proceed to a **HIDA** scan.

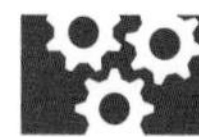

MNEMONIC

Risk factors for cholecystitis–

The 5 F's

Female
Fertile
Fat
Forties
Familial

TREATMENT

- **Acute cholecystitis:**
  - IV antibiotics (generally a third-generation cephalosporin plus metronidazole in severe cases); IV fluids, electrolyte repletion.

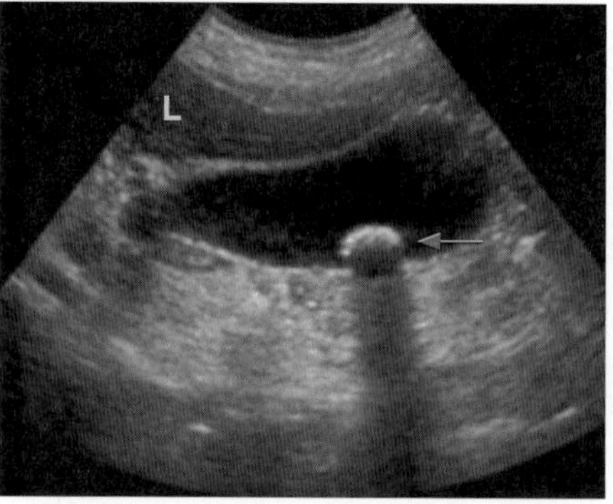

A

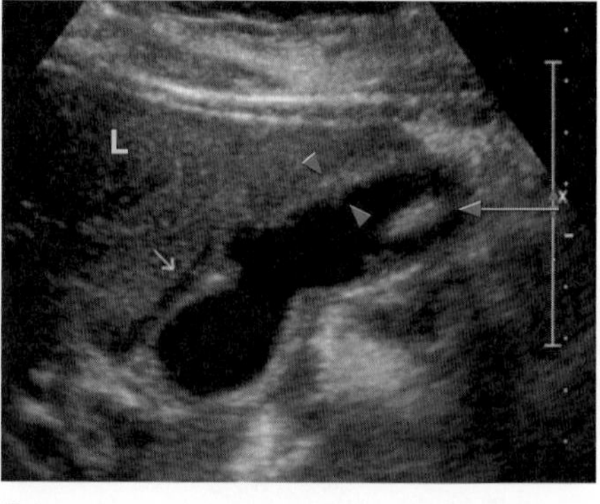

B

FIGURE 7-13. Gallstone disease. (A) **Cholelithiasis.** Ultrasound image of the gallbladder shows a gallstone (arrow) with posterior shadowing. **(B) Acute cholecystitis.** Ultrasound image shows a gallstone (red arrow), a thickened gallbladder wall (arrowheads), and pericholecystic fluid (white arrow). L = liver. (Reproduced with permission from USMLERx.com.)

- Early cholecystectomy within 72 hours with an intraoperative cholangiogram to look for common bile duct stones. If the patient is a high-risk surgical candidate, elective surgery may be appropriate if the clinical condition allows.
- If the patient is not a candidate for surgery, consider a percutaneous biliary drain.
- **Cholangitis:**
  - Admission, NPO, hydration, pressors if needed, **IV antibiotics** (ciprofloxacin is preferred).
  - **For very ill patients who are not responsive to medical treatment, urgent next-day ERCP with endoscopic sphincterotomy** may be needed. Other emergency options are ERCP with stent placement, percutaneous transhepatic drainage, and operative decompression.

Viral and Nonviral Hepatitis

A 59-year-old man comes to your clinic for a checkup. He lived in Vietnam until the age of 32 and has not seen a primary care physician since that time. He is concerned that many of the people in his Vietnamese community have had hepatitis B. Which labs should be ⊕ if this patient has chronic hepatitis B?

HBsAg, HBeAg, and HBcAb IgG.

May be acute and self-limited or chronic and symptomatic. May not be detected until years after the initial infection.

Symptoms/Exam

- In **acute** cases, patients may present with anorexia, **nausea,** vomiting, malaise, and fever but are frequently **asymptomatic.**
- Exam is often normal but may reveal an enlarged and tender liver, dark urine, and jaundice.

Differential

- In the setting of a **high level of transaminase elevation** (> **10–20 times the upper limit of normal),** consider acute viral infection as well as ischemia ("shock liver"), acute choledocholithiasis, or toxins (acetaminophen).
- With **moderate transaminase elevation,** consider the most common cause of nonalcoholic fatty liver disease. Also consider chronic viral infection, autoimmune disorders, mononucleosis, CMV, 2° syphilis, drug-induced illness, and Budd-Chiari syndrome.
- With mild transaminase elevation, also consider hemochromatosis, celiac disease, IBD, and right-sided heart failure.

Diagnosis

Diagnose on the basis of the following:

- The presence of hepatitis based on clinical presentation as well as ↑ transaminases.
- Serology and/or PCR testing confirming a specific virus (see Tables 7-1 and 7-2).
- Biopsy showing hepatocellular inflammation (rarely indicated).

TABLE 7-1. Viral Hepatitis and Serologic Tests

TYPE OF VIRAL HEPATITIS	⊕ SEROLOGY
Acute HAV	Anti-HAV IgM.
Previous HAV	Anti-HAV IgG.
Acute HBV	HBsAg; HBeAg; HBcAb IgM.
Acute HBV, window period	HBcAb IgM only.
Chronic active HBV	HBsAg, HBeAg, HBcAb IgG.
Recovery HBV	HBsAb IgG, HBcAb IgG, normal ALT.
Immunized HBV	HBsAb IgG.
Acute HCV with recovery	HCV RNA early; anti-HCV Ab; recombinant immunoblot assay (RIBA); ALT elevated early.
Acute HCV with chronic infection	HCV RNA, anti-HCV Ab, RIBA, elevated/normal ALT.
Recovery HCV	Anti-HCV Ab and normal ALT.

- An RUQ ultrasound may be performed to see if the liver is enlarged in acute hepatitis (vs. cirrhotic nodular liver in the advanced disease state).

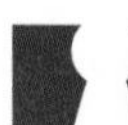

KEY FACT

There is an ↑ (25–40%) risk of cirrhosis and hepatocellular carcinoma with chronic HBV.

TREATMENT

Treat according to subtype as outlined in Table 7-1. Additional guidelines are as follows:

- Rest during the acute phase.
- Avoid hepatotoxic agents; avoid morphine; avoid elective surgery.
- Although most symptoms resolve in 3–16 weeks, LFTs may remain elevated for much longer.

TABLE 7-2. **Etiologies, Diagnosis, and Treatment of Viral Hepatitis**

Subtype	Transmission	Clinical/Lab Findings	Treatment	Other Key Facts
HAV	Transmitted via contaminated food, water, milk, and shellfish. Known day-care-center outbreaks have been identified. **Fecal-oral transmission;** has a six-day to six-week incubation period. Virus is shed in stool up to two weeks before symptom onset.	No chronic infection.	Supportive; generally no sequelae.	Give **immunoglobulin** to close contacts without HAV infection or vaccination.
HBV	Transmitted by **infected blood,** through **sexual contact,** or **perinatally.** Incubation is six weeks to six months. HDV can coinfect persons with HBV.	High prevalence in men who have sex with men, prostitutes, and IV drug users. Fewer than 1% of cases are fulminant. Adult acquired infection usually does not become chronic. Much more common in Asian countries and immigrants from that region.	Interferon and other nucleotide/ nucleoside analogs. (The goal is to ↓ viral load and improve liver histology; cure is uncommon.)	Vaccinate patients with chronic HBV against HAV. Associated with arthritis, glomerulonephritis, and **polyarteritis nodosa.** Chronic infection can result in hepatocellular carcinoma.
HCV	Transmitted through **blood transfusion or IV drug use** as well as through intranasal cocaine use or body piercing. Incubation is 6–7 weeks.	Illness is often mild or asymptomatic and is characterized by **waxing and waning aminotransferases.** HCV antibody is not protective. Antibody appears six weeks to nine months after infection. Diagnose acute infection with HCV RNA. More than 70% of infections become chronic.	Interferon + **ribavirin** combination therapy.	Vaccinate patients with HCV against HAV and HBV. Complications include **cryoglobulinemia** and membranoproliferative glomerulonephritis, as well as hepatocellular carcinoma in patients with cirrhosis.
HDV	Requires a coexistent **HBV** infection. Percutaneous exposure. Usually found in **IV drug users** and high-risk **HBsAg carriers.**	Anti-HDV IgM is present in acute cases. Immunity to HBV implies immunity to HDV.	Similar to HBV infection.	If acquired as a superinfection in chronic HBV, there is an ↑ in the severity of the infection. Fulminant hepatitis or severe chronic hepatitis with rapid progression to cirrhosis can occur. Associated with an ↑ risk of **hepatocellular carcinoma.**
HEV	Fecal-oral transmission.	Will test ⊕ on serology for HEV.	Supportive.	Self-limited; endemic to India, Afghanistan, Mexico, and Algeria. Carries a 10–20% mortality rate in **pregnant** women.

Cirrhosis and Ascites

Chronic irreversible changes of the hepatic parenchyma, including fibrosis and regenerative nodules. The most common cause in the United States is alcohol abuse, followed by chronic viral hepatitis.

SYMPTOMS/EXAM

- Cirrhosis can be asymptomatic for long periods. Symptoms reflect the **severity** of hepatic damage, **not** the underlying etiology of the liver disease (see Figure 7-14).
- ↓ hepatic function leads to jaundice, edema, coagulopathy, and metabolic abnormalities.
- Fibrosis and distorted vasculature lead to portal hypertension, which leads in turn to gastroesophageal varices and splenomegaly.
- ↓ hepatic function and portal hypertension result in ascites and hepatic encephalopathy.

DIAGNOSIS

Cirrhosis is diagnosed as follows:

- **Labs:**
  - Laboratory abnormalities may be absent in quiescent cirrhosis.
  - ALT/AST levels are elevated during active hepatocellular injury. However, levels may not be elevated in cirrhosis because a large portion of the liver is replaced by fibrous tissue, and little new cell injury may be occurring.

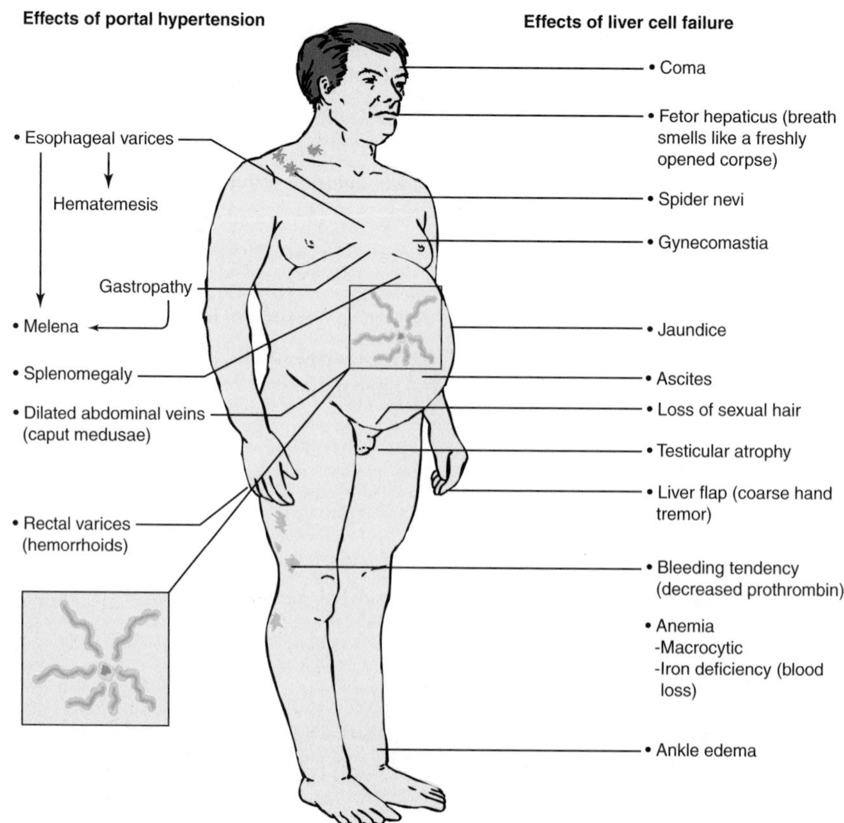

FIGURE 7-14. Clinical effects of cirrhosis. (Modified with permission from Chandrasoma P, Taylor CE. *Concise Pathology,* 3rd ed. Originally published by Appleton & Lange. Copyright © 1998 by The McGraw-Hill Companies, Inc.)

- Additional lab findings include anemia from suppressed erythropoiesis; leukopenia from hypersplenism or leukocytosis from infection; thrombocytopenia from alcoholic marrow suppression; ↓ hepatic thrombopoietin production and splenic sequestration; and a prolonged PT from failure of hepatic synthesis of clotting factors.
- **Imaging:**
  - **Ultrasound:** Used to assess liver size and surface contour and to detect ascites or hepatic nodules. Doppler ultrasound can establish the patency of the splenic, portal, and hepatic veins. Commonly used in the setting of chronic liver disease without known cirrhosis (see Figure 7-15).
  - **CT or MRI with contrast:** Used to characterize hepatic nodules. A biopsy may be needed to rule out malignancy.
  - Liver biopsy is the most accurate means of assessing disease severity.

Ascites is diagnosed in the following manner:

- **Ultrasound** and **paracentesis:** Check cell count, differential, albumin, and bacterial cultures +/– acid-fast stain and +/– cytology. The etiology of the ascites can be further characterized as follows:
  - **Related to portal hypertension (serum-ascites albumin gradient [SAAG] ≥ 1.1):** Cirrhosis, heart failure, Budd-Chiari syndrome (hepatic vein thrombosis).
  - **Unrelated to portal hypertension (SAAG < 1.1):** Peritonitis (eg, TB), cancer, pancreatitis, trauma, nephrotic syndrome.
- If a patient with cirrhosis and established ascites presents with worsening ascites, fever, altered mental status, renal dysfunction, or abdominal pain, think of **spontaneous bacterial peritonitis (SBP).**

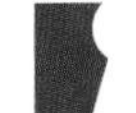

KEY FACT

Diagnose spontaneous bacterial peritonitis with ⊕ cultures or a peritoneal fluid neutrophil count > 250.

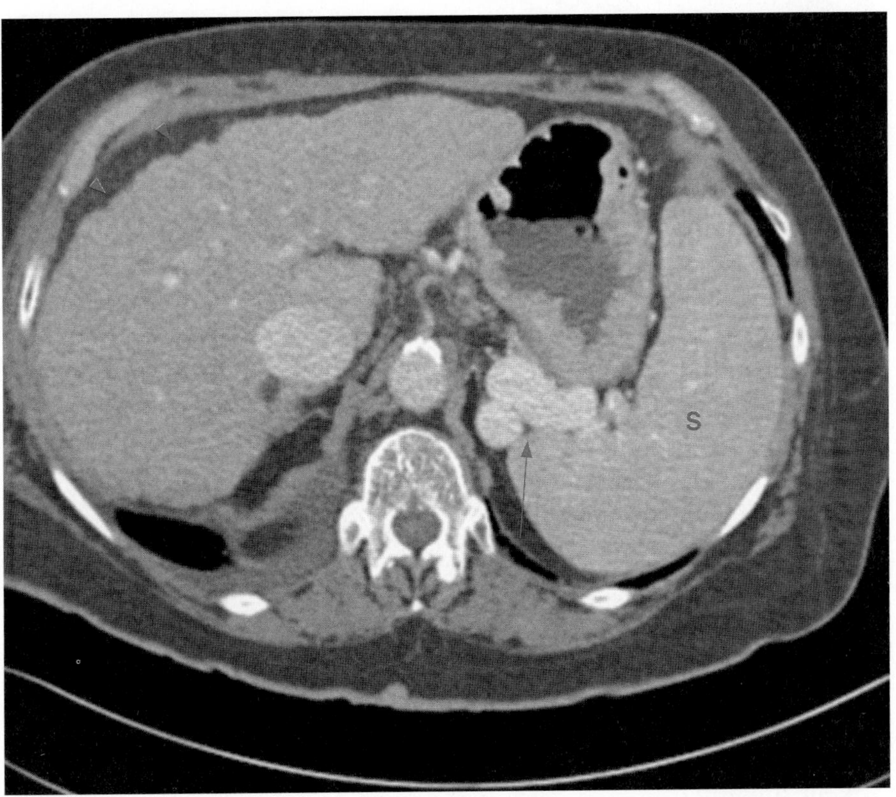

FIGURE 7-15. Cirrhosis. Transaxial image from contrast-enhanced CT shows a nodular liver contour (arrowheads) and the stigmata of portal hypertension, including splenomegaly (S) and perisplenic varices (arrow). (Reproduced with permission from USMLERx.com.)

TREATMENT

Treatment for **cirrhosis** is as follows:

- Abstain from alcohol.
- The diet should include ample protein. Dietary protein should not be restricted except occasionally in refractory hepatic encephalopathy.
- Restrict fluid intake to 800–1000 mL/day if the patient is hyponatremic.
- Treat hypoprothrombinemia with vitamin K and FFP if clinically indicated.
- Treat anemia with iron (in iron-deficiency anemia) or folic acid (in alcoholics).
- Liver transplantation is required in the setting of progressive liver disease.

Treatment for **ascites** includes the following:

- **Portal hypertension:**
  - **Sodium restriction** to < 2 g/day.
  - **Diuretics:** Furosemide and spironolactone in combination.
  - Large-volume paracentesis for ascites that is refractory to diuretics.
  - TIPS can be used in refractory cases, but this ↑ the rate of encephalopathy.
  - Ultimately, liver transplantation if the patient is a candidate.
- **No portal hypertension:**
  - Treat the underlying disorder.
  - Therapeutic paracentesis also can be performed.
- Treat SBP with a **third-generation cephalosporin** (first-line therapy) or a fluoroquinolone. Often recurs.

KEY FACT

Treat hepatic encephalopathy with lactulose, rifaximin (Xifaxan), and neomycin.

Acetaminophen Toxicity

Within 2–4 hours of an acute overdose, patients present with nausea, vomiting, diaphoresis, and pallor. Within 24–48 hours, hepatotoxicity is manifested by RUQ tenderness, hepatomegaly, and ↑ transaminases.

TREATMENT

- Supportive measures; oral administration of activated charcoal or cholestyramine within 30 minutes of ingestion to prevent absorption of residual drug.
- Begin **N-acetylcysteine** administration up to 36 hours after ingestion if the acetaminophen level is > 200 µg/mL measured at 4 hours or > 100 µg/mL at 8 hours after ingestion or if the time of ingestion is unknown and ↑ levels are seen (see Figure 7-16). Even late treatment can be helpful.

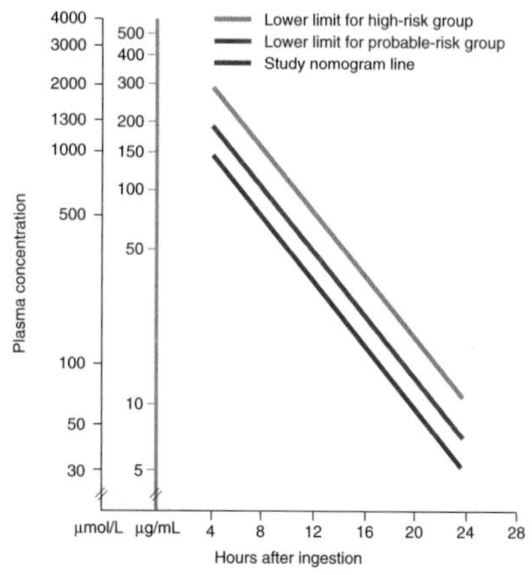

FIGURE 7-16. Estimation of the severity of acetaminophen ingestion.

Hereditary Hemochromatosis

- An **autosomal recessive** disorder of **iron overload.** Usually affects **middle-aged Caucasian men** at a rate of 1 in 300.
- **Sx/Exam:** Presents with **mild transaminitis, DM, arthritis, infertility,** and heart failure.
- **Dx:** Diagnosis is made with ↑ iron saturation (> 60% in men and > 50% in women), ↑ ferritin, ↑ transferrin saturation, and the presence of the **HFE gene mutation.**
- **Tx:** Treat with **phlebotomy** to ↓ the iron burden. Genetic counseling is useful to assess the likelihood of transmission.

Wilson's Disease

- An **autosomal recessive** disorder of **copper overload.**
- **Sx/Exam:** Exam may reveal **Kayser-Fleischer rings** and **neuropsychiatric** disorders.
- **Dx:** Labs reveal ↑ urinary copper, ↓ serum **ceruloplasmin,** and ↑ hepatic copper content on liver biopsy.
- **Tx:** Treatment is via **chelation** with penicillamine and trientine.

α_1-Antitrypsin Disorder

- Usually affects the **liver** (cirrhosis) and the **lung** (emphysema).
- **Dx:** Diagnosed by the quantitative absence of α_1-antitrypsin on serum protein electrophoresis (SPEP) as well as by genotype analysis (autosomal recessive).
- **Tx:** Treatment is via **liver transplantation** and α_1-antitrypsin replacement for the lung.

Autoimmune Hepatitis

- Primarily affects **young women;** usually suspected when transaminases are elevated.
- **Dx:** Hypergammaglobulinemia is seen on SPEP; autoantibodies are sometimes seen (**ANA**, anti–smooth muscle antibody [**ASMA**], liver/kidney microsomal antibody [**LKMA**]). Ultimately, a **liver biopsy** is needed to confirm the diagnosis.
- **Tx:** Treat with **corticosteroids and azathioprine.** A significant number of patients relapse when off therapy and thus require long-term treatment.

1° Biliary Cirrhosis

A 46-year-old woman presents to your clinic with scleral icterus, pruritus, and abnormal LFTs. Her AST, ALT, and alkaline phosphatase are 48, 56, and 603 U/L, respectively. What lab test will reveal the likely diagnosis?

A ⊕ antimitochondrial antibody will reveal the likely diagnosis of 1° biliary cirrhosis.

- **Autoimmune** destruction of microscopic intrahepatic bile ducts. Usually associated with other autoimmune diseases. More commonly occurs in **women.**
- **Sx/Exam:** Presents with fatigue, **pruritus, jaundice,** fat **malabsorption,** and **osteoporosis.**
- **Dx:** Suggested by markedly ↑ alkaline phosphatase, ↑ bilirubin (late), and **antimitochondrial antibody (AMA).** Confirmed by biopsy.
- **Tx:** Ursodeoxycholic acid, fat-soluble vitamins, cholestyramine for pruritus, and transplantation.

1° Sclerosing Cholangitis

- **Idiopathic** intra- and extrahepatic fibrosis of the bile ducts. Affects **men** 20–50 years of age; associated with **IBD, usually ulcerative colitis.**
- **Sx/Exam:** Can present with **RUQ pain** and pruritus but is often **asymptomatic.**
- **Dx:** Look for ↑ bilirubin and alkaline phosphatase; ⊕ **ASMA;** ⊕ **p-ANCA;** and multiple areas of beaded bile duct strictures on ERCP (see Figure 7-17).
- **Tx:** Treat with ursodeoxycholic acid, cholestyramine, fat-soluble vitamins, stenting of the strictures, and ultimately liver transplantation.

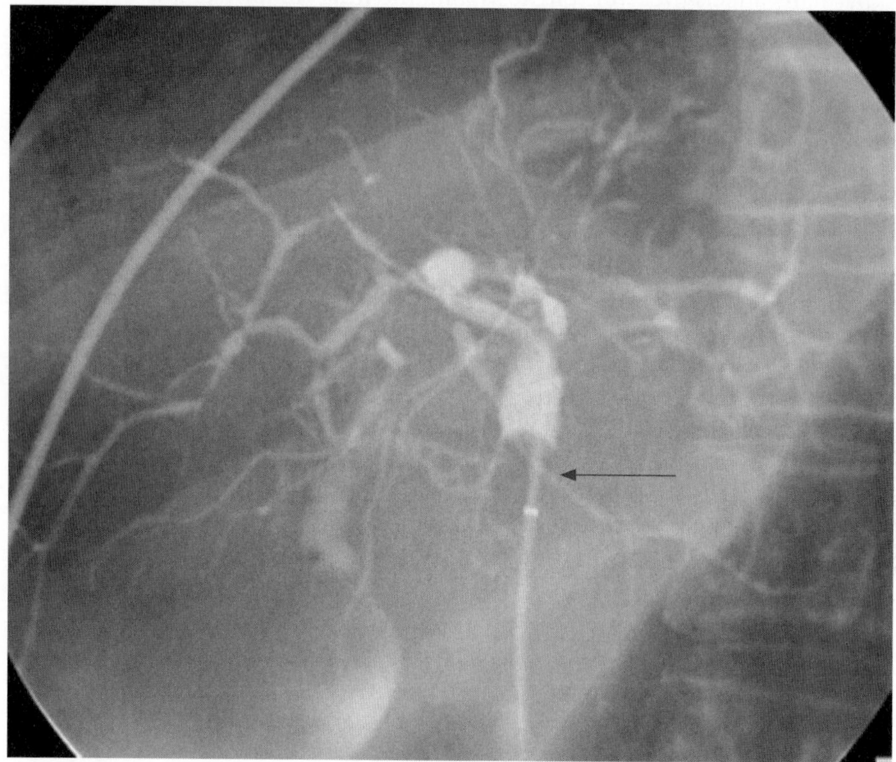

FIGURE 7-17. Primary sclerosing cholangitis. ERCP image following contrast injection through a catheter in the common bile duct with the balloon (blue arrow) inflated. Multifocal structuring and dilation of the intrahepatic bile ducts can be seen. (Reproduced with permission from USMLERx.com.)

CHAPTER 8

HEMATOLOGY

Anemia

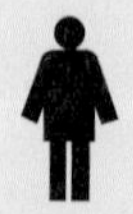

A nine-year-old boy who was recently treated for meningitis in a developing country develops purpura and then pallor. He is found to have a platelet count of 42,000/µL, a hematocrit of 26%, and a WBC count of 1700. Which antibiotic that is now rarely used in the United States is known to cause pancytopenia?

Chloramphenicol.

Anemia can be classified by the size of the red cell (mean corpuscular volume, or MCV) as microcytic, normocytic, or macrocytic:

- **Microcytic:** MCV < 80 fL.
- **Normocytic:** MCV 80–100 fL.
- **Macrocytic:** MCV > 100 fL.

DIAGNOSIS

- Initially, order a CBC, an MCV, a blood smear, and a reticulocyte count.
- On the basis of the initial results, order 2° tests such as iron studies (serum ferritin, serum iron, TIBC, % transferrin saturation), serum folate, TSH, serum B_{12}, hemolysis labs (LDH, unconjugated bilirubin, haptoglobin, Coombs' test), and a DIC panel (D-dimer, fibrinogen, blood smear, soluble fibrin monomer complex). Serum ferritin studies may be less accurate in patients with acute illness or chronic inflammatory/chronic liver disease.
- Look for a bleeding source, and order a type and cross if the patient is actively bleeding or symptomatic from anemia.
- Look for **pancytopenia.** Etiologies include toxins, drugs, infection, myelodysplasia, malignancy, radiation, vitamin B_{12}/folate deficiency, SLE, and congenital causes.

KEY FACT

Normal hemoglobin and hematocrit values for pediatric patients are lower than those for adults, so check age-standardized ranges.

KEY FACT

If possible, check all necessary lab studies pertaining to anemia **prior** to transfusion.

TREATMENT

Patients with severe anemia and those who are symptomatic initially require fluid resuscitation and RBC transfusion. Transfuse to keep serum hemoglobin > 7 g/dL, or > 8 g/dL for CAD patients. Identify the cause of the anemia and treat the underlying disorder.

MICROCYTIC ANEMIA

Anemia with an MCV of < 80 fL. Anemia with an **MCV of > 70 fL** is due to either iron-deficiency anemia or thalassemia. Other causes include anemia of chronic disease and sideroblastic anemia (see the mnemonic **TICS**).

MNEMONIC

Causes of microcytic anemia–

TICS

Thalassemia
Iron deficiency
Chronic disease
Sideroblastic anemia

SYMPTOMS/EXAM

- Iron-deficient patients may have **pica.**
- Ask about melena and blood in the stools, and check for fecal occult blood. Ask female patients about heavy menstrual periods. A family history of anemia should raise suspicion for thalassemia.

- The Mentzer index can be used to help distinguish iron-deficiency anemia from thalassemia:

$$\text{Mentzer index} = \text{MCV/RBC count}$$

If the Mentzer index is > 13, the condition is more likely to be iron-deficiency anemia.

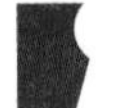

KEY FACT

In iron-deficiency anemia, first RDW widens and then MCV ↓.

DIAGNOSIS

- Examine iron studies, a blood smear, and a CBC to identify the cause of the microcytic anemia (see Table 8-1).
- Suspect **colorectal cancer** in elderly patients with microcytic anemia, and refer these patients for a colonoscopy.

KEY FACT

Serum ferritin, a measure of iron stores, is ↓ in iron-deficiency anemia but is ↑ in infection and inflammation (anemia of chronic disease). Low serum ferritin is highly specific but not sensitive for iron deficiency.

TREATMENT

- If iron-deficiency anemia is the cause, identify the site of blood loss and initiate oral iron supplementation (patients intolerant of oral therapy and those with GI disease may need parenteral therapy). **To help replenish stores, treatment should be continued 3–6 months after lab values have normalized.**

TABLE 8-1. Causes of Microcytic Anemia

	Iron-Deficiency Anemia	Thalassemia	Anemia of Chronic Disease (Late)	Sideroblastic Anemia
Serum ferritin	↓ (may be normal in inflammatory states, including cancer).	Normal to ↑	↑ (may be normal in early stages).	↑
Serum iron	↓	Normal to ↑	Slightly ↓	↑
Iron-binding capacity	↑	Normal to ↑	**Normal to ↓**	Normal or ↓
Other tests	**Wide RDW.**	**Normal RDW.** Order hemoglobin electrophoresis to confirm the diagnosis.		Smear shows normal and dimorphic RBCs with basophilic stippling. Confirm the diagnosis with bone marrow biopsy (shows erythroid hyperplasia and ringed sideroblasts).
Comments	Etiologies include malabsorption, chronic blood loss, and malnutrition. Thrombocytosis is common.	Characterized by ↓ or absent production of one or more globin chains in the hemoglobin. Also marked by an elevated MCHC and a Mentzer index of < 13.	Etiologies include chronic inflammation, infection, and malignancy.	Etiologies include chronic alcohol use, drugs (antitubercular, chloramphenicol), and lead poisoning. Has ↑ transferrin levels. Order lead levels if lead toxicity is suspected.

- Erythropoietin (**Epogen**) should be administered to patients with anemia of chronic disease, particularly those with chronic kidney disease.
- The treatment of thalassemia is outlined separately in the discussion below.

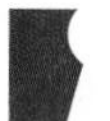

KEY FACT

Clinically significant α-thalassemia can present at birth because the α chain is made in fetal and neonatal hematopoiesis, but β-thalassemia won't present until the α-chain predominance (present in fetal hemoglobin) changes to the β chain in infancy.

Thalassemia

A group of disorders resulting from ↓ synthesis of α- or β-globin protein subunits. α-thalassemia is most common among **Asians** and African Americans; β-thalassemia is most frequently found in people of **Mediterranean** origin as well as in Asians and African Americans.

Symptoms/Exam

Clinical presentation varies according to subtype:

- **α-thalassemia:** If **all four** α alleles are affected, babies are stillborn with **hydrops fetalis** or die shortly after birth. **HbH** disease with **three** affected alleles leads to **chronic hemolytic microcytic anemia and splenomegaly.** Carriers of one or two affected alleles are usually asymptomatic.
- **β-thalassemia: β-thalassemia major** (homozygous; no β-globin production and hence no HbA) presents in the first year of life as the fraction of HbF declines. Manifestations include growth retardation, **bony deformities,** hepatosplenomegaly, and jaundice. **β-thalassemia minor** (heterozygous) is usually less severe and is diagnosed by an ↑ HbA_2 on electrophoresis.

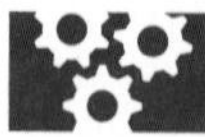

MNEMONIC

Features of β-thalassemia major—

BETA THAL D

Basophilic stippling
Excess iron from transfusions
Transplant, bone marrow
Hb**A** decreased
Tower skull and bony abnormalities
Heart failure
Anisocytosis
Liver and spleen enlargement
Deferoxamine

Diagnosis

CBC reveals severe microcytic anemia with a normal RDW and an ↑ **RBC count** (vs. iron deficiency). Hemoglobin electrophoresis is the definitive diagnostic test.

Treatment

- Although an emerging treatment for patients with severe thalassemia is allogeneic bone marrow transplantation, blood transfusions should be given as necessary for symptomatic control, and patients must receive folate supplementation.
- To prevent 2° hemosiderosis due to iron overload, deferoxamine, an iron chelator, is usually given concomitantly.
- Prenatal diagnosis is now available, and genetic counseling should be offered to high-risk families.

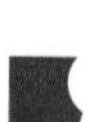

KEY FACT

With a severely low MCV, a Mentzer index of < 13, microcytic anemia not responsive to iron supplementation, or familial anemia, suspect thalassemia and order a hemoglobin electrophoresis.

MACROCYTIC ANEMIA

A 32-year-old woman with Crohn's disease and a history of partial bowel resection, including resection of the terminal ileum, comes to you for fatigue and is found to have a hematocrit of 29% and an MCV of 104 fL. Why is she at risk for vitamin B_{12} deficiency?

Intrinsic factor receptors are located in the terminal ileum. Patients with B_{12} absorption deficiencies, such as those with intestinal disease or pernicious anemia, should be treated with injected vitamin B_{12}.

Anemia with an MCV of > 100 fL. The most common etiologies include the following:

- **Folate deficiency:** Common causes include poor dietary intake (including that which occurs with **alcoholism**) and **drugs** (eg, phenytoin, zidovudine, TMP-SMX, methotrexate, and other chemotherapeutic agents).
- **B_{12} deficiency:** Commonly caused by a strict vegan diet, **pernicious anemia**, gastrectomy, PPIs (which inhibit B_{12} absorption), and ileal dysfunction (IBD, surgical resection). B_{12} deficiency can cause **neurologic deficits** (paresthesias, gait disturbance, and mental status changes).
- **Other:** Liver disease, hypothyroidism, alcohol abuse, myelodysplasia, reticulocytosis.

KEY FACT

An MCV of > 110 fL is usually due to vitamin B_{12} or folate deficiency.

DIAGNOSIS

- Initial diagnostic labs should include a serum B_{12} level, an RBC folate level, and a **blood smear** to look for megaloblastic anemia, which shows **oval macrocytes** and hypersegmented neutrophils (see Figure 8-1).
- If B_{12} deficiency is suspected, check intrinsic factor antibody and anti–parietal cell antibody for pernicious anemia. A Schilling test may be used to confirm the cause.
- Elevated methylmalonic acid levels will confirm the diagnosis in patients with borderline levels.

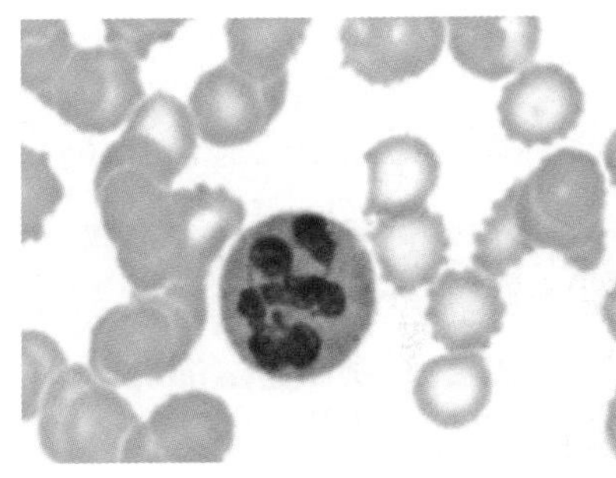

FIGURE 8-1. Hypersegmented neutrophil seen in megaloblastic anemia. (Reproduced with permission from USMLERx.com.)

TREATMENT

- Treat B_{12} deficiency with monthly B_{12} shots; treat folate deficiency with oral replacement.
- Discontinue any medications that could be contributing to megaloblastic anemia; minimize alcohol use.

NORMOCYTIC NORMOCHROMIC ANEMIA

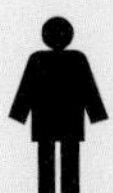

While evaluating a 59-year-old woman for dyspnea on exertion, you find that she has a hematocrit of 31% with an MCV of 89 fL. What are your next steps?

Check a blood smear, a reticulocyte count, renal function tests (creatinine), LDH, haptoglobin, and indirect bilirubin, and look for possible bleeding sites.

Anemia with an MCV of 80–100 fL. Can be due to **blood loss (hemorrhage), hemolysis,** or **↓ production.**

SYMPTOMS/EXAM

Look for evidence of acute bleeding on history and exam. Patients with **hemolytic anemia** may present with jaundice and dark urine from unconjugated hyperbilirubinemia as well as with pigment gallstones and splenomegaly.

DIAGNOSIS

The initial workup should focus on reticulocyte count, creatinine, hemolysis labs, and blood smear.

- **Normal reticulocyte count:** Anemia of chronic disease or chronic kidney disease.
- **↑ reticulocyte count with normal hemolysis labs:** Hemorrhage.

- ↑ **reticulocyte count,** ↑ **LDH,** ↑ **unconjugated bilirubin,** and ↓ **haptoglobin: Hemolysis.** Causes include the following:
  - **Microangiopathic hemolytic anemia:** Schistocytes or helmet cells are seen on blood smear (see Figure 8-2 and the subtopic below). These RBC fragments are thought to be due to RBC shearing through partially coagulated capillaries.
  - **Hereditary spherocytosis:** Characterized by spherocytes, a ⊕ family history, and a ⊖ Coombs' test.
  - **Autoimmune hemolytic anemia:** Marked by spherocytes with a **⊕ Coombs' test.**
  - **Cold agglutinin disease:** Acrocyanosis in cold exposure. The cold agglutinin test is ⊕. Seen with mycoplasmal infection and mononucleosis.
  - **Sickle cell anemia:** See the subtopic below.
  - **G6PD deficiency:** Hemolysis in the presence of infection or drugs (most commonly sulfa drugs). Peripheral blood smear may show characteristic bite cells (which have the appearance of a bite taken out from the periphery). G6PD levels may be normal during hemolytic episodes but are ↓ thereafter.
  - **Myelofibrosis:** A myeloproliferative disorder of abnormally activated marrow fibroblasts, with subsequent medullary fibrosis and anemia. Most commonly idiopathic or 2° to polycythemia vera or hematologic malignancy. Extramedullary hematopoiesis causes **hepatosplenomegaly.** Labs show reticulocytosis, **teardrop RBCs,** and elevated LDH. Marrow biopsy is diagnostic. See Table 8-2 for lab features differentiating myelofibrosis from other myeloproliferative disorders.
  - **Paroxysmal nocturnal hemoglobinuria (PNH): An acquired disorder with intravascular hemolysis** (with ensuing hemoglobinuria) and **recurrent thrombosis.** May involve pancytopenia. Diagnosed by **flow cytometry.**

MNEMONIC

Patients with PNH have morning FITS of pink urine:

Flow cytometry to diagnose
Intravascular hemolysis
Thrombosis
Supportive treatment for complications

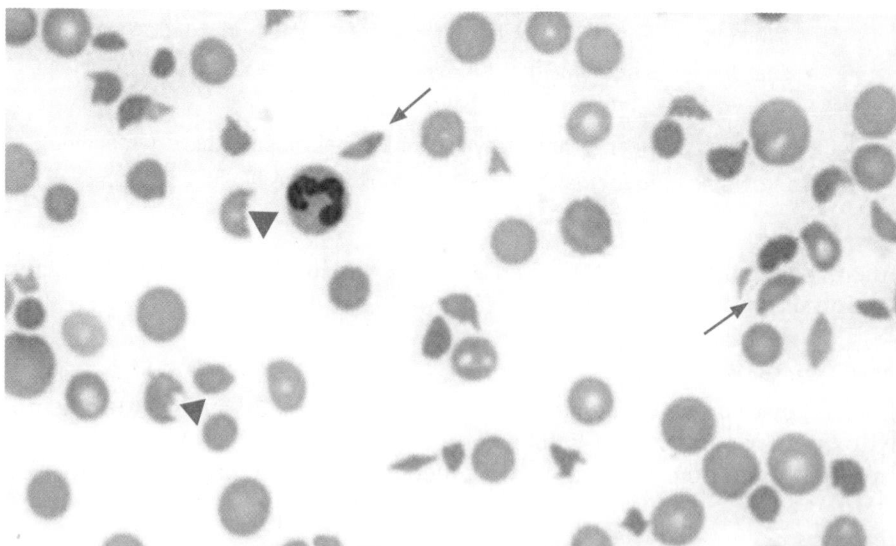

FIGURE 8-2. Schistocytes (arrows) and helmet cells (arrowheads) in a patient with DIC. (Reproduced with permission from USMLERx.com.)

TABLE 8-2. Laboratory Features of Myeloproliferative Disorders

	WBC COUNT	HEMATOCRIT	PLATELET COUNT	RBC MORPHOLOGY
CML	↑↑	Normal	Normal or ↑	Normal
Myelofibrosis	Normal or ↓/↑	Normal or ↓	Normal or ↓/↑	**Abnormal**
PCV	Normal or ↑	↑	Normal or ↑	Normal
Essential thrombocytosis	Normal or ↑	Normal	↑	Normal

(Reproduced with permission from Tierney LM et al [eds]. *Current Medical Diagnosis & Treatment: 2004.* New York: McGraw-Hill, 2004: 481.)

TREATMENT

- Patients who are hemorrhaging must be resuscitated with fluids and RBC transfusions. The cause of the bleeding must be identified and treated.
- **Hereditary spherocytosis** usually responds to **splenectomy.** Remember to vaccinate against encapsulated organisms (*Neisseria meningitidis, Streptococcus pneumoniae, Haemophilus influenzae* type b).
- Treatment for **autoimmune hemolytic anemia** includes **steroids,** immunosuppressive agents, IVIG, and, if necessary, splenectomy.

Microangiopathic Hemolytic Anemia

An eight-year-old boy eats at a local burger joint at which meat was later found to be contaminated with bacteria. Two days after his fast-food meal, he develops bloody diarrhea and is hospitalized. On day 4 he is noted to have dark urine. Labs reveal a hemoglobin level of 8.5 g/dL, a platelet count of 41,000/μL, a creatinine level of 5.6 mg/dL, and schistocytes on blood smear. You diagnose HUS. What is the treatment for his renal failure?

Hemodialysis.

Defined as the presence of **intravascular hemolysis with fragmented RBCs** (**schistocytes and helmet cells** on blood smear). Constitutes a **medical emergency.** Distinguished as follows (see also Table 8-3):

- **DIC:** Overwhelming systemic activation of the coagulation system stimulated by serious illness. Causes include sepsis, shock, malignancy, obstetric complications, and trauma.
- **HUS:** The triad of hemolytic anemia, thrombocytopenia, and ARF. Causes include viral illness and ***E coli* O157:H7. Most common in children > 10 years of age.**
- **TTP:** Presents as a **pentad** of the HUS triad plus fever and fluctuating neurologic signs, although patients may not have all five. Causes include HIV, pregnancy, and OCP use.

TREATMENT

- **DIC:** Treat the underlying condition; transfuse platelets; give protein C concentrate or cryoprecipitate (to replace fibrinogen) and FFP (to replace coagulation factors).

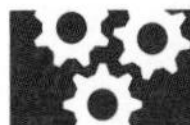

MNEMONIC

The pentad of TTP, a medical emergency—

Run FAST!

Renal failure
Fever
Anemia (microangiopathic hemolytic anemia)
Seizure (CNS dysfunction)
Thrombocytopenia

KEY FACT

Differentiate HUS and TTP by the presence of neurologic signs in TTP. The treatment of choice for TTP is plasmapheresis; that for HUS is dialysis.

TABLE 8-3. Differential of Microangiopathic Hemolytic Anemia

	PLATELETS	PT/PTT	D-DIMER	OTHER FINDINGS
TTP or HUS	↓↓↓	Normal	Normal	ARF, CNS dysfunction.
DIC	↓↓	↑	↑↑	↑ fibrin split products, ↓ fibrinogen, ↑ D-dimer.
Mechanical valve	Normal	Normal	Normal	Heart murmur.
Severe vasculitis, severe hypertension, HELLP	↓	Normal	Normal	Elevated liver enzymes in HELLP.

- **HUS:** Treat with dialysis for ARF.
- **TTP:** The treatment of choice is **plasmapheresis.** In urgent situations, give FFP until plasmapheresis becomes available. Do not give platelets, as this may exacerbate the TTP.

Sickle Cell Anemia

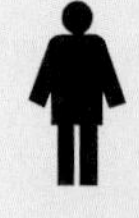

A five-year-old girl with sickle cell disease is in a kindergarten class with a child who recently came down with a facial rash and was diagnosed with fifth disease. The girl's mother calls you for advice. What complication is a concern?

Aplastic crisis due to parvovirus B19.

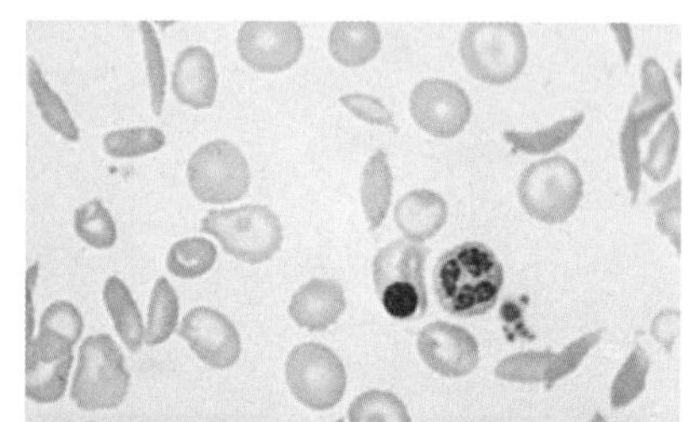

FIGURE 8-3. Sickled red blood cells. The elongated and crescent-shaped RBCs seen on this smear represent circulating irreversibly sickled cells. Target cells and a nucleated red blood cell are also seen. (Reproduced with permission from Fauci AS et al. *Harrison's Principles of Internal Medicine,* 17th ed. New York: McGraw-Hill, 2008, Fig. 99-4.)

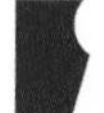

KEY FACT

Hydroxyurea is a chemotherapeutic agent that ↓ HbS and ↑ fetal hemoglobin, HbF. It should be considered in patients with frequent pain crises and a history of strokes or other serious complications.

An autosomal recessive disease resulting from the substitution of valine for glutamic acid at the sixth position in the globin chain.

Symptoms/Exam

Seen predominantly among African Americans, who often have a family history. Clinical features include stigmata of chronic hemolysis such as gallstones, poorly healing ulcers, jaundice, splenomegaly (usually during childhood), and CHF.

Diagnosis

Blood smear reveals sickled cells (see Figure 8-3), Howell-Jolly bodies, and evidence of hemolysis. **Hemoglobin electrophoresis** is the definitive diagnostic test.

Treatment

- Vaccinate all patients for *S pneumoniae, H influenzae,* HBV, and the influenza virus in the appropriate season.
- Give folic acid supplementation.
- Consider transfusions for severe anemia, sickle cell crisis, and priapism.
- Instruct patients to avoid dehydration, hypoxia, intense exercise, and high altitudes.
- In patients with frequent pain crisis, hydroxyurea or bone marrow transplantation should be considered.

COMPLICATIONS

The complications of sickle cell disease include the following (see also Figure 8-4):

- **Pain (vaso-occlusive) crisis:**
  - Sickled cells cause occlusion of arterioles, leading to tissue ischemia and/or infarction.
  - Characterized by pain in the back, limbs, abdomen, and ribs; precipitated by dehydration, acidosis, infection, fever, or hypoxia.
  - Treat with hydration, analgesia, and supplemental O_2.
- **Aplastic crisis:** A sudden ↓ in hemoglobin and reticulocyte count caused by parvovirus B19. Support with transfusions.
- **Acute chest syndrome:**
  - Presumed to be due to a combination of factors, including infection, infarction, and pulmonary fat embolism.
  - Clinical findings include fever, chest pain, cough, wheezing, tachypnea, and new pulmonary infiltrate on CXR.
  - Treat with O_2, analgesia, transfusions, and antibiotics (a second- or third-generation cephalosporin with a macrolide such as erythromycin).
- **Lungs:** Pulmonary infarcts can cause pulmonary hypertension.
- **Heart:** Sickle cell cardiomyopathy may lead to heart failure.
- **GI tract:** Cholecystitis, splenic infarcts.
- **Kidneys:** Sickling of cells can cause infarcts, leading to papillary necrosis and ARF (particularly in sickle cell trait).
- **Genital:** Priapism, impotence in males.
- **Infections:** The absence of a functional spleen predisposes patients to encapsulated organisms, including *S pneumoniae, H influenzae, N meningitidis*, and gram-⊖ bacterial infections.

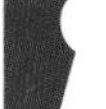

KEY FACT

As in thalassemia, sickle cell patients who receive frequent transfusions need prophylactic treatment of hemosiderosis with iron chelators such as deferoxamine.

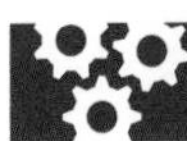

MNEMONIC

Treatment of acute chest syndrome–

TO AID

Transfusion
Oxygen
Antibiotics
Incentive spirometry
Dilators (bronchodilators)

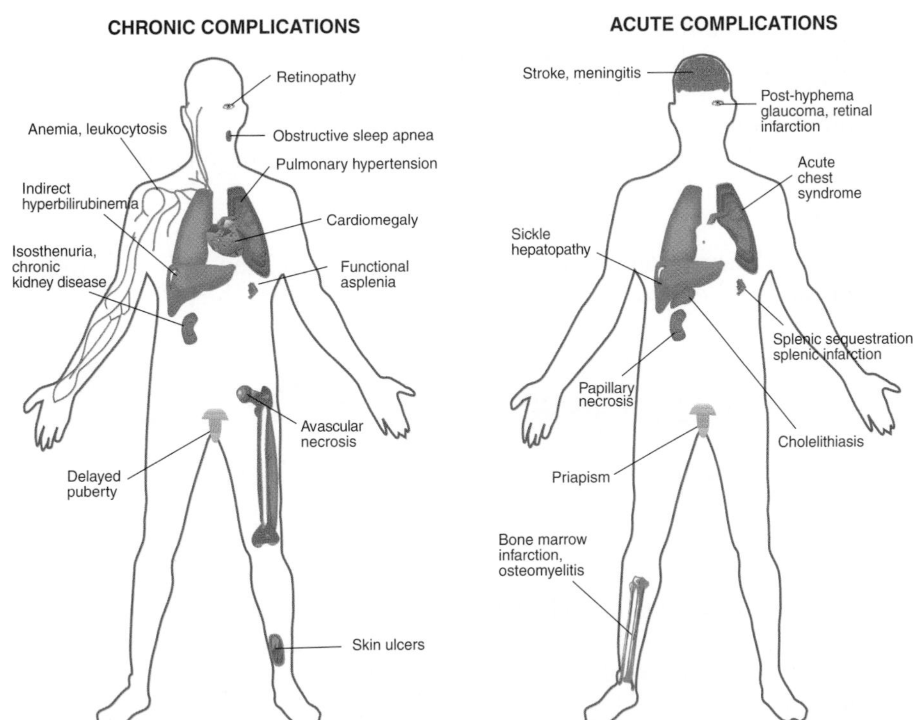

FIGURE 8-4. Complications of sickle cell disease.

- **Bones:** Avascular necrosis, *Salmonella* osteomyelitis.
- **CNS:** Stroke is one of the most devastating complications.
- **Pregnancy:** Patients are at ↑ risk of spontaneous abortions.

Polycythemia Vera (PCV)

A myeloproliferative syndrome in which the predominant abnormality is ↑ RBCs. Classically affects males > 60 years of age. Remember, the most common cause of erythrocytosis is **chronic hypoxia** 2° to lung disease rather than 1° PCV.

SYMPTOMS/EXAM

- Patients present with malaise, fever, pruritus (especially after a warm shower), and signs of vascular sludging (eg, **stroke,** angina, MI, claudication, hepatic vein thrombosis, headache, and blurred vision).
- Exam may reveal **plethora,** large retinal veins on funduscopy, and **splenomegaly.**

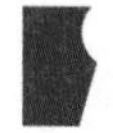

KEY FACT

Distinguish polycythemia vera from other causes of 2° polycythemia through an erythropoietin level. An elevated erythropoietin level excludes the diagnosis of PCV.

DIAGNOSIS

- Labs show ↑ **hematocrit** (≥ 50%), ↑ RBC mass, and a normal **erythropoietin** level (↑ in chronic hypoxia-induced polycythemia). Basophilia suggests proliferative myelopoiesis. JAK-2 ⊕.
- Establish the diagnosis by bone marrow biopsy, which shows a hypercellular marrow.
- Table 8-2 outlines the laboratory features of PCV in contrast to those of other myeloproliferative disorders.

TREATMENT

- Treatment includes **serial phlebotomy** until hematocrit is < 45 (men) and < 42 (women) along with **daily ASA.**
- Hydroxyurea is appropriate for those at high risk of thrombosis (age > 70, prior thrombosis, platelet count > 1,500,000/μL, presence of cardiovascular risk factors). Anagrelide can be used to ↓ platelets in refractory patients.

COMPLICATIONS

PCV, like other myeloproliferative syndromes, is associated with an ↑ **risk of conversion** to other myeloproliferative syndromes or AML.

Bleeding Disorders

Disorders in **coagulation or platelets** that predispose patients to bleed (see Table 8-4).

DIAGNOSIS

- Initial tests to order include PT/PTT, CBC, platelet count, and a DIC panel (D-dimer, fibrinogen, blood smear). Use these laboratory data to determine if the cause of the bleeding is 2° to a coagulopathy or a platelet problem.
  - Think **thrombocytopenia** when the platelet count is < 90,000 cells/μL (see the discussion of platelet pathology below).
  - Think **coagulopathy** if the PT or PTT is ↑ (see the discussion of coagulopathies).

TABLE 8-4. Coagulopathy vs. Platelet Disorders

Clinical Feature	Platelet Disorder	Coagulopathy
Amount of bleeding after surface cuts	Excessive, prolonged.	Normal to slightly ↑.
Onset of bleeding after injury	Immediate bleeding.	Delayed bleeding after surgery or trauma. Spontaneous bleeding into joints or hematoma.
Clinical presentation	Superficial and mucosal bleeding (GI tract, gingival, nasal). Petechiae, ecchymosis.	Deep and excessive bleeding into joints, muscles, GI tract, and GU tract.

- If platelet count and PT/PTT are normal, check bleeding time (PFA-100 test) and thrombin time. An ↑ bleeding time suggests a **platelet dysfunction.** An ↑ thrombin time suggests a **defect in the cross-linking of fibrin** such as that in **dysfibrinogenemia** or **DIC.**

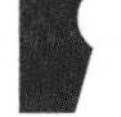

KEY FACT

Petechiae = **P**latelet deficiency.
Cavity/joint bleeding = **C**lotting factor deficiency.

TREATMENT

- Patients who are hemodynamically unstable need immediate resuscitation with IV fluids. The source of hemorrhage should be identified and stopped.
- Blood transfusions should be given to maintain a hemoglobin of > 8 g/dL. FFP should be given to normalize PTT and PT. Platelets should be given as needed.

PLATELET DISORDERS

You are called to the ICU to evaluate a 64-year-old woman who was admitted six days ago, following cardiac surgery, for a "black" rash. On exam, you find necrotic patches of skin on the distal extremities. The woman's medications include furosemide, enoxaparin, enalapril, amlodipine, insulin, and ASA. Her platelet count is 36,000/μL with ⊕ PF-4 antibodies. You diagnose heparin-induced thrombocytopenia (HIT). What condition accounts for the patient's skin necrosis?

HIT causes platelet activation and thrombosis.

Disorders associated with a ↓ in the number of platelets (**thrombocytopenia**) or a ↓ in the functioning of platelets that predisposes patients to bleed (**platelet dysfunction**). Look for petechiae and easy bruising. In addition to TTP and HUS, common platelet disorders include the following:

- **Drug-induced thrombocytopenia:** One of the most common causes of mild asymptomatic thrombocytopenia. Common drugs include quinine, antibiotics, sulfa drugs, and glycoprotein IIb/IIIa inhibitors. Usually resolves within one week of stopping the implicated drug.

- **ITP/autoimmune thrombocytopenia:** Severe thrombocytopenia due to **platelet-associated IgG** antibodies. A diagnosis of exclusion. DIC panel is ⊖. Treatment involves **prednisone** and, if the patient is unresponsive to steroids, splenectomy.
- **HIT: Immune-mediated** thrombocytopenia occurring 4–14 days after the initiation of heparin. Platelet factor-4 (PF-4) antibodies are used for diagnosis. Treat by stopping heparin immediately and starting an alternative anticoagulant such as lepirudin, argatroban, or danaparoid sodium (**not** warfarin).
- **Acquired disease:** Platelet proliferation and function can be impaired as a result of severe liver disease, severe renal disease, or multiple myeloma. ASA impairs platelet function. Treat with desmopressin, OCPs for menorrhagia, and FFP or cryoprecipitate for major bleeding. Do not use ASA.
- **Inherited disease:** Includes Bernard-Soulier syndrome, Glanzmann's thrombasthenia, and storage pool disease. Treatment is the same as that for acquired disease.
- **Platelet dysfunction:** Normal platelet count.

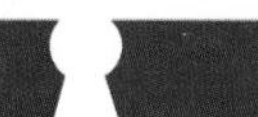

KEY FACT

Idiopathic **T**hrombocytopenic **P**urpura: **T**reat with **P**rednisone.

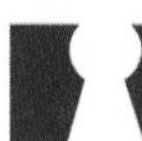

KEY FACT

Generally, treat with platelet transfusion if platelet count is:

- < 90,000 before neurosurgery
- < 50,000 before a general procedure
- < 50,000 in a symptomatic/bleeding patient
- < 20,000 in an asymptomatic patient with fever/sepsis
- < 10,000 in an asymptomatic patient

Diagnosis

- First confirm or disprove the presence of thrombocytopenia (ie, recheck platelets in citrated blood).
- Then obtain a CBC, a peripheral blood smear, and a one-hour posttransfusion platelet count to distinguish between low platelet production (pancytopenia; small platelets; ↑ platelet count following platelet transfusion) and ↑ platelet destruction (large platelets; no significant ↑ in platelet count following platelet transfusion).
- Obtain a bone marrow biopsy in cases of severe thrombocytopenia.

Treatment

See above.

COAGULOPATHIES

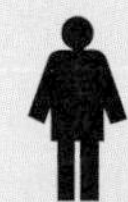

A seven-year-old boy with hemophilia A comes to the ER after having fallen on his knee two hours ago. His knee is now red, warm, and held in partial flexion due to an effusion. What medication should be used to reverse his coagulopathy?

Recombinant factor VIII. Adjunctive treatments include joint rest, ice, analgesia (but avoid salicylates and NSAIDs), and sometimes joint aspiration.

Conditions in which a defective clotting cascade predisposes patients to bleeding. Ask about medications that predispose to bleeding (eg, warfarin, enoxaparin, heparin); note factors that predispose to **vitamin K** deficiency (eg, malnutrition, antibiotic use, alcoholism). A history of recurrent spontaneous bleeding suggests a factor deficiency. A history of delayed bleeding after trauma or surgery (classically after the umbilical cord falls off) suggests factor XIII deficiency.

Diagnosis

- Look for evidence of liver disease on exam, and order LFTs to look for evidence of liver dysfunction.
- Defects in the clotting cascade can be due to defects in the intrinsic pathway, the extrinsic pathway, or the common pathway.
  - **Intrinsic pathway:** Involves **factors VIII, IX, XI, and XII.** Abnormality results in an ↑ in **aPTT. Impaired in patients with hemophilia A or B.**
  - **Extrinsic pathway:** Involves **factor VII.** Abnormality leads to an ↑ in **PT (INR). Prolonged by warfarin.**
  - **Combined pathway:** Involves **factors V, X, and II (fibrinogen).** Abnormality leads to an ↑ in **both aPTT and PT (INR).** Thrombin time or reptilase time assesses the function of fibrin cross-linking; both are abnormal in **fibrinolytic disorders.**
- A diagnostic approach toward patients with coagulation disorders is summarized in Figure 8-5.

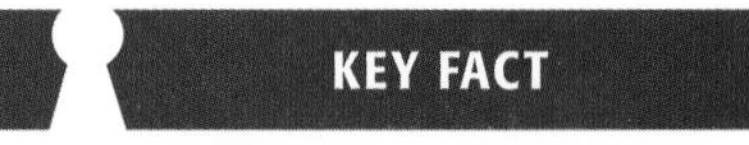

The **EX-PAT** (**EX**trinsic **PAT**hway) went to **WAR**(farin).

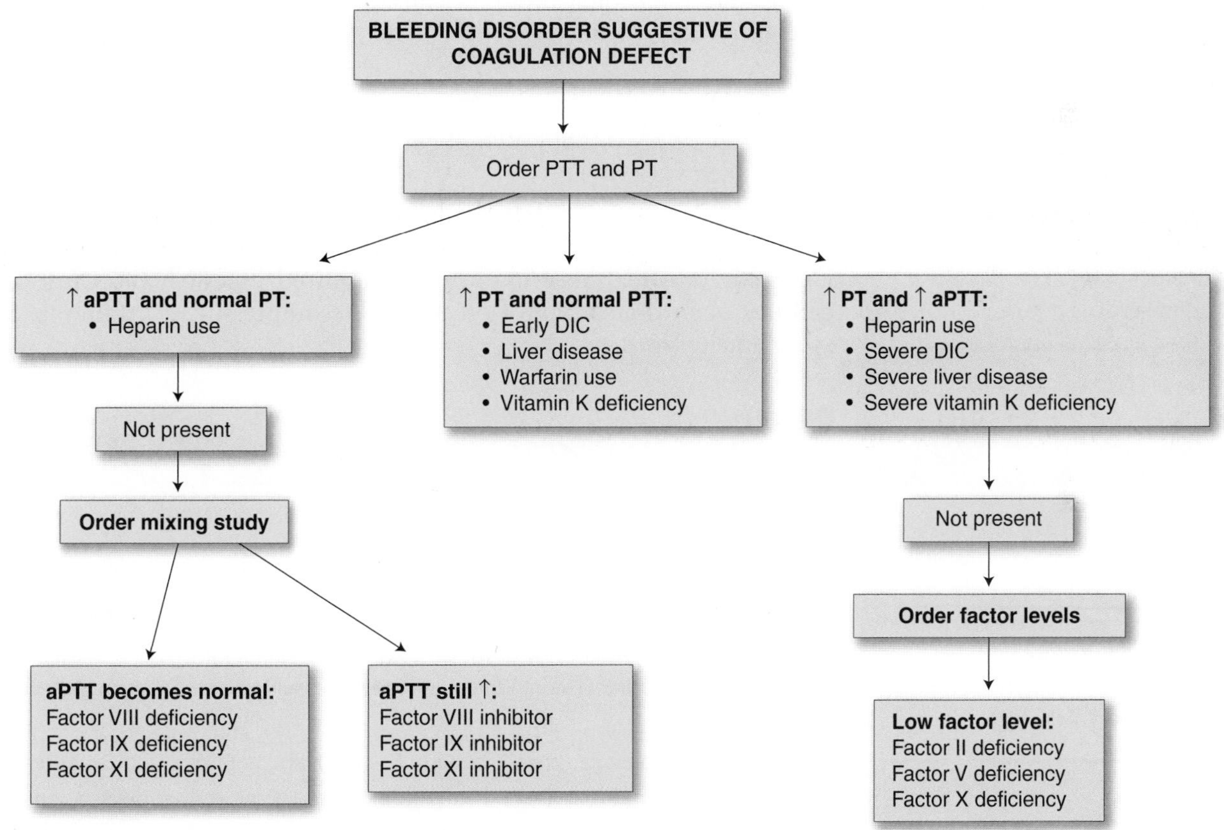

FIGURE 8-5. Approach to patients with bleeding disorders suggestive of a coagulation defect.

Treatment

- Coagulopathic patients who are actively bleeding need **FFP** to normalize their PT and PTT levels. Heparin and warfarin must be stopped.
- If vitamin K deficiency is suspected, it is reasonable to empirically give a patient 10 mg of oral vitamin K for three days to see if the PT normalizes.
- Patients with hemophilia A or B require **factor VIII** (either recombinant factor VIII or as cryoprecipitate) or **factor IX** replacement, respectively.

von Willebrand's Disease (vWD)

An autosomal dominant condition that represents the most common bleeding disorder. It is characterized by low levels of von Willebrand's factor (vWF), which is involved in the transport of factor VIII and also helps platelets form a hemostatic plug.

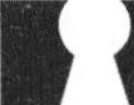

KEY FACT

Desmopressin, also known as ADH, ↑ circulating concentrations of factor VIII and vWF while also improving platelet adhesion. Classic uses are to reverse coagulopathic hemorrhage in vWD and hemophilia.

Symptoms/Exam

Clinical features can mimic platelet dysfunction (causing mucocutaneous bleeds and ↑ bleeding time) as well as hemophilia (joint bleeds, ↑ aPTT), depending on the subtype.

Diagnosis

Diagnosed by ↓ levels of vWF antigen and/or by abnormal vWF activity (ristocetin cofactor activity).

KEY FACT

von **W**illebrand's **D**isease: Treat **W**ith **D**esmopressin.

Treatment

Generally, **no treatment is routinely required except before surgical procedures or in the setting of bleeding. Desmopressin** is first-line therapy in symptomatic cases.

KEY FACT

Factor V Leiden deficiency, the most common inherited hypercoagulable disorder, is screened with an activated protein C (APC) resistance assay and is confirmed with a factor V Leiden genotypic mutation assay. Remember: **factor Vee**—check **APC.**

Hypercoagulable State (Thrombophilia)

A 28-year-old G2P1 at 28 weeks' gestation comes to a routine pregnancy check complaining of unilateral ankle swelling. You find her left leg to be > 2 cm larger in girth than her right, and ultrasound shows a noncompressible left popliteal vein. Which anticoagulant will you start, and for what duration?

Start low-molecular-weight heparin (LMWH), and continue until 24 hours prior to delivery (more easily done if you are inducing). Restart after delivery, and continue anticoagulation four weeks after pregnancy. Although a known teratogen, warfarin is considered safe for nursing mothers and is an option postpartum.

KEY FACT

Virchow's triad of factors allowing for venous thrombosis are vessel wall trauma, venous stasis, and alterations in coagulation.

A group of conditions that predispose patients to blood clotting. Common causes of thrombophilia include the following:

- **Inherited:** Includes factor V Leiden deficiency, prothrombin 20210 mutation, protein C or S deficiency, anti–thrombin III deficiency, homocystinemia, and fibrinolysis defects.
- **Acquired:** Associated with prolonged rest, immobilization, smoking, OCP use, pregnancy, nephrotic syndrome, cancer, DIC, and lupus anticoagulant.

Diagnosis

Two weeks after the completion of anticoagulation, look for possible 1° **causes of hypercoagulability** in the following patients:

- Those with a history of a first venous thrombotic event before age 50.
- Those with recurrent thrombotic episodes.
- Those who have had a thrombotic event as well as a first-degree relative who experienced a thromboembolic event before age 50.
- Screening should include APC resistance, prothrombin mutation, antiphospholipid antibody, plasma homocysteine, antithrombin deficiency, protein C deficiency, and protein S deficiency.

Treatment

- Acute thrombosis must be treated with at least six months of anticoagulation with warfarin.
- Indications for **lifelong warfarin use** include > 2 spontaneous thromboses, antithrombin deficiency, antiphospholipid syndrome, spontaneous life-threatening thrombosis, and thrombosis in an unusual site (eg, the mesenteric or cerebral vein).
- Warfarin takes 3–5 days to reach its therapeutic effect; can lead to serious skin necrosis in people with protein C deficiency; and can initially be thrombotic. Thus, bridge with heparin.
- Pregnant women with a history of hypercoagulable state need to be treated with LMWH.
- Homocystinemia can be treated with vitamin B_{12} and folate.

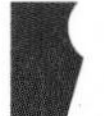

KEY FACT

Bridge the initiation of warfarin therapy with heparin for 3–5 days until INR rises to the therapeutic goal.

Transfusion

The complications of transfusion-related reactions are listed in Table 8-5.

TABLE 8-5. Transfusion Complications

	Clinical	Tests	Management
Major/minor hemolytic reaction	Chills, fever, SOB, nausea, chest/flank pain, hypotension, flushing. Complications: ARF (from hemoglobinuria), DIC.	⊕ Coombs' test, agglutination of RBC on smear, low haptoglobin (best test). UA for hemoglobinuria (⊕ urine dip for hematuria in the setting of few RBCs on microscopy).	Stop transfusion. Maintain BP and urine output with IV fluids; give patient furosemide (Lasix) if urine output is < 100 mL/hr. Type and cross RBCs just transfused.
Delayed hemolysis	Onset 4–14 days posttransfusion. Jaundice, anemia, hemoglobinuria, fever.	↑ LDH, unconjugated hyperbilirubinemia, ↓ haptoglobin.	Type and screen blood before future transfusions. Acetaminophen for fever.
Febrile, nonhemolytic reaction	Onset within two hours posttransfusion. Fever, rigors, nausea, vomiting, chills.	Rule out biochemical evidence of hemolysis.	For future transfusions, use leukocyte-reduced RBCs. Avoid transfusion when febrile.
Anaphylaxis	↑ risk in patients with congenital IgA deficiency. Sudden onset, flushing, hypertension followed by hypotension, edema, respiratory distress, shock, wheezing, chest pain.	None.	IV epinephrine. Use saline-washed packed RBCs in future RBC transfusions.
Urticaria	Rash, pruritus.		Stop transfusion; monitor for anaphylaxis. Give diphenhydramine (Benadryl). Resume transfusion at a slower rate when symptoms resolve.
Transfusion-related acute lung injury (TRALI)	Occurs 1–6 hours posttransfusion. Like ARDS of lung. Acute respiratory distress, cyanosis, fever; gone in 24 hours. DDx: Fluid overload.	CXR shows bilateral pulmonary infiltrates without CHF.	Ventilation (O_2, intubation), diuretics, steroids.
Bacterial infection	More likely with platelets. Fever, hypotension; onset within four hours.	Culture remaining blood product.	Antibiotics.

(Reproduced with permission from Le T et al. *First Aid for the USMLE Step 2,* 4th ed. New York: McGraw-Hill, 2003: 202.)

CHAPTER 9

ONCOLOGY

Hematologic Malignancies

LEUKEMIA

Defined as malignant proliferations of hematopoietic cells. Categorization is based on cellular origin (ie, myeloid or lymphoid) and on the level of differentiation.

- **Acute leukemia:** Proliferation of minimally differentiated cells (myeloblasts, lymphoblasts); defined as > 20% blasts in bone marrow (< 20% blasts is defined as myelodysplastic syndrome).
- **Chronic leukemia:** Proliferation of more mature differentiated cells (metamyelocytes/myelocytes, lymphocytes).

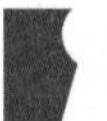

KEY FACT

Patients with Down syndrome have an ↑ risk of malignancy, especially leukemias.

Acute Lymphocytic Leukemia (ALL)

Most common in children; has an ↑ incidence in those with Down syndrome.

Symptoms/Exam

- The symptomatology can be explained by the infiltration of bone marrow and other tissues by malignant cells.
- Often presents as a **viral-like prodrome** of fever, sore throat, and lethargy.
- Children may present with limpness and refusal to walk together with **bone pain, easy bruising,** and **fever.**
- Exam may reveal pallor, widespread **petechiae/purpura,** multiple ecchymoses, and bleeding.
- Patients often have signs of **extramedullary spread** with adenopathy, **hepatosplenomegaly,** and testicular/CNS involvement.

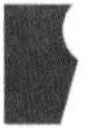

KEY FACT

Lymphadenopathy, splenomegaly, and CNS involvement are common in ALL but are rare in AML.

Diagnosis

- The leukocyte count may be ↑ or ↓. Look for ↓↓ platelets and ↑ **LDH and uric acid.**
- Peripheral blood smear shows a predominance of lymphoblasts.
- **Bone marrow biopsy** is necessary to confirm the diagnosis and is superior to blood for cytogenetic studies (CALLA ⊕, TdT ⊕).
- Obtain a CXR, an LP, and a CT scan to rule out mediastinal involvement and brain metastases.
- Cytogenetic tests are very important for obtaining key prognostic information.

KEY FACT

Recombinant human hematopoietic growth factors (G-CSF or GM-CSF) can be used to treat neutropenia.

Treatment

- Treat with **chemotherapy.**
- The prognosis is largely determined by age of onset and cytogenetic studies. Nearly all children achieve complete remission, and 80% achieve long-term leukemia-free survival. For adults, these numbers are lower.
- Phases of treatment and their objectives are as follows:
  - **Induction therapy: To induce remission (ie, to destroy all blasts).** Usually involves vincristine + prednisone + daunorubicin.
  - **Consolidation therapy: To kill any residual leukemia.** High-dose methotrexate is used.
  - **Maintenance therapy: To maintain remission.** Involves daily methotrexate, 6-mercaptopurine (6-MP), or both.

KEY FACT

Before initiating chemotherapy, administer allopurinol to patients with acute leukemia to prevent tumor lysis syndrome.

Acute Myelogenous Leukemia (AML)

Most cases occur in adults, with the incidence increasing with each decade of life.

SYMPTOMS/EXAM

- Similar to ALL, presenting with **fatigue, easy bruising, anemia,** fever, leukemia cutis (small, raised, painless skin lesions), and a history of **frequent infections.**
- May also present with **DIC, gingival hyperplasia,** or CNS involvement.
- Exam reveals fever, lethargy, bleeding, and **petechiae/purpura.**

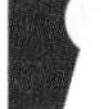

KEY FACT

AML is associated with exposure to smoking, benzene, radiation, and chemotherapeutic agents.

DIFFERENTIAL

Leukemoid reactions (ie, prominent leukocytosis) due to infection, stress, chronic inflammation, and certain neoplasms can result in WBC counts of 40,000–100,000 cells/μL but lack the cytogenetic changes and ↓ leukocyte alkaline phosphatase (LAP) seen with AML and CML.

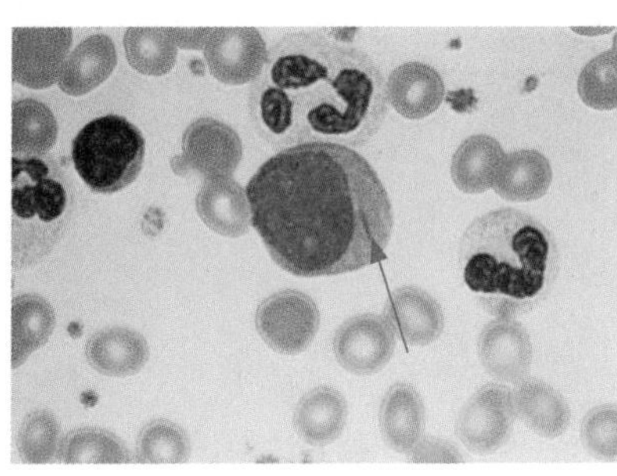

FIGURE 9-1. Leukemic myeloblast with an Auer rod. Note the large, prominent nucleoli. (Reproduced with permission from Fauci AS et al. *Harrison's Principles of Internal Medicine,* 17th ed. New York: McGraw-Hill, 2008, Fig. 104-1B.)

DIAGNOSIS

- In addition to ↑ myelocytic cell lines, there is ↓ **LAP. Hyperuricemia is often seen from ↑ cell turnover.**
- Peripheral blood smear shows a predominance of myeloblasts, distinguished by the presence of **Auer rods** (see Figure 9-1).
- **Bone marrow biopsy** is necessary to confirm the presence of blasts by ⊕ **myeloperoxidase staining,** Auer rods, and cytogenetic tests.

TREATMENT

- The prognosis depends on subtype, but generally 70–80% of adults < 60 years of age achieve complete remission.
- Treatment phases consist of induction (generally with cytosine arabinoside [Ara-C] + anthracycline) and consolidation chemotherapy. Exceptions are as follows:
  - **All-*trans*-retinoic acid** is used for induction and maintenance therapy for the promyelocytic form (AML M3).
  - Allogeneic **bone marrow transplantation (BMT)** is considered for patients with poor prognostic factors for long-term disease-free survival as well as for those < 60 years of age.

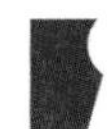

KEY FACT

Cytoplasmic Auer rods are diagnostic for AML.

Chronic Lymphocytic Leukemia (CLL)

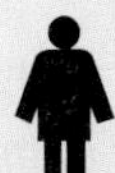

A 70-year-old man presents with fatigue. His physical exam is unrevealing, but a routine CBC reveals lymphocytosis with a normal hematocrit and platelet count. What is the next step in diagnosis?

Obtain a peripheral smear.

Malignancy of mature lymphocytes, typically seen in patients > 65 years of age.

SYMPTOMS/EXAM

- Usually an **indolent disease;** many patients are diagnosed by the incidental finding of lymphocytosis.
- **Lymphadenopathy,** fatigue, and hepatosplenomegaly may be present on exam.

Diagnosis

- **Isolated lymphocytosis** with a normal hematocrit and platelet count is seen on CBC.
- Peripheral blood smear shows a predominance of small lymphocytes.
- Bone marrow biopsy is necessary for confirmation (infiltrated with lymphocytes). Aberrant **CD5+** expression (T-cell marker) is characteristic, and **smudge cells** may be present on peripheral smear.

KEY FACT

Although symptomatic CLL does not require treatment, it may transform to intermediate- or high-grade lymphoma (Richter's transformation) or may be complicated by autoimmune hemolytic anemia, which requires splenectomy +/– steroids.

Treatment

- **No treatment is indicated for asymptomatic patients.**
- Anemia and thrombocytopenia are associated with ↓ survival and are treated symptomatically or with fludarabine.
- CLL may be associated with autoimmune hemolytic anemia and immune thrombocytopenia, which are treated with splenectomy and/or steroids.

Chronic Myelogenous Leukemia (CML)

Malignancy of myeloid cells that is seen in middle-aged adults. CML can occur de novo or may result from other myeloproliferative disorders. It is often stable for several years (chronic phase) and then transforms into an acute leukemia (**blast crisis**) that typically proves fatal within a few months. CML is associated with prior radiation and benzene exposure.

Symptoms/Exam

- CML is typically diagnosed on a routine CBC that demonstrates **leukocytosis** with myeloid precursors.
- Patients may have mild, nonspecific symptoms such as **fatigue, fever, malaise,** ↓ exercise tolerance, weight loss, and night sweats.
- **Blast crisis** presents as fever, bone pain, weight loss, and **splenomegaly.**

Differential

Hairy cell leukemia can be another cause of pancytopenia in the elderly. It is a malignancy of B lymphocytes that is characterized by cells with hairy cytoplasmic projections and **CD11c positivity.** In addition to aplastic anemia and myelofibrosis, it is a common cause of a "dry bone marrow tap."

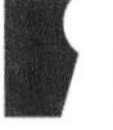

KEY FACT

The Philadelphia chromosome is pathognomonic for CML and forms the target of imatinib (Gleevec), the new first-line therapy for CML.

Diagnosis

- Peripheral smear reveals an ↑↑ WBC count (median of 150,000 cells/μL at the time of diagnosis) and prominent myeloid cells with basophilia.
- Also seen are ↓ **LAP** and ↑↑ B_{12} levels.
- Confirm the diagnosis through detection of the **t(9;22) Philadelphia chromosome bcr-abl gene** by karyotyping, PCR, or fluorescence in situ hybridization (FISH) analysis of blood or bone marrow aspirate.

Treatment

- **Imatinib mesylate (Gleevec), currently the first-line therapy for CML,** specifically targets and inhibits **bcr-abl** tyrosine kinase and eliminates the CML clone, leading to rapid hematologic and cytogenetic remission.
- **Allogeneic BMT,** if performed while the patient is in the **chronic phase** (within one year of diagnosis), may result in long-term survival. Although the best results are achieved in patients < 40 years of age, treatment can be complicated by graft-versus-host disease.

LYMPHOMA

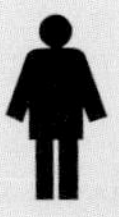

A 30-year-old man presents with a temperature of 38.7°C (101.7°F), drenching night sweats, and weight loss of six months' duration. Physical exam reveals cervical lymphadenopathy. What is the next step in diagnosis?

Lymph node biopsy.

Lymphomas result from monoclonal proliferation of cells of lymphocyte lineage. Approximately 90% are derived from B cells, 9% from T cells, and 1% from monocytes or natural killer (NK) cells.

Hodgkin's Lymphoma

Malignancy of neoplastic Reed-Sternberg (RS) cells (see Figure 9-2), which are of B-cell origin. EBV infections play a role in the pathogenesis of this disease. Usually affects young adults.

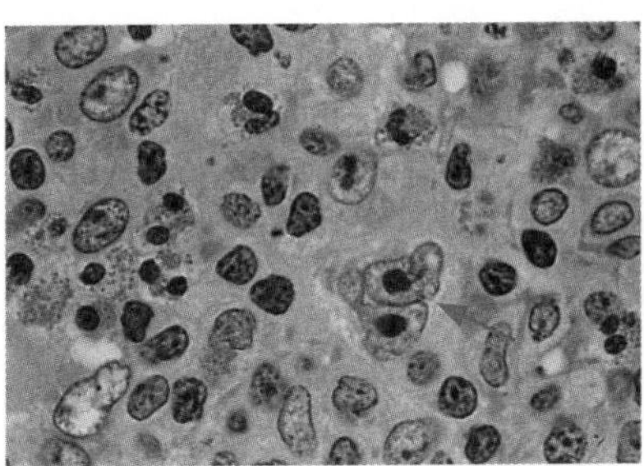

FIGURE 9-2. Hodgkin's lymphoma. A Reed-Sternberg cell—a large cell with a bilobed nucleus and prominent nucleoli, giving an "owl's eye" appearance—can be seen near the center of the image (arrow). (Reproduced with permission from Fauci AS et al. *Harrison's Principles of Internal Medicine,* 17th ed. New York: McGraw-Hill, 2008, Fig. 105-11.)

Symptoms/Exam

- Usually presents with cervical lymphadenopathy and spreads in a predictable manner along the lymph nodes. The spleen is the most commonly involved intra-abdominal site.
- "B symptoms" are defined as **10% weight loss in six months, night sweats requiring a change of clothes, and fever > 38.5°C (101.3°F).** These symptoms indicate bulky disease and a worse prognosis.

Diagnosis

- Diagnosis is usually based on biopsy of an enlarged lymph node that demonstrates the presence of RS cells.
- Staging is predicated on the anatomically based **Ann Arbor system** and on the presence of prognostic factors. Chest and abdominal/pelvic CT as well as bilateral bone marrow biopsies and aspirates are routine.

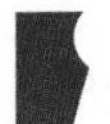

KEY FACT

EBV is a common cause of aggressive lymphoma in patients with immune deficiencies.

Treatment

Treat with chemotherapy consisting of doxorubicin, bleomycin, vinblastine, and dacarbazine (**ABVD cocktail**) with or without radiation of the involved field.

Non-Hodgkin's Lymphoma (NHL)

Classified as low, intermediate, or high grade on the basis of histologic type. Associated with infections—EBV with Burkitt's lymphoma; HIV with CNS lymphoma; HTLV with T-cell lymphoma; and *H pylori* with gastric MALToma.

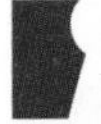

KEY FACT

Reed-Sternberg cells ("owl's eye" nuclei) are pathognomonic for Hodgkin's lymphoma.

Symptoms

Symptoms are similar to that of other lymphomas, including B symptoms.

Diagnosis

Diagnosis is similar to that of other lymphomas. LDH is a prognostic marker.

TREATMENT

- Treat with chemotherapy consisting of cyclophosphamide, hydroxydoxorubicin, vincristine, and prednisone (**CHOP** therapy).
- The addition of **rituximab** (monoclonal anti-CD20) to the chemotherapeutic regimen improves outcomes **(R-CHOP).**
- The treatment of **high-grade NHL** may be complicated by **tumor lysis syndrome,** which consists of **hyperkalemia, hyperphosphatemia, hyperuricemia, and hypocalcemia. Treat with aggressive hydration and allopurinol.**
- Gastric MALTomas can be treated with antibiotics for *H pylori* as initial therapy.
- All HIV-related NHL requires immediate institution of antiretroviral therapy (HAART).

KEY FACT

Treatment of lymphoma:

- Hodgkin's—think **ABVD** cocktail.
- Non-Hodgkin's—think **CHOP/ R-CHOP.**

MULTIPLE MYELOMA

A 65-year-old woman presents with back pain and fatigue. Routine lab testing reveals anemia and renal failure. A diagnosis of multiple myeloma is suspected. What is the next step in management?

Testing for serum protein electrophoresis (SPEP) and urine protein electrophoresis (UPEP).

A malignancy of **plasma cells** within bone marrow, often with unbalanced, excessive production of immunoglobulin heavy/light chains. Typically seen in **older adults.**

SYMPTOMS/EXAM

- Symptoms include **back pain** (the presenting symptom in 80% of patients), **hypercalcemic symptoms** ("stones, bones, abdominal moans, and psychiatric overtones"), **pathologic fractures,** fatigue, and frequent infections (2° to dysregulation of antibody production).
- Exam may reveal pallor, fever, bone tenderness, and lethargy.

DIFFERENTIAL

Waldenström's macroglobulinemia is a plasma cell disorder that is similar to multiple myeloma but has a predominance of IgM as well as a higher incidence of cold agglutinins and hyperviscosity syndrome (visual disturbance, dizziness, headache). The latter is treated with urgent plasmapheresis.

DIAGNOSIS

- Critical tests to evaluate for the presence of multiple myeloma (and to distinguish it from Waldenström's) include **UPEP** (to examine for **Bence Jones protein**) **and SPEP** (to look for monoclonal immunoglobulin, most commonly **IgG, > 3 g/dL**).
- **Bone marrow aspirate** can enumerate **plasma cells** (> **10%**), and a **full-body skeletal survey** can demonstrate **punched-out osteolytic lesions** of the skull and long bones (see Figure 9-3).
- LAP levels are normal (lesions are osteolytic, not osteoblastic).

KEY FACT

Plain radiographs of the axial skeleton show the characteristic lytic lesions of multiple myeloma. Bone scans are not helpful, since they show blastic activity.

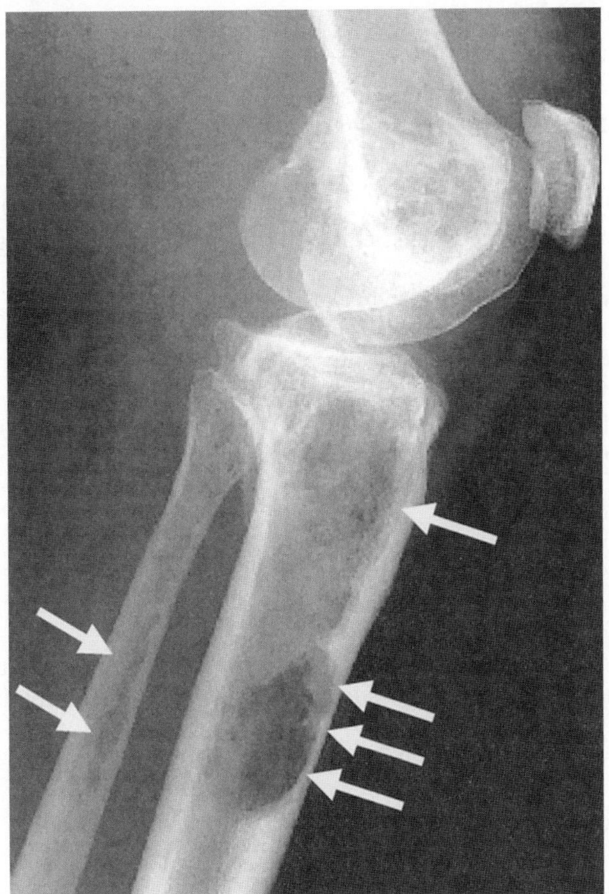

FIGURE 9-3. Multiple myeloma. Lateral view of the tibia and fibula shows the typical radiographic appearance of focal lytic lesions resulting from multiple myeloma (arrows). (Reproduced with permission from Lichtman MA et al. *Williams Hematology,* 7th ed. New York: McGraw-Hill, 2006, Fig. 100-10A.)

TREATMENT

- Treatment is aimed at reducing tumor burden, relieving symptoms, and preventing complications. β-microglobulin is a prognostic marker.
- **Chemotherapy involves use of melphalan and steroids** +/– **thalidomide or bortezomib. Autologous stem cell transplantation** is used for patients who are < 60 years of age and in advanced stages of disease.
- Treatment measures aimed at alleviating symptoms or preventing complications include the following:
  - **Hypercalcemia:** Treat with hydration, glucocorticoids, and diuresis.
  - **Bone pain/destruction/fractures:** Treat with bisphosphonates and local radiation.
  - **Renal failure:** Give hydration to aid in the excretion of light-chain immunoglobulins.
  - **Infections:** Vaccinate against preventable infections; diagnose early and treat aggressively.
  - **Anemia:** Administer erythropoietin.

Breast Cancer

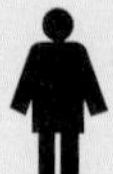

A 62-year-old woman presents with a suspicious breast mass. Mammography reveals clusters of microcalcifications and stellate lesions. A biopsy confirms invasive cancer. What is the next step in management?

Testing for estrogen and progesterone receptor status and HER2/neu status.

The most common cancer and the second most common cause of cancer death in women in the United States (after lung cancer). Routine annual or biennial mammography is recommended after age 50 (or earlier for high-risk cases and patients with a family history of breast cancer). Routine mammography for those who are 40–50 years of age and are not at high risk is controversial. Risk factors include the following:

- Female gender.
- Older age.
- Breast cancer in first-degree relatives.
- A prior history of breast cancer.
- A history of atypical ductal or lobular hyperplasia or carcinoma in situ.
- Early menarche, early menopause, or late first full-term pregnancy (before age 35).
- HRT use for > 5 years.
- Obesity.
- Prior radiation (eg, for treatment of Hodgkin's lymphoma).

KEY FACT

Women should be tested for BRCA-1 and BRCA-2 mutations if they have a "genetic" risk—ie, a strong family history of breast and/or ovarian cancer.

Symptoms/Exam

- Most masses are discovered by the patient and present as a **hard, irregular, immobile, painless breast lump,** possibly with nipple discharge.
- **Skin changes** (dimpling, erythema, ulceration) and **axillary adenopathy** indicate more advanced disease.
- Any breast mass in postmenopausal women is breast cancer until proven otherwise. The most common location is the **upper outer quadrant.**

Diagnosis

- The diagnosis is suggested by a palpable mass or by **mammographic abnormalities** (eg, microcalcifications, hyperdense regions, irregular borders) and is confirmed by biopsy.
- In clinically suspicious cases involving patients > 35 years of age with any breast lump, a ⊖ mammogram should be followed by **ultrasound** (to look for cysts vs. solid masses), **FNA** (for palpable lumps), **stereotactic** core biopsy (for nonpalpable lesions), or **excisional biopsy** until convincing evidence has been gathered to support the absence of cancer.
- In clinically suspicious cases involving patients < 35 years of age and those with dense breasts, the initial workup should also include ultrasound. Be wary of biopsying lesions too early; sometimes the correct course of action is to watch and observe. A mass that fluctuates with menstruation is likely benign in this age group.
- Biopsied specimens should be tested for prognostic factors such as estrogen/progesterone receptors (**ER/PR**) and **HER2.**

- Special forms of breast cancer include the following:
  - **Inflammatory breast cancer:** A highly aggressive, rapidly growing cancer that invades the lymphatics and causes skin inflammation (ie, mastitis). Has a poor prognosis.
  - **Paget's disease:** Ductal carcinoma in situ (DCIS) of the nipple with unilateral itching, burning, and nipple erosion. May be mistaken for infection; associated with a focus of invasive carcinoma.

KEY FACT

The sensitivity of mammography for breast cancer is 75–80%, so do not stop workup with a ⊖ mammogram in clinically suspicious cases.

Treatment

- **Intraductal carcinoma (DCIS):** Warrants **only local therapy** (either mastectomy or wide excision plus radiation therapy).
- **Lobular carcinoma in situ (LCIS):** Associated with a high risk (up to 20%) of developing a subsequent infiltrating breast cancer, including cancer in the contralateral breast. Therapy options include close monitoring, mastectomy, or the use of tamoxifen for prophylaxis.
- **Invasive cancer:** The choice of treatment for invasive breast cancer is based on **lymph node status, tumor size,** and **hormone receptor status:**
  - Those with **node-⊖ disease** (stage I) can be treated with **breast conservation therapy** (wide tumor excision) or **modified radical mastectomy with radiation therapy.**
  - **Adjuvant chemotherapy** (two or more agents such as 5-FU, methotrexate, doxorubicin, cyclophosphamide, or epirubicin for 3–6 months) is usually given for **tumors > 2 cm or those with axillary lymph node involvement (stages II–III).**
  - **Endocrine** therapy such as tamoxifen, raloxifene, or aromatase inhibitors (anastrozole) is beneficial only for patients with **ER-⊕** or **PR-⊕ tumors.**
  - Trastuzumab (Herceptin) is beneficial for those with HER2-neu-⊕ tumors.

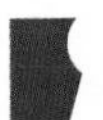

KEY FACT

ER/PR-⊕ status is a good prognostic indicator in breast cancer, and such patients should be treated with hormonal therapy.

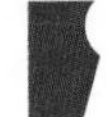

KEY FACT

Breast conservation therapy is generally as effective as modified radical mastectomy in patients with a unifocal tumor size of < 4 cm.

Lung Cancer

Once a diagnosis of lung cancer is suspected, which imaging studies can aid in the completion of staging?

Chest and abdominal CT with contrast, bone scan, and CT or MRI of the head.

The **leading cause of cancer death.** The major risk factor is **tobacco** use. Other risk factors include radon and asbestos exposure. Subtypes are described in Table 9-1.

Symptoms/Exam

- In some cases, an asymptomatic lesion is discovered incidentally on either CXR or chest CT (see Figure 9-4).
- Most patients develop signs that herald a problem—eg, chronic **cough, hemoptysis, weight loss, or postobstructive pneumonia.**
- Less frequently, patients may present late with **complications of a large tumor burden:**
  - **Pancoast's syndrome:** Presents with shoulder pain, Horner's syndrome (miosis, ptosis, anhidrosis), and lower brachial plexopathy.

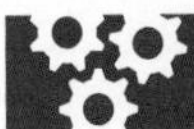

MNEMONIC

The 3 C's of squamous cell carcinoma of the lung:

Central
Cavitary
Hyper**C**alcemia

TABLE 9-1. Classification of Lung Cancers

SUBTYPE	CHARACTERISTICS	TREATMENT
Small cell lung cancer (SCLC)	Highly related to **cigarette exposure.** Usually **centrally** located and always presumed to be **disseminated** at the time of diagnosis.	**Chemotherapy** is the treatment of choice.
Non–small cell lung cancer (NSCLC)	**Adenocarcinoma:** The most common lung cancer; has a **peripheral** location. More common in women than in men. **Adenocarcinoma, bronchoalveolar subtype:** Associated with multiple nodules, bilateral lung infiltrates, and metastases late in the disease course. **Squamous cell carcinoma:** Presents **centrally** and is **usually cavitary.** **Large cell carcinoma:** Least common.	**Potentially curable with resection of localized disease, but only modestly responsive to chemotherapy.** Patients are classified into one of three clinical groups at the time of diagnosis: ▪ **Stages I and II:** Early-stage disease. Represents candidacy for surgical resection. ▪ **Locally or regionally advanced disease** (supraclavicular or mediastinal lymphadenopathy or chest wall/pleural/pericardial invasion): Treated with combination chemotherapy and radiation; surgery is not indicated. ▪ **Distant metastases:** The goal of any chemotherapy or radiation is **palliation only.**

- **Superior vena cava syndrome:** Characterized by swelling of the face and arm, most often on the right side, and elevated JVP. Treated with radiation therapy.
- **Hoarseness:** Vocal cord paralysis from entrapment of the recurrent laryngeal nerve, most often on the left.

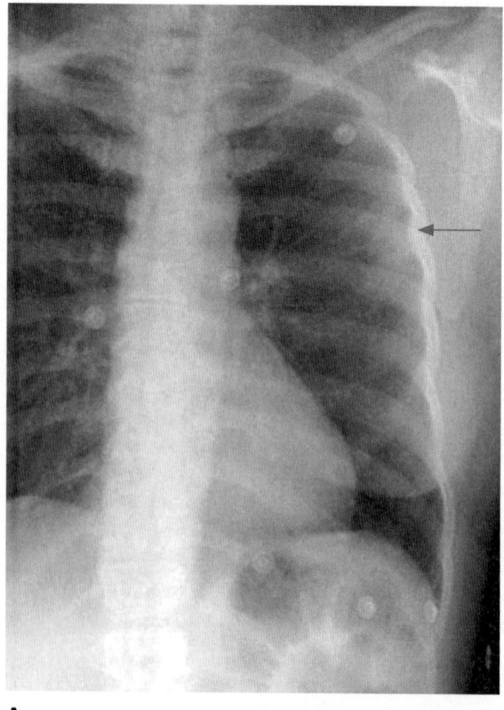

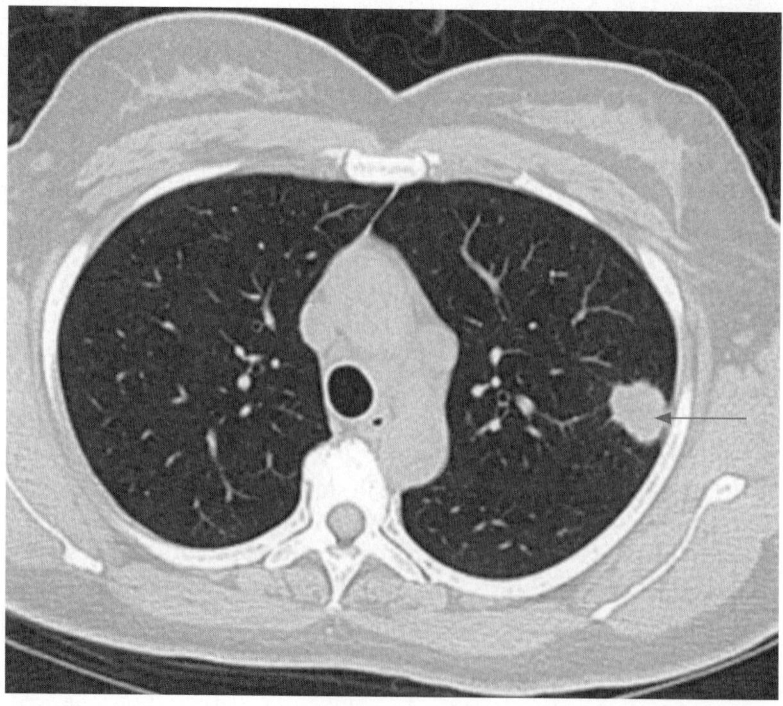

FIGURE 9-4. Lung cancer. Lung cancer (arrows) on (A) frontal CXR and (B) transaxial CT. (Reproduced with permission from USMLERx.com.)

- **Hypercalcemia:** Most often seen with squamous cell carcinoma. Treat with bisphosphonates.
- **Hyponatremia/SIADH:** Small cell carcinoma.
- **Lambert-Eaton syndrome: Similar to myasthenia gravis,** except that **muscle fatigue improves with repeated stimulation** (vs. myasthenia gravis, in which such measures yield no improvement).

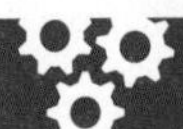

MNEMONIC

Paraneoplastic syndromes–

CLASH

Carcinoid
Lambert-Eaton syndrome
ACTH
SIADH
Hypercalcemia

Differential

- Other common causes of lung masses include TB/other granulomatous diseases, fungal disease (aspergillosis, histoplasmosis), lung abscess, metastasis, benign tumors (bronchial adenoma), and hamartoma.
- Serial CXRs are useful for distinguishing benign lesions from malignant ones. Lesions that remain stable over > 2 years are generally not cancerous. Other features suggestive of benign lesions include young age, smooth margins, small size (< 2 cm), and the presence of satellite lesions. However, any lung nodule in a smoker or an ex-smoker should be evaluated for the presence of cancer.

Diagnosis

- If there is a palpable lymph node (axillary, supraclavicular), consider biopsy of the node first. If not, order a CXR initially, and in doubtful/suspicious cases, obtain a **chest CT and, if needed, bronchoscopy.**
- If mediastinal lymph nodes are enlarged, consider a PET scan and mediastinoscopy for proper staging.
- **Centrally** located cancers can be diagnosed by **bronchoscopy** or **sputum cytology.**
- **Staging** includes chest and abdominal CT with contrast, bone scan, and CT or MRI of the head.

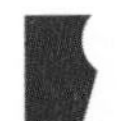

KEY FACT

All supraclavicular lymph nodes should be biopsied.

Treatment

See Table 9-1.

GI Tumors

PANCREATIC CANCER

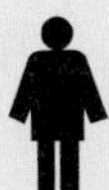

A 60-year-old woman presents with painless obstructive jaundice and weight loss. What is the most likely location of the obstructing mass?

The pancreatic head.

Typically seen in patients > 50 years of age. **Ductal adenocarcinoma** accounts for 90% of 1° tumors; > 50% arise in the head of the pancreas. Risk factors include smoking, chronic pancreatitis, and diabetes mellitus (DM). **Trousseau's syndrome,** a hypercoagulable state seen with adenocarcinoma, was first described in association with pancreatic cancer.

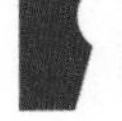

KEY FACT

Painless jaundice and/or a palpable gallbladder—think pancreatic cancer.

Symptoms/Exam

Common symptoms include **nausea, anorexia, lumbar back pain, new-onset DM, venous thromboembolism,** and **painless obstructive jaundice** (associated with adenocarcinoma in the **head** of the pancreas).

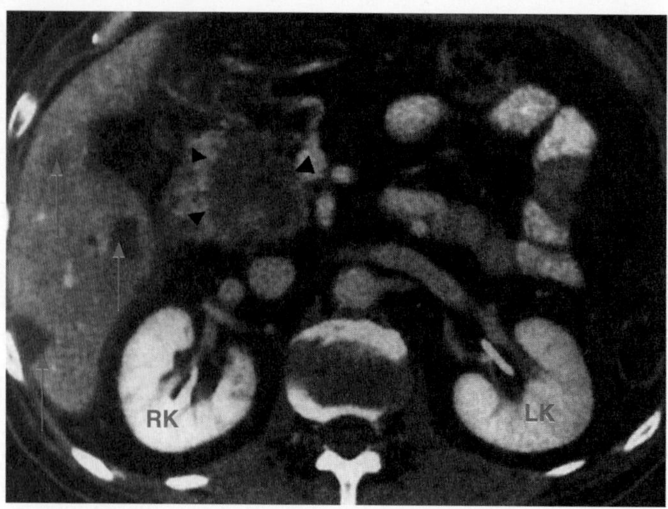

FIGURE 9-5. Pancreatic adenocarcinoma. Transaxial contrast-enhanced CT shows a mass in the head of the pancreas (arrowheads) and multiple liver metastases (arrows). RK = right kidney; LK = left kidney. (Reproduced with permission from Chen MY et al. *Basic Radiology.* New York: McGraw-Hill, 2004, Fig. 11-72.)

DIAGNOSIS

- Characterized by ↑ bilirubin, ↑ aminotransferases, and normocytic normochromic anemia.
- **Ultrasound** is useful as an initial diagnostic test. Abdominal/pelvic CT can evaluate the extent of disease; a **thin-section helical CT** through the pancreas (see Figure 9-5) can determine if the mass is resectable.
- **Endoscopic ultrasonography** yields excellent anatomic detail and can help confirm if the tumor is resectable.

TREATMENT

- **Pancreaticoduodenectomy** (Whipple procedure) is appropriate for patients with resectable tumors.
- **Chemotherapy** or **radiation** is used for **palliative care** in patients with advanced or unresectable disease.

HEPATOCELLULAR CANCER (HEPATOMA)

Risk factors for hepatocellular cancer (HCC) include viral hepatitis (HBV, HCV), alcoholic cirrhosis, aflatoxin, hemochromatosis, and α_1-antitrypsin deficiency. OCPs are associated with benign hepatic adenoma (vs. HCC).

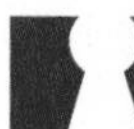
KEY FACT

2° liver tumors (metastases) are more common than 1° liver tumors.

SYMPTOMS/EXAM

Presents with abdominal discomfort together with laboratory abnormalities (↑ aminotransferases, ↑ bilirubin, coagulopathy) that warrant abdominal imaging (see Figure 9-6).

TREATMENT

- Surgical resection and liver transplantation can yield long-term survival.
- Alternatives for unresectable tumors include percutaneous alcohol injections, arterial chemoembolization, radiofrequency ablation, and chemotherapeutic agents such as sorafenib.

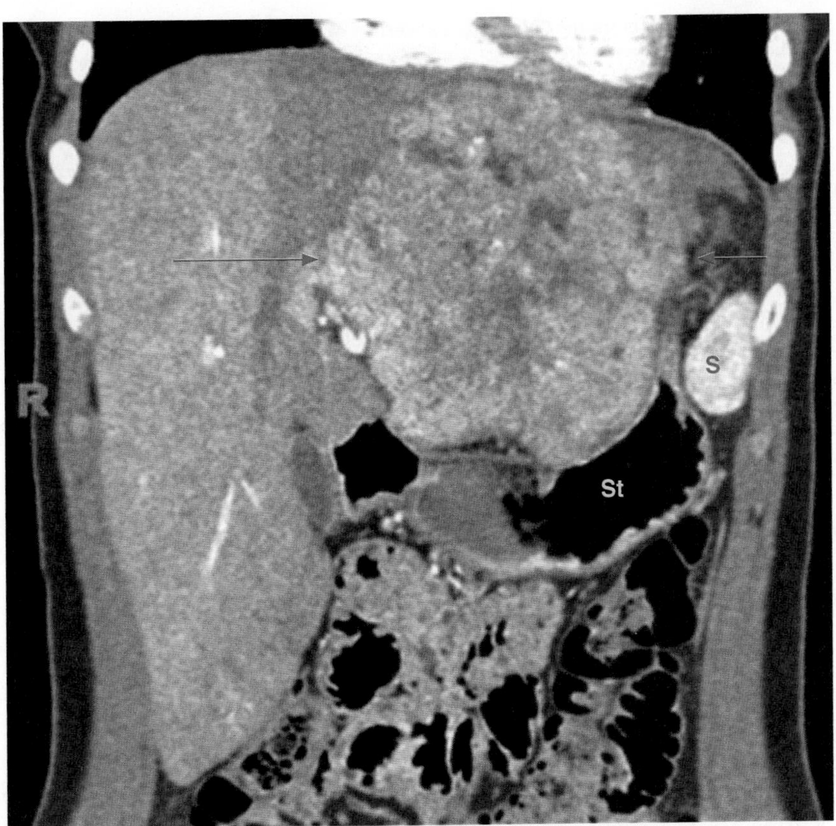

FIGURE 9-6. Hepatocellular carcinoma. Coronal reformation from a contrast-enhanced CT shows a large HCC in the left hepatic lobe (arrows). St = stomach; S = spleen. (Reproduced with permission from USMLERx.com.)

COLORECTAL CANCER

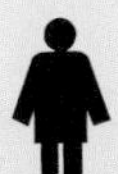

A 60-year-old man with a known diagnosis of colon cancer in remission is found to have a CEA level that is ↑ from baseline. What does this indicate?

Cancer recurrence.

Most cases occur after age 50. Suspect hereditary nonpolyposis colorectal cancer (HNPCC) in a younger person with colon cancer and a family history of colon, ovarian, and endometrial cancer. Table 9-2 discusses risk factors. Screen all asymptomatic individuals > 50 years of age with annual fecal occult blood testing (FOBT) and flexible sigmoidoscopy every 5 years, or with colonoscopy every 10 years.

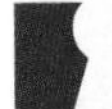

KEY FACT

If there is a family history of polyps or colorectal cancer, start screening when the patient is 10 years younger than the age of the affected relative at the time of diagnosis.

Symptoms/Exam

Symptoms depend on the site of the 1° tumor and may include a change in bowel habits, melena, bright red blood per rectum, weight loss, fatigue, vomiting, and abdominal discomfort.

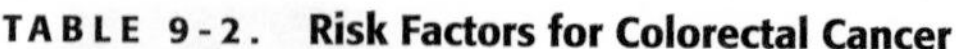

TABLE 9-2. Risk Factors for Colorectal Cancer

		Family History	
Patient Age	Personal History	Colorectal Cancer or Adenomatous Polyps	Hereditary Colorectal Cancer Syndromes
> 50 years	Previous colorectal cancer Adenomatous polyps IBD, particularly ulcerative colitis	One first-degree relative < 60 years of age or two first-degree relatives of any age	Familial adenomatous polyposis (FAP) HNPCC Hamartomatous polyposis syndromes

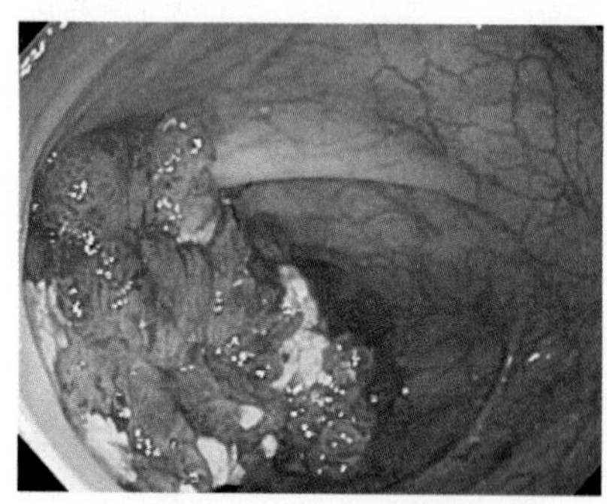

FIGURE 9-7. Colon cancer. Colonoscopy reveals an adenocarcinoma growing into the lumen of the colon. (Reproduced with permission from Fauci AS et al. *Harrison's Principles of Internal Medicine,* 17th ed. New York: McGraw-Hill, 2008, Fig. 285-6.)

Diagnosis

- Diagnosed by a mass palpated by DRE or detected by FOBT.
- Iron-deficiency anemia or ↑ transaminases may be seen.
- Confirm the diagnosis via colonoscopy and biopsy in suspected cases (see Figure 9-7).

Treatment

- Treatment decisions are influenced by tumor stage at diagnosis. 1° surgical resection involves resection of the bowel segment with adjacent mesentery and regional lymph nodes. Solitary liver/lung metastases can be resected.
- Stage I patients have an excellent prognosis with surgery alone (90% survival at five years).
- **Adjuvant chemotherapy (5-FU based)** is warranted for patients at stage III and above.

MNEMONIC

Esophageal cancer risk factors—

ABCDEF

Achalasia
Barrett's esophagus
Corrosive esophagitis
Diverticulitis
Esophageal web
Familial

MISCELLANEOUS GI TUMORS

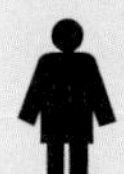

A 65-year-old man with a history of GERD presents with a 10-lb weight loss, dysphagia, and epigastric pain. What will biopsy results from EGD most likely reveal?

Esophageal adenocarcinoma.

Esophageal Tumors

- **Sx/Exam:** The classic symptom is **dysphagia in the elderly,** especially in smokers and alcoholics; tumors are usually squamous in nature. Esophageal adenocarcinoma can arise from long-standing esophageal reflux with Barrett's disease.
- **Dx:** Confirm the diagnosis by EGD with biopsy (see Figure 9-8).
- **Tx:** Treatment involves resection for localized disease and radiation therapy with chemotherapy for advanced disease.

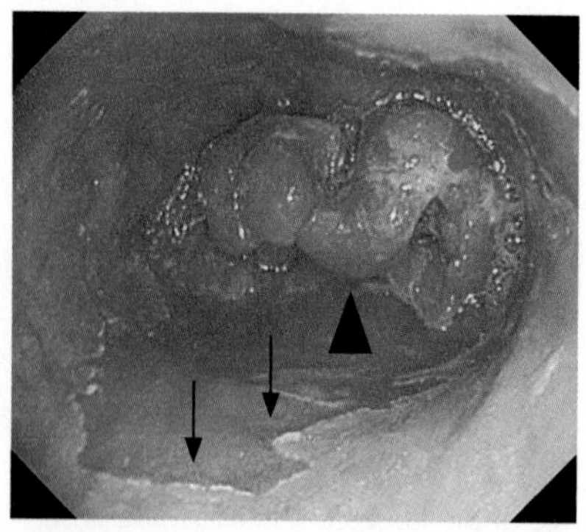

FIGURE 9-8. Esophageal cancer. An esophageal adenocarcinoma (arrowhead) is seen on endoscopy against a background of the pink tongues of Barrett's esophagus (arrows). (Reproduced with permission from Fauci AS et al. *Harrison's Principles of Internal Medicine,* 17th ed. New York: McGraw-Hill, 2008, Fig. 285-3D.)

Gastric Tumors

- More common among those of Asian ethnicity.
- **Sx/Exam:** Classically presents as **iron-deficiency anemia with vague abdominal pain in the elderly.**

- **Dx:** Confirm the diagnosis via EGD with biopsy (see Figure 9-9).
- **Tx:** Treatment involves resection for localized disease and radiation therapy with chemotherapy for advanced disease.

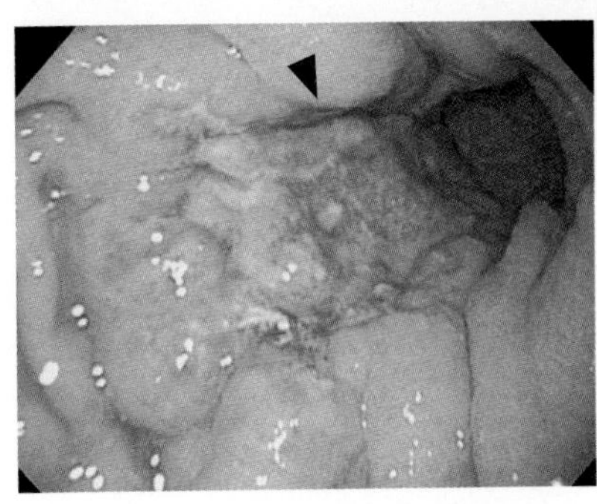

FIGURE 9-9. Gastric cancer. A malignant gastric ulcer (arrowhead) involving the greater curvature of the stomach is seen on endoscopy. (Reproduced with permission from Fauci AS et al. *Harrison's Principles of Internal Medicine,* 17th ed. New York: McGraw-Hill, 2008, Fig. 285-2B.)

Carcinoid Tumors

- Usually occur in the appendix or small bowel.
- **Sx/Exam:** Clinical features include flushing, abdominal pain, diarrhea, and tricuspid regurgitation (carcinoid syndrome).
- **Dx:** Diagnosed by **elevated levels of 5-HIAA** or chromogranin A.
- **Tx:** Surgical resection is curative in localized disease. Consider **octreotide for symptomatic control.**

Islet Cell Tumors

- **Sx/Exam:** Presentation depends on tumor type.
  - **Insulinoma (elevated proinsulin, C-peptide, and insulin levels):** Should be suspected with a triad consisting of hypoglycemic symptoms, a fasting blood glucose level of < 40 mg/dL, and immediate relief with glucose administration.
  - **VIPoma (elevated VIP levels):** Suspect in the setting of profuse watery diarrhea that causes hypokalemia.
  - **Glucagonoma (elevated glucagon levels):** Characterized by persistent hyperglycemia with necrolytic erythema (intertriginous and perioral rash).
- **Dx:** Islet cell tumors and their metastases (liver is most common) can be localized by somatostatin receptor scintigraphy.
- **Tx:** Options vary according to tumor type. Treatment includes surgical resection, debulking, chemotherapy, and somatostatin analogs with glucagonomas and VIPomas.

Genitourinary Tumors

BLADDER CANCER

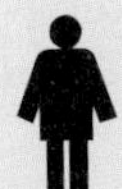

A 60-year-old man with a 35-pack-year smoking history presents with pink-colored urine. UA reveals macrohematuria. CT urogram reveals no abnormalities of the kidneys or ureters. What is the diagnostic test of choice?

Cystoscopy with possible biopsy.

The **most common** malignant tumor of the urinary tract; usually **transitional cell carcinoma.** Risk factors include **smoking,** exposure to aniline (rubber) dyes, and chronic bladder infections (eg, **schistosomiasis**).

Symptoms/Exam

Gross hematuria is the most common presenting symptom. Other urinary symptoms, such as frequency, urgency, and dysuria, may also be seen.

DIAGNOSIS

- **UA** is the most basic diagnostic modality and often shows hematuria (macro- or microscopic). Lack of dysmorphic RBCs helps distinguish this from glomerular bleeding. Cytology may show dysplastic cells (a first-morning specimen is best).
- **CT urography** or **IVP** can examine the upper urinary tract as well as defects in bladder filling.
- **Cystoscopy with biopsy is diagnostic.**

TREATMENT

Treatment depends on the extent of spread beyond the bladder mucosa.

- **Carcinoma in situ:** Intravesicular chemotherapy.
- **Invasive cancers without metastases:** Aggressive surgery, radiation therapy, or both.
- **Distant metastases:** Chemotherapy alone.

PROSTATE CANCER

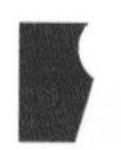

KEY FACT

Incidental asymptomatic prostate cancer is especially common among men > 80 years of age and does not always need treatment.

The most common cancer in men. Ninety-five percent are adenocarcinomas. Risk ↑ linearly with age.

SYMPTOMS/EXAM

- Many patients are asymptomatic and are incidentally diagnosed either by **DRE** or by a **PSA** level that is obtained for screening purposes.
- If symptomatic, patients may present with **urinary urgency/frequency/hesitancy** and, in late or aggressive disease, with anemia, hematuria, or low back pain.
- Screening with **DRE** or **PSA** should be done in patients > 50 years of age with > 10 years of life expectancy; it is not routinely recommended in patients > 75 years of age.

DIAGNOSIS

- Ultrasound-guided needle biopsy of the prostate allows for both diagnosis and staging.
- The **Gleason score (2–10)** remains the best predictor of tumor biology. It sums the scores of the two most dysplastic biopsy samples on a scale of 1–5 (well differentiated to poorly differentiated).

TREATMENT

- Treatment choice is based on the aggressiveness of the tumor and on the patient's risk of dying from the disease.
- **Watchful waiting** may be the best approach for elderly patients with low Gleason scores.
- Consider **radical prostatectomy** or **radiation therapy** (eg, brachytherapy or external beam) for node-⊖ disease. Treatment is associated with an ↑ risk of incontinence and/or impotence.
- Treat node-⊕ and metastatic disease with **androgen ablation** (eg, GnRH agonists, orchiectomy, flutamide) +/– chemotherapy.

TESTICULAR CANCER

The most common solid malignant tumor in men 20–35 years of age. It is highly treatable and often curable. Risk factors include **cryptorchid testis** and Klinefelter's syndrome. Ninety-five percent are germ cell tumors.

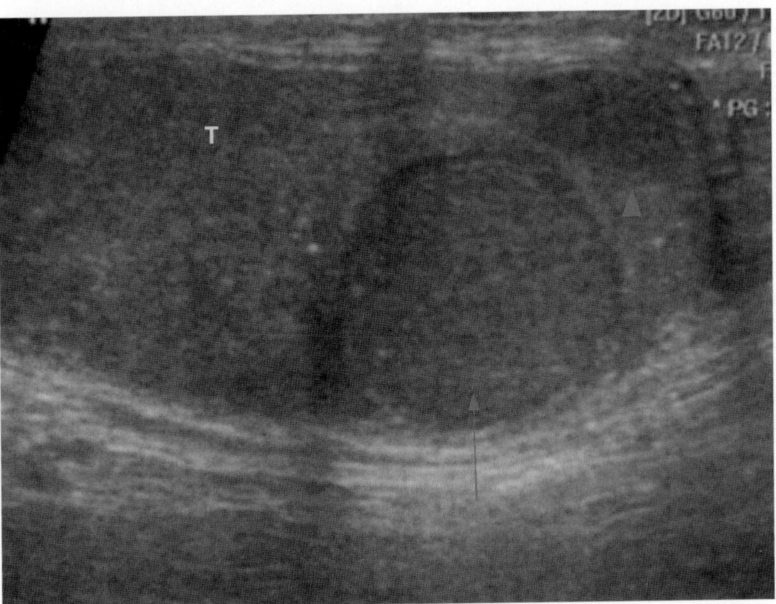

FIGURE 9-10. Seminoma. Longitudinal ultrasound image of testicle (T) shows a homogeneous intratesticular mass (arrow) and an additional smaller focus of tumor (arrowhead). (Reproduced with permission from USMLERx.com.)

Symptoms/Exam

- A **unilateral scrotal mass is testicular cancer until proven otherwise.**
- Other presentations include testicular discomfort or swelling suggestive of orchitis or epididymitis.

Diagnosis

- Serum levels of **α-fetoprotein (AFP), LDH,** and **β-hCG** should be measured.
- Scrotal ultrasound is also a useful means of differentiating cancer from non-neoplastic lesions (eg, hydrocele, spermatocele, infection) (see Figure 9-10).
- Definitive diagnosis is made by radical inguinal orchiectomy.
- Staging evaluation (TNM is widely used) should include serum LDH, AFP, β-hCG, and CT of the chest/abdomen and pelvis.

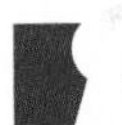

KEY FACT

Do not do a scrotal biopsy to diagnose testicular cancer, as this may result in seeding of the biopsy tract.

Treatment

Radical inguinal orchiectomy +/– **chemotherapy/radiation therapy** is the treatment of choice.

RENAL CELL CARCINOMA

The most common cause of kidney cancer in adults. The cause is unknown, but risk factors include **cigarette smoking,** von Hippel–Lindau disease, tuberous sclerosis, and cystic kidney disease.

Symptoms/Exam

- Generally asymptomatic in the early stages, but symptoms can include hematuria, flank pain, a palpable mass, fevers, night sweats, anemia, or symptoms of disseminated disease such as dyspnea and bone pain.
- Paraneoplastic effects such as erythrocytosis, hypercalcemia, and hypertension may be seen.

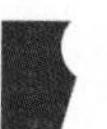

KEY FACT

Do not do a biopsy to diagnose renal cell carcinoma unless disseminated disease or another 1° tumor is suspected. Risks include false negatives, bleeding, and tumor seeding.

Diagnosis

CT with contrast is the modality of choice for diagnosis and operative planning.

Treatment

- **Local disease: Partial vs. radical nephrectomy** vs. cryoablation/radiofrequency ablation.
- **Disseminated disease:** Medical therapy with chemotherapeutic agents (eg, sorafenib, sunitinib) or biologic response modifiers (eg, IL-2, IFN-α) +/– nephrectomy.

OVARIAN CANCER

More than 90% are adenocarcinomas. Risk factors include age, use of infertility drugs, and familial cancer syndromes (eg, BRCA-1, BRCA-2). Risk is ↓ with sustained use of OCPs, having children, breast-feeding, bilateral tubal ligation, and TAH-BSO.

Symptoms/Exam

- Usually **asymptomatic** until the disease has reached an advanced stage.
- Patients may have abdominal pain, bloating, pelvic pressure, urinary frequency, early satiety, constipation, vaginal bleeding, and systemic symptoms (fatigue, malaise, weight loss).
- Exam findings may include a palpable solid, fixed, nodular pelvic mass; ascites; and pleural effusion (Meigs' syndrome). **An ovarian mass in postmenopausal women is ovarian cancer until proven otherwise.**

Diagnosis/Treatment

- Evaluate adnexal masses with **pelvic ultrasound** and possibly CT or **MRI;** obtain serum **CA-125** and a **CXR.**
- Staging is surgical and includes **TAH-BSO, omentectomy,** and **tumor debulking.**

CERVICAL CANCER

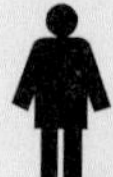

A 25-year-old woman is noted to have dysplastic cells on a routine screening Pap smear. What test is required to confirm a diagnosis of cervical cancer?

Colposcopy and biopsy.

KEY FACT

Infection with HPV types 16, 18, and 31 ↑ the risk of cervical cancer. An HPV vaccine has been approved for the prevention of cervical cancer.

Despite the **screening Pap smear,** cervical cancer remains the third most common gynecologic malignancy. Risk factors include **HPV infection, tobacco use,** early onset of sexual activity, multiple sexual partners, immune compromise (eg, HIV), and STDs. An **HPV vaccine** has recently been approved by the FDA for the prevention of cervical cancer.

Symptoms/Exam

- Patients are usually asymptomatic and are diagnosed on routine **Pap smear.**
- If symptomatic, patients may present with menorrhagia and/or metrorrhagia, **postcoital bleeding,** pelvic pain, and vaginal discharge.

DIAGNOSIS

- **Colposcopy** and biopsy in patients with an abnormal Pap smear or visible cervical lesions.
- Cancers are categorized as **invasive cervical carcinoma** (depth > 3 mm, width > 7 mm) or **cervical intraepithelial neoplasia (CIN).**

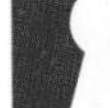

KEY FACT

In suspicious cases, the Pap smear should be followed by colposcopy and biopsy.

TREATMENT

- **CIN I (mild dysplasia or low-grade squamous intraepithelial lesion [LGSIL]):** Most regress spontaneously. Reliable patients can be observed with Pap smears and colposcopy every three months for one year.
- **CIN II/III:** Treat with **cryosurgery,** laser surgery, or **LEEP.**
- **Invasive cancer:** Early-stage disease can be treated with **radical hysterectomy and lymph node dissection.** Advanced disease requires **radiation and chemotherapy.**

Skin Tumors

The differences in appearance of the three most common dermatologic malignancies are depicted in Figures 9-11 and 9-12.

MELANOMA

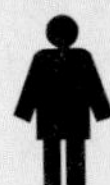

A patient presents for evaluation of a pigmented skin lesion. Biopsy reveals melanocytes with marked atypia characteristic of melanoma. What feature is the most important prognostic factor?

Depth of invasion of the melanoma.

An aggressive malignancy of melanocytes and the **leading cause of death** from skin disease. Risk factors include **sun exposure,** fair skin, a family history, a large number of nevi, and the presence of dysplastic nevi.

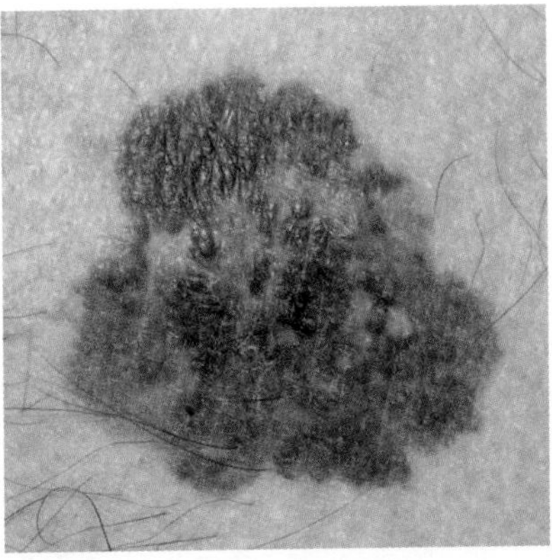

FIGURE 9-11. Melanoma. Lesion illustrating the ABCDs of melanomas: asymmetry, border irregularity, color variegation, and a diameter greater than 6 mm. (Reproduced with permission from Wolff K et al. *Fitzpatrick's Dermatology in General Medicine,* 7th ed. New York: McGraw-Hill, 2008, Fig. 124-1A.)

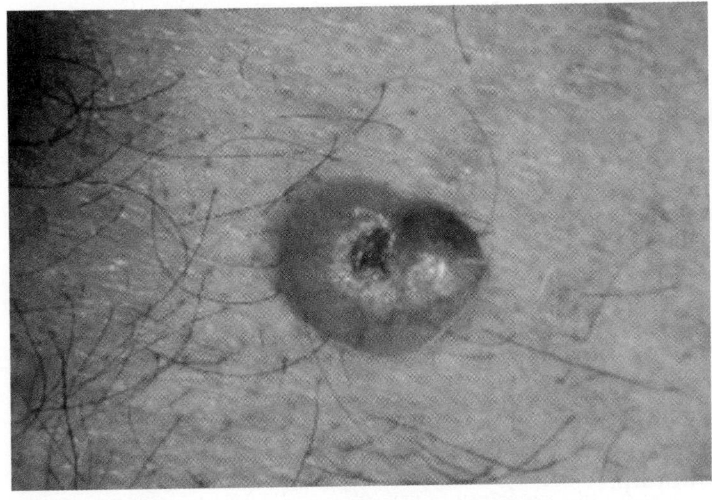

A

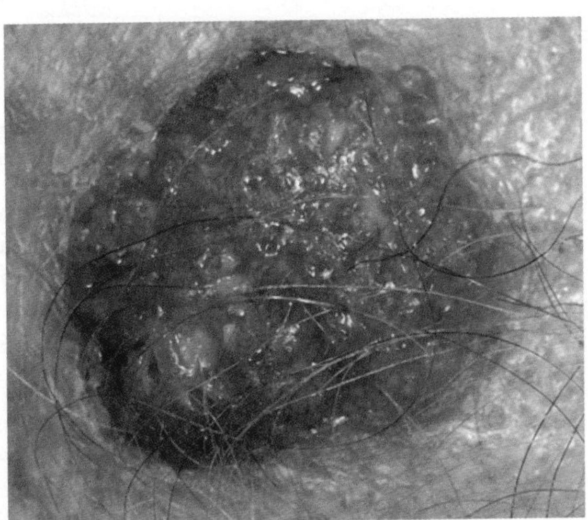

B

FIGURE 9-12. Basal cell and squamous cell carcinomas. (**A**) Basal cell carcinoma showing a characteristic "pearly" appearance. (**B**) Undifferentiated squamous cell carcinoma consisting of a circular, dome-shaped, reddish nodule with a partly eroded surface. (Image A reproduced with permission from USMLERx.com. Image B reproduced with permission from Wolff K, Johnson RA. *Fitzpatrick's Color Atlas & Synopsis of Clinical Dermatology,* 6th ed. New York: McGraw-Hill, 2009, Fig. 11-9.)

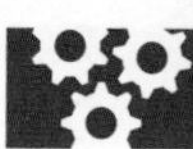

MNEMONIC

The ABCDEs of melanoma:

Asymmetric shape
Borders irregular
Color variegated
Diameter > 6 mm
Enlargement of any lesion

Symptoms/Exam

- **A pigmented skin lesion that has recently changed in size or appearance should raise concern.**
- Lesions are characterized by the **ABCDEs** of melanoma (see mnemonic) and may occur **anywhere** on the body. They are most commonly found on the **trunk for men** and on the **legs for women.**

Diagnosis

Skin biopsy shows **melanocytes with marked cellular atypia** and melanocytic invasion into the dermis.

Treatment

- **Surgical excision** is the treatment of choice. **The thickness of the melanoma (depth of invasion)** is the most important prognostic factor.
- Depending on depth, lymph node dissection may be necessary. Systemic **chemotherapy** is used for metastatic disease.

BASAL CELL CARCINOMA

The **most common skin cancer;** associated with excessive sun exposure.

Symptoms/Exam

- Exam reveals a **pearl-colored papule** of variable size. The external surface is frequently covered with fine **telangiectasias** and appears **translucent.**
- Lesions may be located anywhere on the body but are most commonly found on **sun-exposed** areas, **particularly the face.** Large ulcers are described as "**rodent ulcers.**"

Diagnosis

Skin biopsy shows characteristic basophilic **palisading cells with retraction.**

Treatment

- Therapy depends on the size and location of the tumor, the histologic type, the history of prior treatment, the underlying health of the patient, and cosmetic considerations.
- Options include curettage, surgical excision, cryosurgery, and radiation.

SQUAMOUS CELL CARCINOMA

Risk factors include exposure to the **sun** or to ionizing radiation, prior **actinic keratosis, immunosuppression,** arsenic exposure, and exposure to industrial carcinogens.

Symptoms/Exam

- Lesions are usually slowly evolving and **asymptomatic;** occasionally, bleeding or pain may develop.
- Exam reveals small, red, **exophytic nodules** with varying degrees of scaling or crusting. Lesions are commonly found in **sun-exposed areas, particularly the lower lip.**

Diagnosis

Biopsy shows irregular masses of anaplastic epidermal cells proliferating down to the dermis.

Treatment

- **Surgical excision** is necessary for larger lesions and for those involving the periorbital, periauricular, perilabial, genital, and perigenital areas.
- **Mohs' micrographic surgery** may be performed for recurrent lesions and on areas of the face that are difficult to reconstruct.
- **Radiation** may be necessary in cases in which surgery is not a viable option.

CNS Tumors

1° brain tumors make up < 2% of all tumors diagnosed. Meningioma, glioma, vestibular schwannoma, pituitary adenoma, and 1° CNS lymphoma are the most common CNS tumors in adults and can occur in association with AIDS.

MENINGIOMA

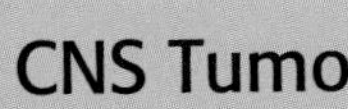

A 60-year-old woman is involved in a motor vehicle accident in which she sustains head trauma. Aside from some minor bruising of the forehead, her physical exam is unrevealing and includes a nonfocal neurologic exam. Routine imaging reveals a 9-mm calcified lesion. What is the most likely diagnosis?

Benign meningioma.

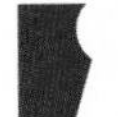

KEY FACT

MRI is superior to CT for viewing skull-base/cerebellar lesions but is less reliable for detecting calcifications.

- The **most common** tumor of the brain; **usually benign.**
- **Sx/Exam:** Most tumors are small, asymptomatic, and discovered incidentally. When symptoms are present, they usually consist of **progressive headache** or a **focal neurologic deficit** reflecting the location of the tumor.
- **Dx:** CT or MRI of the head typically demonstrates a partially **calcified, homogeneously enhancing extra-axial mass adherent to the dura** (see Figure 9-13). **Craniopharyngioma** is another highly calcified tumor in

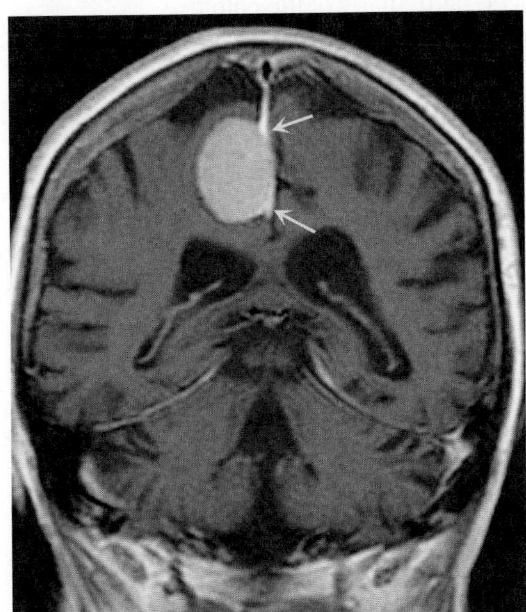

FIGURE 9-13. Meningioma. Coronal postcontrast T1-weighted MRI demonstrates an enhancing extra-axial mass arising from the falx cerebri (arrows). (Reproduced with permission from Fauci AS et al. *Harrison's Principles of Internal Medicine,* 17th ed. New York: McGraw-Hill, 2008, Fig. 374-5.)

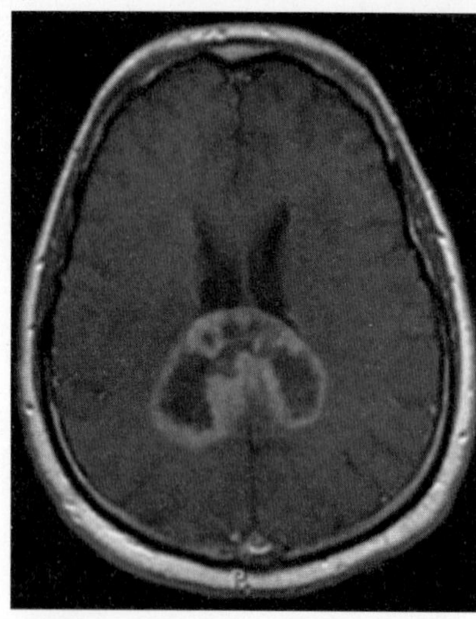

FIGURE 9-14. Glioblastoma multiforme. Transaxial contrast-enhanced image shows an enhancing intra-axial mass with central necrosis crossing the corpus callosum ("butterfly glioma"). (Reproduced with permission from USMLERx.com.)

children but is present **around the pineal gland** and can cause bitemporal hemianopia.

- Tx: Surgical resection is appropriate for large or symptomatic tumors; **observation with serial scans** is the preferred approach for **small or asymptomatic lesions.**

GLIAL TUMORS

- Include astrocytomas, oligodendrogliomas, mixed gliomas, and ependymomas.
- **Sx/Exam:**
  - Headache is the most common symptom and may be generalized or unilateral; often **awakens** the patient from sleep and induces **vomiting;** and **worsens with the Valsalva maneuver.**
  - Tumors appear as a **diffusely infiltrating area** of low attenuation on CT or an ↑ T2 signal on MRI.
  - **Glioblastoma multiforme** is usually a **unifocal and centrally necrotic** enhancing lesion with surrounding edema and mass effect (see Figure 9-14).
- Dx: **Biopsy** is required for definitive diagnosis.
- Tx: **Surgical resection** followed by **external beam radiation** is used for high-grade tumors. Chemotherapy is reserved for high-grade gliomas.

Tumor Markers

Usually sensitive but not specific. Thus, they are most useful for monitoring of recurrence and disease activity following resection. However, tumor markers can also be useful in diagnosis if they are supported by clinical evidence. Common tumor markers and associated malignancies include the following:

- CA 125: Ovarian cancer.
- CA 15-3: Breast cancer.
- CA 19-9: Pancreatic cancer.
- CEA: GI cancer, particularly of the colon.
- AFP: Liver, yolk sac (testicular) cancer.
- hCG: Choriocarcinoma (testicular/ovarian).
- PSA: Prostate cancer.
- LDH: Lymphoma.
- **Calcitonin:** Medullary thyroid carcinoma.
- **Chromogranin A:** Carcinoid tumor.

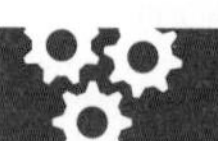

MNEMONIC

Common tumor markers:

CEA = **C**olon cancer
hCG = **Ch**oriocarcinoma
PSA= **P**ro**S**tate
L**D**H = Lymp**H**oma

CHAPTER 10

INFECTIOUS DISEASE

Soft Tissue Infections

Soft tissue infections are infections of the dermis, subcutaneous fat, and/or fascia. Patients with diabetes, HIV or other immunosuppressed states, peripheral vascular disease, and edema are at ↑ risk.

CELLULITIS

Infection of the dermis that may be associated with an identifiable portal of entry—eg, cuts, tinea pedis, animal/insect bites, ulcers, or injection sites.

Symptoms/Exam

- Presents with **warm, erythematous, and tender skin.** The erythema usually has well-demarcated borders.
- Patients may also present with fever, chills, regional lymphadenopathy, or lymphangitis (seen as red streaks).

Differential

Stasis dermatitis, necrotizing fasciitis, allergic reactions.

Diagnosis

- Primarily a clinical diagnosis.
- Consider getting blood cultures, CBC, ESR, and radiographs if there is a possibility of deeper infection such as necrotizing fasciitis or osteomyelitis.
- Lower extremity cellulitis can also be associated with DVT. If clinically indicated, ultrasound may be useful for evaluation.

Treatment

- Demarcate borders and select the antimicrobial and route on the basis of patient risk factors and clinical severity.
- For most patients, a first-generation cephalosporin or a second-generation penicillin is appropriate, but consider pseudomonal coverage in diabetics, and weigh the possibility of methicillin-resistant *S aureus* (MRSA).

NECROTIZING FASCIITIS

Rapidly spreading infection of the subcutaneous fat and fascia, with risk factors including diabetes, other immunosuppressed states, IV drug use, and peripheral vascular disease.

Symptoms/Exam

- Presents with erythematous, warm, tender, and edematous skin that may rapidly progress to dark, indurated skin with bullae. Patients are typically more toxic appearing than those with simple cellulitis.
- Assess for compartment syndrome by checking for distal symptoms and signs, including **P**ulselessness, **P**ain, **P**allor, **P**aresthesias, **P**oikilothermia, and **P**aralysis (the **6 P's**).

Differential

Cellulitis, myonecrosis.

Diagnosis

Clinical diagnosis can be difficult. Obtain radiographs and a CT or an MRI to look for gas and soft tissue involvement.

Treatment

- A penicillin is best for group A strep coverage, with clindamycin used to shut down toxin production. Vancomycin can be added for MRSA coverage.
- If mixed infection is possible, a broad-spectrum penicillin with anaerobic coverage (piperacillin/tazobactam) should be used. Obtain a surgery consult for debridement and fasciotomy.

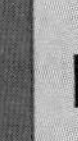

KEY FACT

If necrotizing fasciitis is suspected, prompt medical **and** surgical management is imperative.

Complications

If it is not treated early, the condition may rapidly progress to compartment syndrome, shock, multiorgan failure, and death.

Periorbital/Orbital Infections

- Differentiating between periorbital and orbital infection is critical. A periorbital infection can be treated as a simple cellulitis. However, an **orbital infection** may require **surgical intervention** to prevent **blindness, meningitis,** and **cavernous sinus thrombosis.**
- **Sx/Exam:** Patients with orbital cellulitis can present with oculomotor dysfunction, proptosis, chemosis, ↓ visual acuity, and significant lid erythema.
- **Dx:** Obtain a CT, blood cultures, and a CBC.
- **Tx:** Start broad-spectrum IV antimicrobials and request a surgical consult.

Acute Osteomyelitis

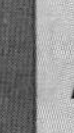

A 23-year-old woman is diagnosed with osteomyelitis. She is an IV heroin user and has a past medical history that is significant for sickle cell anemia. While you are awaiting culture results, she needs to begin empiric antibiotic treatment. In addition to *S aureus,* what other organisms is this patient at risk for?

Her IV drug use puts her at risk for *Pseudomonas* infection, and her sickle cell anemia puts her at risk for *Salmonella.*

Infection of the bone that is spread hematogenously or, more commonly, by direct inoculation. Those with peripheral vascular disease, diabetes, and recent orthopedic surgery are at ↑ risk.

Symptoms/Exam

Presents with pain with overlying erythema, edema, and tenderness. Patients may also have an overlying ulcer or skin interruption. Systemic symptoms include fevers, chills, and fatigue.

Differential

Cellulitis, necrotizing fasciitis.

Encephalitis

Usually involves the brain parenchyma. HSV is the leading cause. Patients may have nonspecific complaints that are initially consistent with a viral prodrome (eg, fever, malaise, body aches) and may then go on to develop confusion, seizures, and focal neurologic deficits (eg, weakness, cranial nerve/sensory deficits). Headaches, photophobia, and meningeal signs can be seen in meningoencephalitis.

HERPES SIMPLEX VIRUS (HSV) ENCEPHALITIS

- The majority of cases are due to HSV-1 reactivation.
- **Sx/Exam:** Think of HSV encephalitis when patients present with bizarre behavior, speech disorders, gustatory or olfactory hallucinations, or acute hearing impairment.
- **Dx:** Key CSF studies include **HSV polymerase chain reaction (PCR) tests and HSV culture.** MRI will show a characteristic pattern in the temporal lobes, usually bilaterally.
- **Tx:** Treat empirically with IV acyclovir.

WEST NILE ENCEPHALITIS

- Suspect in anyone presenting with an acute febrile illness in late spring, summer, or early autumn.
- **Sx/Exam:** Patients have fever +/– a maculopapular rash. Look for acute flaccid paralysis suggestive of Guillain-Barré syndrome.
- **Dx:** CSF findings resemble those of **viral meningitis.** Test serum or CSF by ELISA for IgM antibody to West Nile virus or a rise in IgG titer.
- **Tx:** Treatment is supportive (eg, fluids).

Bacterial Meningitis

A 33-year-old man with HIV/AIDS and a CD4 count of 20 is admitted to the ER with a 12-hour history of fever, photophobia, and headache. A major trauma has just arrived in the ER, so his LP will be delayed by two hours. What medications should the patient be given before the LP is performed?

Vancomycin, ampicillin, cefepime, and dexamethasone. Given that the patient's immunocompromised status and clinical presentation raise concern for bacterial meningitis, he should be covered for both gram-⊕ and gram-⊖ organisms. Additionally, he should be given a dose of dexamethasone 10 minutes before his first dose of antibiotics. This may be discontinued if the Gram stain is not consistent with *Streptococcus pneumoniae*.

Common causative organisms vary with age group (see Table 10-1).

TABLE 10-1. Common Causes of Bacterial Meningitis by Age

PREDISPOSING FACTORS	TYPICAL BACTERIAL PATHOGEN
Neonates (0–4 weeks)	**Group B strep, *E coli, Listeria.***
Infants (1–23 months)	***Streptococcus pneumoniae,*** *Neisseria meningitidis, Haemophilus influenzae.*
Age 2–50 years	***S pneumoniae, N meningitidis.***
Elderly (> 50 years)	*S pneumoniae, N meningitidis,* ***Listeria monocytogenes.***

SYMPTOMS/EXAM

- Typical symptoms include fever, malaise, headaches, photophobia, and neck stiffness. Patients may also complain of nausea and vomiting.
- Be sure to look for fever, nuchal rigidity, and Kernig's or Brudzinski's sign.
- Funduscopic exam may reveal papilledema, indicating ↑ ICP.

DIAGNOSIS

Obtain an LP in any patient suspected of having meningitis. When clinical features suggest a possible intracranial mass or ↑ ICP, obtain a head CT prior to LP. See Table 10-2 for common CSF findings in meningitis.

TREATMENT

- **Begin empiric therapy immediately** in anyone suspected of having bacterial meningitis, as even a short delay will ↑ mortality.
- Consider the patient's **risk factors,** and then choose an antimicrobial regimen that will cover the most likely organisms (see Table 10-3).

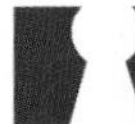

KEY FACT

Treat suspected meningitis immediately; don't wait for CT or LP results! Therapy can always be tailored later.

TABLE 10-2. Common CSF Findings in Meningitis

CSF PARAMETER	BACTERIAL	VIRAL	TB
Opening pressure (mmH_2O)	200–500	< 250	180–300
Cell type	PMNs	Lymphocytes	Lymphocytes
Glucose (mg/dL)	Low	Normal	Low to normal
Protein (mg/dL)	High	Normal	Normal to high

TABLE 10-3. Antibiotic Regimens for Bacterial Meningitis

Pathogen	Therapy of Choice
S pneumoniae	Vancomycin + third-generation cephalosporin +/– dexamethasone.
N meningitidis	Ampicillin or third-generation cephalosporin.
L monocytogenes	Ampicillin **(not cephalosporins).**
Streptococcus agalactiae	Ampicillin.
H influenzae type b	Third-generation cephalosporin.

Upper Respiratory Tract Infections

ACUTE SINUSITIS

- Defined as inflammation of the mucosal lining of the paranasal sinuses. Viruses are the most common cause. The most common bacterial organisms include *S pneumoniae, H influenzae,* and *Moraxella catarrhalis.* Anaerobes and rhinoviruses may also be implicated.
- **Sx/Exam:** Look for acute onset of **fever, headache, facial pain, or swelling.** Most cases involve cough and purulent postnasal discharge. Patients with bacterial sinusitis are typically febrile and have unilateral tenderness over the affected sinus.
- **Dx:** Diagnosis is based on clinical findings. Radiographic imaging or CT may help (air-fluid level, inflammation of tissues).
- **Tx:** If symptoms persist after seven days or are suggestive of bacterial sinusitis, empiric therapy consists of a 10-day course of amoxicillin +/– clavulanate or cefpodoxime. If the patient has diabetes or is immunocompromised, it may be necessary to evaluate for **fungi such as *Mucor* or atypical bacteria such as *Pseudomonas.***

CHRONIC SINUSITIS

- Defined as sinus symptoms lasting > 4 weeks.
- **Dx:** A noncontrast dedicated sinus CT with bone windows is the imaging modality of choice.
- **Tx:**
  - Amoxicillin +/– clavulanate × 21 days.
  - Intranasal corticosteroids, saline irrigation, mucolytics, and decongestants can provide symptomatic relief.
  - Refractory cases require endoscopic surgery.

OTITIS MEDIA

- Causative agents are similar to those of acute sinusitis.
- **Sx/Exam:**
  - Typical features include **fever** and unilateral **ear pain.**
  - There may also be hearing loss, and children may be irritable or may tug at their ears.
  - The tympanic membrane is typically erythematous, lacks a normal light reflex, and may be bulging. Look for perforation of the tympanic membrane along with pus in the ear canal.
- **Tx:**
  - First-line treatment is with amoxicillin or TMP-SMX × 10 days. However, many recent studies suggest that a five- to seven-day course may be adequate if the patient is > 2 years of age and has no history of recurrent otitis media.
  - Patients who do not respond to antimicrobial therapy and develop hearing loss should have tympanostomy tubes placed.

OTITIS EXTERNA

- Predisposing factors include **swimming,** eczema, hearing aid use, and mechanical trauma (eg, cotton swab insertion). In most patients, the causative organism is *Pseudomonas. S aureus* is implicated in acute otitis externa.
- **Sx/Exam:**
  - Patients have a painful ear along with foul-smelling drainage. The **external ear canal** will be swollen and erythematous. There may also be pus.
  - Patients have tenderness upon **movement of the pinna** or tragus.
- **Tx:** Remove any foreign material from the ear canal and start a topical antimicrobial (typically **ofloxacin**) with **steroids.**

PHARYNGITIS

A 28-year-old man with a past medical history significant for IV drug use presents to his primary care physician with sore throat, myalgia, fever, and night sweats of 10 days' duration. He has cervical lymphadenopathy. In addition to being screened for group A streptococcus, what should this patient be evaluated for?

He should also be evaluated for acute HIV infection. The symptoms of acute HIV are nonspecific but usually arise 2–4 weeks postexposure. Symptoms last anywhere from a few days to 10 weeks.

Typically due to **viral causes** such as rhinovirus or adenovirus. **Group A streptococcus** is implicated in up to 25% of cases. Untreated group A streptococcal infection can result in acute pyogenic complications and **rheumatic fever.**

Symptoms/Exam

Symptoms include sore throat and fever +/– cough. Look for tonsillar exudates and tender anterior cervical adenopathy.

DIAGNOSIS

- Think about infectious mononucleosis in patients with lymphadenopathy and malaise.
- In adults with pharyngitis, always consider HIV infection and acute retroviral syndrome.
- In children, think about epiglottitis (febrile patients with complaints of severe sore throat and dysphagia with minimal findings on exam).
- For streptococcal infection, check a rapid antigen test (good sensitivity and specificity) as well as a throat swab for culture.

TREATMENT

- Treat group A streptococcal infections with penicillin. Use a macrolide for patients with penicillin allergy.
- Chronic carriers (ie, those who have a ⊕ throat culture or are asymptomatic) should be treated with clindamycin for eradication.

Pneumonia

COMMUNITY-ACQUIRED PNEUMONIA (CAP)

Pneumonia still ranks as the sixth leading cause of death overall and is the leading cause of death from infection. Etiologies are as follows:

- **Typical pathogens:** *S pneumoniae, H influenzae, S aureus* (in the setting of influenza virus).
- **Atypical pathogens:** *Mycoplasma, Chlamydia, Moraxella, Legionella.*

SYMPTOMS/EXAM

- Think of pneumonia in any patient with acute onset of fever, **chills, productive cough,** and **pleuritic chest pain.**
- **Atypical organisms** present with low-grade fever, nonproductive cough, and myalgias ("walking pneumonia").
- Look for evidence of consolidation (dullness to percussion, crackles, bronchial breath sounds) on lung exam.

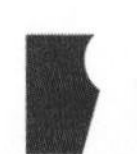

KEY FACT

Think of *Legionella* infection in a smoker with pneumonia, diarrhea, and elevated LDH.

DIAGNOSIS

- There should be radiographic evidence of an infiltrate in all immunocompetent patients (see Figure 10-3) as well as recovery of a pathogenic organism from blood, sputum, or pleural fluid.
- **Urine *Legionella* antigen** should be sent in patients with risk factors.
- Remember to check an ABG to determine the acid-base status of patients who appear to be in distress.
- If the patient is hospitalized, check blood cultures.

TREATMENT

- Decide whether the patient needs to be hospitalized based on clinical risk factors. Admit patients who are > 50 years of age or those who have chronic underlying disease (eg, COPD, CHF, cancer), unstable vital signs, or a high fever.

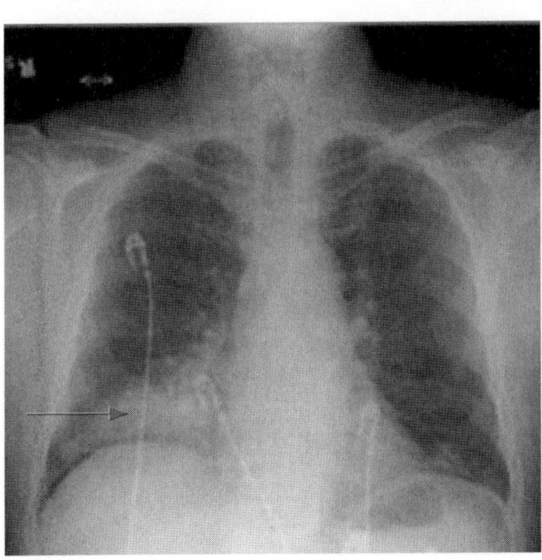

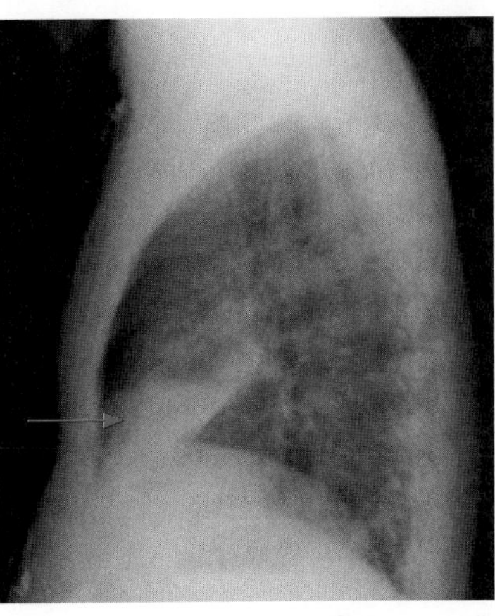

FIGURE 10-3. Community-acquired pneumonia. Frontal (**A**) and lateral (**B**) radiographs show airspace consolidation in the right middle lobe (red arrows) in a patient with community-acquired pneumonia. (Reproduced with permission from USMLERx.com.)

- Initiate empiric antimicrobial therapy based on the patient's risk factors (eg, community-dwelling and healthy vs. diabetic). **Think about MRSA** in patients with a history of colonization or in those who have been hospitalized (see Table 10-4).

TABLE 10-4. Empiric Antibiotic Treatment Strategies for CAP

PATIENT PROFILE	INCLUDE COVERAGE FOR	EMPIRIC ANTIBIOTIC CHOICE
Community-dwelling outpatients	*S pneumoniae* *H influenzae* Atypicals	Azithromycin PO
Patients with comorbidities (age > 60, DM, EtOH use, COPD)	*S pneumoniae* *Klebsiella* *Legionella*	Fluoroquinolone or azithromycin PO
Inpatient (severe or multilobar pneumonia)	As above	Ceftriaxone IV + azithromycin IV
Nursing home–acquired CAP	Gram-⊖ rods *Pseudomonas* MRSA	Ceftriaxone IV + azithromycin IV +/– vancomycin
Patients with cystic fibrosis	*Pseudomonas*	Ceftazidime IV + levofloxacin IV + aminoglycoside
Aspiration	Anaerobes Gram-⊖ rods *S aureus*	Ceftriaxone IV + azithromycin IV + clindamycin IV

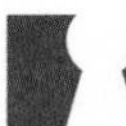

KEY FACT

The sputum sample should have < 10 epithelial cells.

VENTILATOR-ASSOCIATED PNEUMONIA

- Dx: Typical agents in this setting include methicillin-sensitive S *aureus*, MRSA, ***Pseudomonas***, ***Legionella***, ***Acinetobacter***, and other gram-⊖ rods.
- **Tx: Always obtain sputum cultures before starting or changing antimicrobials.** Tailor empiric therapy as soon as culture data become available.

PNEUMOCYSTIS JIROVECI PNEUMONIA

Formerly known as *Pneumocystis carinii* pneumonia (PCP). Can occur as an opportunistic infection in HIV-⊕ patients (usually when CD4 count < 200) as well as in anyone on immunosuppressive therapies such as high-dose steroids.

SYMPTOMS/EXAM

- Presents with fever, nonproductive cough, and dyspnea on minimal exertion that resolves quickly at rest.
- Patients may have findings consistent with atypical pneumonia, or there may be few physical exam findings. Look for pneumothorax.

DIAGNOSIS

- CXR ranges from normal to bilateral interstitial or alveolar infiltrates. The classic appearance is that of "ground-glass" infiltrates (see Figure 10-4).
- Other findings include ↑ LDH.
- Obtain a silver stain of sputum or bronchoalveolar lavage to look for PCP.

TREATMENT

- First-line therapy is with IV TMP-SMX. Alternatives include IV pentamidine.
- Use **concomitant prednisone if PaO_2 is < 70 mm Hg** or if the patient has an alveolar-arterial (A-a) oxygen gradient of > 35 mm Hg on room air.

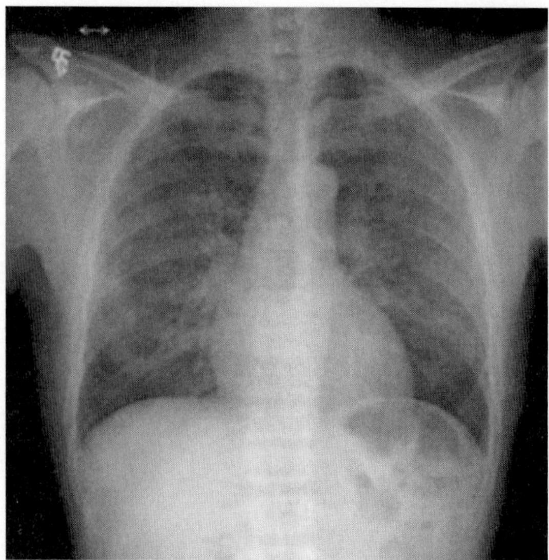

FIGURE 10-4. *Pneumocystis jiroveci* pneumonia. Frontal CXR shows diffuse "ground-glass" lung opacities characteristic of PCP in this patient with AIDS and a CD4 count of 26. (Reproduced with permission from USMLERx.com.)

Bronchitis

Infection of the upper airways (bronchi), with risk factors including cigarette smoking and COPD.

SYMPTOMS/EXAM

Presents with cough with or without sputum production, dyspnea, fever, and chills. The lungs are clear with possible upper airway noise.

DIFFERENTIAL

URI, pneumonia, allergic rhinitis.

DIAGNOSIS

CBC, CXR, sputum Gram stain and culture.

TREATMENT

- Depending on comorbidities and severity, patients may need hospitalization.
- If a bacterial etiology is suspected, give antimicrobials to cover *S pneumoniae* and atypicals.

Tuberculosis (TB)

Caused primarily by *Mycobacterium tuberculosis*. May be 1°, latent, extrapulmonary, or reactivation (see Figure 10-5). Only about 10% of those infected with the bacterium develop active disease.

SYMPTOMS/EXAM

- **1° TB:** Symptoms include fevers and a dry cough. 1° TB usually involves the middle or lower lung zones and is associated with hilar adenopathy (Ghon complex) and radiographic abnormalities. The infection usually resolves, but reactivation occurs in 50–60% of patients.
- **Latent TB infection (LTBI):** Nonactive and noninfectious, but reactivation occurs in about 10% of patients, typically involving the upper lungs and cavitation. Latent infection can be detected by a ⊕ PPD. If the PPD is ⊕, the next step is to evaluate for possible active disease with a CXR (see Figure 10-6).
- **Extrapulmonary TB:** Usually associated with HIV-⊕ patients. May involve any organ, but those most commonly affected (in order of frequency) are the lymph nodes, pleura, GU tract, bones and joints, meninges, peritoneum, and pericardium. Symptoms are related to the organ involved. Diagnosis is based on an AFB culture of affected tissue.
- **Reactivation TB:** After 1° infection, TB can cause reinfection. Symptoms include fevers, productive cough, hemoptysis, night sweats, and weight loss. Reactivation TB is characterized by fibrocaseous cavitary lesions. Diagnosis is based on an AFB sputum culture.

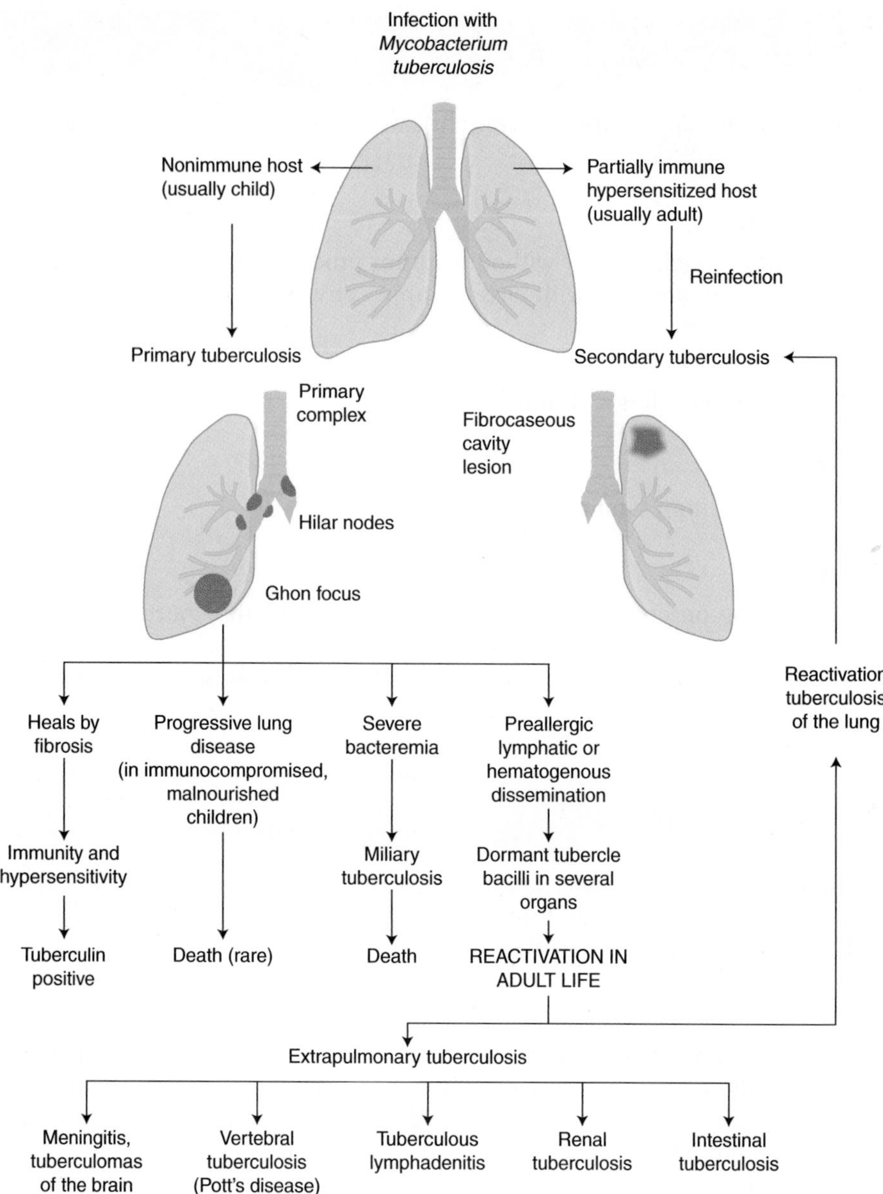

FIGURE 10-5. Evolution of pulmonary tuberculosis. (Modified with permission from Chandrasoma P, Taylor CR. *Concise Pathology,* 2nd ed. Originally published by Appleton & Lange. Copyright © 1995 by The McGraw-Hill Companies, Inc.)

Diagnosis

- Screening by PPD placement should be conducted for LTBI in high-risk groups—eg, immigrants from endemic areas, HIV-⊕ patients, homeless persons, health care workers, IV drug users, and patients with chronic medical conditions (COPD, chronic kidney disease, DM, post-transplant, cancer).
- BCG vaccination status should be disregarded in the interpretation of test results (see Table 10-5).
- Active infection is diagnosed by AFB culture of sputum or tissue involved (see Figure 10-7).

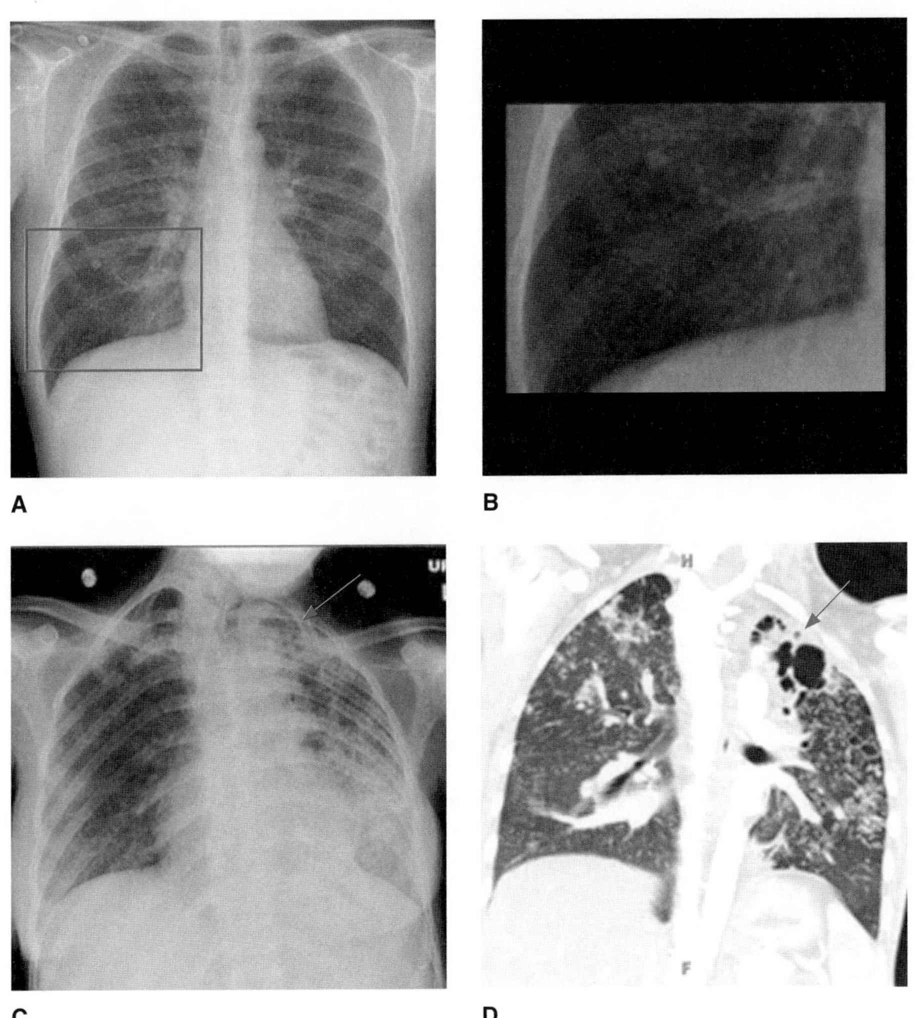

FIGURE 10-6. Pulmonary tuberculosis. (A) Frontal CXR demonstrating diffuse, 1- to 2-mm nodules due to miliary TB. (B) A zoomed-in view corresponding to the area delineated by the red box in Image A. (C) Frontal CXR demonstrating left apical cavitary consolidation (red arrow) and patchy infiltrates in the right and left lung in a patient with reactivation TB. (D) Coronal reformation from a noncontrast chest CT in the same patient as Image C, better demonstrating left apical cavitary consolidation (red arrow) and other areas of parenchymal abnormality corresponding to the endobronchial spread of TB. (Reproduced with permission from USMLERx.com.)

TABLE 10-5. PPD Interpretation

Population	⊕ TB Skin Test
Low risk of disease	≥ 15 mm
Patients with exposure risk (health care workers, immigrants, diabetics)	≥ 10 mm
HIV-⊕, immunocompromised, recent contact with TB, CXR consistent with previous TB infection	≥ 5 mm

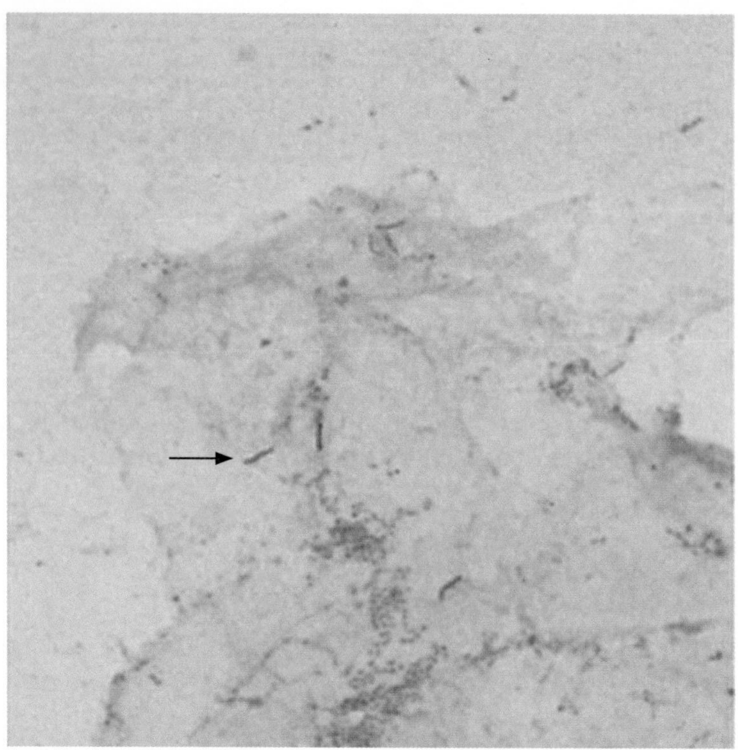

FIGURE 10-7. ***Mycobacterium tuberculosis* on AFB smear.** (Courtesy of the Centers for Disease Control and Prevention, Atlanta, GA, as published in Fauci AS et al. *Harrison's Principles of Internal Medicine,* 17th ed. New York: McGraw-Hill, 2008, Fig. 158-1.)

Treatment

- The most commonly used regimen consists of four drugs described by the mnemonic **RIPE**—**R**ifampin, **I**soniazid (INH), **P**yrazinamide, and **E**thambutol—given daily for eight weeks, followed by INH and rifampin for an additional 16 weeks. Table 10-6 outlines the common side effects of these drugs.
- Treatment of LTBI requires nine months of INH.
- Patients coinfected with TB and HIV should be treated with rifabutin instead of rifampin, as the latter can interact with anti-HIV medications.

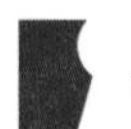

KEY FACT

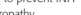

Give vitamin B_6 to prevent INH-associated neuropathy.

TABLE 10-6. Common Side Effects of Tuberculosis Drugs

Drug	Side Effects
Rifampin	Red-orange body fluids, hepatitis.
Isoniazid	Peripheral neuropathy (consider giving pyridoxine, or vitamin B_6, with medication), hepatitis, lupus-like syndrome.
Pyrazinamide	Hyperuricemia, hepatitis.
Ethambutol	Optic neuritis.

Genitourinary Tract Infections

CYSTITIS

- Some 10% of U.S. women have at least one uncomplicated UTI each year. The most common pathogen is *E coli*.
- **Sx/Exam:** Dysuria, urgency, and frequency of urination are the most common complaints.
- **DDx:**
  - Think about urethritis/cervicitis in sexually active patients.
  - Renal stones may also present with colicky pain and dysuria.
- **Dx:** Check a UA for the presence of bacteria, WBCs, leukocyte esterase, and nitrites.
- **Tx:**
  - Give a three-day course of either TMP-SMX or a fluoroquinolone. Cultures are not necessary. A seven-day course is recommended for diabetics, patients with symptoms of > 7 days' duration, and men.
  - Complicated UTIs (eg, hospital-acquired, catheter-associated, and recently treated cases) often require IV antibiotics such as ceftriaxone and a fluoroquinolone.

PYELONEPHRITIS

- **Sx/Exam:**
  - Findings are similar to those of UTI except that patients are more acutely ill.
  - Be sure to check for **CVA tenderness.** Also look for signs of bacteremia such as fever, tachycardia, and hypotension.
- **Dx:** Urine specimens usually demonstrate significant bacteriuria, pyuria, and occasional WBC casts. A urine culture should be sent on all patients. **Always obtain blood cultures on admission, as 15–20% of patients will be bacteremic.**
- **Tx:** Begin a fluoroquinolone IV. If there is no clinical response, look for an intrarenal or perinephric abscess or for foreign bodies such as **renal calculi** with CT or ultrasound.

PROSTATITIS

- **Sx/Exam:**
  - Presenting symptoms include spiking fevers, chills, dysuria, cloudy urine, and even obstructive symptoms if prostate swelling is significant.
  - In patients with chronic infection, low back pain or perineal/testicular discomfort may be present.
  - The gland is exquisitely tender on prostate DRE.
- **Dx:** Obtain urine cultures before and after a prostatic massage to look for gram-⊖ rods.
- **Tx:** Treat with TMP-SMX or a fluoroquinolone × 14 days. Chronic prostatitis may cause more low-grade symptoms. Treatment should be extended to at least one month with a fluoroquinolone or to three months with TMP-SMX.

Sexually Transmitted Diseases (STDs)

SYPHILIS

Caused by *Treponema pallidum.* Transmissible during early disease (1° and 2° syphilis) through exposure to open lesions (loaded with spirochetes!).

Symptoms

- **1° syphilis:** Develops within several weeks of exposure; involves one or more painless, indurated, superficial ulcerations (chancre; see Figure 10-8).
- **2° syphilis:** After the chancre has resolved, patients may develop malaise, anorexia, headache, diffuse lymphadenopathy, or rash (involves the mucosal surfaces, palms, and soles).
- **3° syphilis:** Includes cardiovascular, neurologic, and gummatous disease (eg, general paresis, tabes dorsalis, aortitis, meningovascular syphilis).

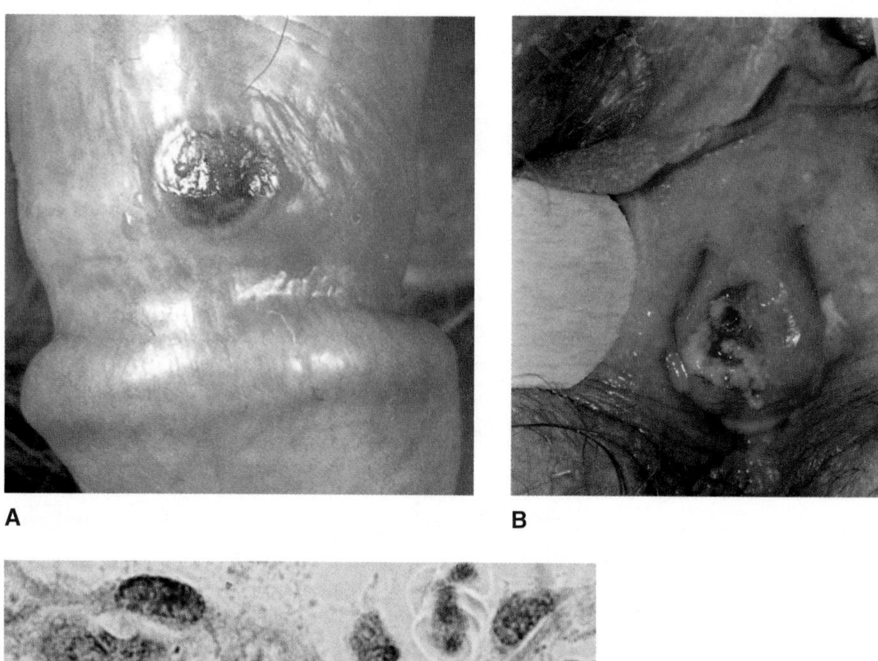

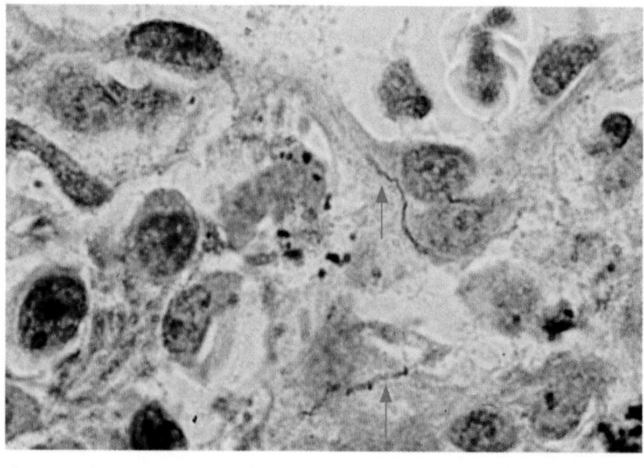

FIGURE 10-8. Syphilis. (A) Male and (B) female genital chancres, respectively, in primary syphilis infection. (C) Silver stain of sample from a chancre showing spiral-shaped spirochetes (arrows). (Reproduced with permission from Wolff K et al. *Fitzpatrick's Dermatology in General Medicine,* 7th ed. New York: McGraw-Hill, 2008, Figs. 200-2, 200-5, and 200-1.)

Exam

Findings depend on the stage of syphilis—the painless chancre for 1° disease; maculopapular rash or diffuse lymphadenopathy for 2° disease; and multiple neurologic and/or cardiovascular signs for 3° disease.

Diagnosis

- 1°: Do a nontreponemal serologic test (RPR or VDRL). Darkfield microscopy of the lesion's exudate will show the spirochetes. Direct antigen tests (MHA-TP or FTA-ABS) are used for confirmation.
- 2°: Diagnosed by the presence of clinical illness and ⊕ serologic tests.
- 3°: Perform an LP when neurologic or ophthalmic signs and symptoms are present; in the setting of treatment failure; or with a VDRL of ≥ 1:32. Correlate with cardiovascular, neurologic, and systemic symptoms.

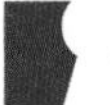

KEY FACT

Patients who have had HIV or syphilis longer than a year should always undergo LP.

Treatment

- 1°/2°: Penicillin G 2.4 MU in a single IM dose. Alternatives include doxycycline or erythromycin × 14 days. If the disease duration is > 1 year, give three doses of penicillin G IM a week apart.
- **Neurosyphilis:** Penicillin G IV × 14 days.

GENITAL HERPES

- Painful grouped vesicles in the anogenital region. Caused by the human herpes simplex virus, usually type 2.
- **Sx/Exam:** Frequently associated symptoms include tender inguinal lymphadenopathy, fever, myalgias, headaches, and aseptic meningitis. Symptoms are usually more pronounced during the initial episode and grow less frequent with recurrences.
- **Dx:** Diagnosis can be confirmed by viral PCR of the vesicle fluid.
- **Tx:**
  - Acyclovir × 7–10 days for 1° infections. Treatment should begin within one week of symptom onset.
  - Severe recurrences may necessitate repeat treatment with either acyclovir or valacyclovir × 5 days. Daily suppressive therapy can be used for frequent recurrences.

KEY FACT

Counsel patients regarding safe-sex practices. HSV transmission can occur even in the absence of visible vesicles.

CERVICITIS/URETHRITIS

- Chlamydial and gonococcal infections often present as cervicitis or urethritis. *Mycoplasma genitalium* is an emerging pathogen in this syndrome.
- **Sx/Exam:** Dysuria, dyspareunia, and a mucopurulent vaginal discharge are frequent complaints in women. In men, dysuria and a purulent penile discharge predominate.
- **Dx:** A ⊕ endocervical or urethral culture or a ⊕ urine PCR for chlamydia/gonorrhea is diagnostic.
- **Tx:**
  - **Always treat for both infections simultaneously, and treat sexual partners.**
  - Treat chlamydia with a single PO dose of azithromycin.
  - Treat gonorrhea with a single PO dose of ofloxacin or ciprofloxacin or with a single IM dose of ceftriaxone.

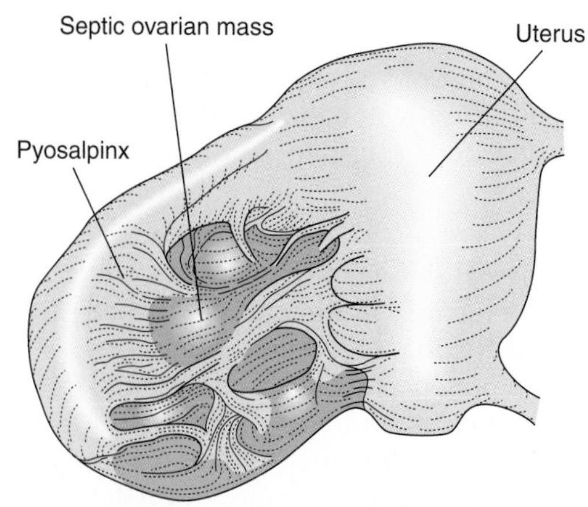

FIGURE 10-9. Tubo-ovarian abscess. (Reproduced with permission from Benson RC. *Handbook of Obstetrics & Gynecology,* 8th ed. Stamford, CT: Appleton & Lange, 1983.)

PELVIC INFLAMMATORY DISEASE (PID)

- An upper genital tract infection in women that is usually a complication of chlamydia and/or gonorrhea infection.
- **Sx/Exam:** Presents with pelvic pain, dyspareunia, vaginal discharge, fever, and menstrual irregularities as well as with lower abdominal tenderness, adnexal tenderness, and cervical motion tenderness.
- **Dx:** A finding of > 10 WBCs/low-power field on Gram stain and endocervical smear is consistent with a diagnosis of PID. Always remember to first rule out pregnancy.
- **Tx:** Treat with a second-generation cephalosporin IV and doxycycline IV. If the patient does not improve, consider imaging (ultrasound) to evaluate for a tubo-ovarian abscess that would require drainage (see Figure 10-9).

KEY FACT

IUDs greatly ↑ the risk of PID and should be removed in women who have been diagnosed with an STD.

HIV Infection

Acute retroviral syndrome occurs in 50–90% of cases. The incubation period is usually 2–6 weeks. Acute symptoms last 1–4 weeks, with an average of two weeks.

Symptoms/Exam

Patients have a typical viral prodrome (eg, malaise, low-grade fever) followed by the development of adenopathy. Unusual presentations include Bell's palsy, peripheral neuropathy, radiculopathy, cognitive impairment, and psychosis.

Diagnosis

- HIV serology (ELISA) detects antibody to HIV. Serology becomes ⊕ 2–3 months after exposure, with > 95% seroconversion at six months. Send a confirmatory Western blot in patients with a ⊕ ELISA screen.
- For patients with suspected acute retroviral syndrome, check a viral load, as the ELISA may not have had time to turn ⊕.

TREATMENT

- Begin highly active antiretroviral therapy (HAART) in any of the following situations:
  - In symptomatic patients (any CD4 or viral load).
  - In asymptomatic patients with a CD4 of < 350 and any viral load.
  - In pregnant women.
  - In the setting of a needle stick involving blood from an HIV-⊕ patient.
- Regimens should include three drugs, **preferably from different categories** (see Table 10-7).

COMPLICATIONS

Complications are numerous and typically involve opportunistic infections and side effects from drugs. See Table 10-8 for prophylaxis indications.

TABLE 10-7. Categories of Antiretroviral Drugs

Major Antiretroviral Classes	Examples	Common Side Effects
Nucleoside reverse transcriptase inhibitors (NRTIs)	Zidovudine (AZT)	Myopathy and bone marrow suppression.
	Didanosine (ddI)	Pancreatitis.
	Abacavir	Hypersensitivity reactions (eg, fever, chills, dyspnea).
	Emtricitabine (FTC) and lamivudine (3TC)	Diarrhea, nausea, and headache.
	Tenofovir (TNV)	Renal toxicity.
Non-nucleoside reverse transcriptase inhibitors (NNRTIs)	Efavirenz	CNS toxicity and teratogenicity.
	Nevirapine	Rash and hepatic failure.
Protease inhibitors (PIs)	Atazanavir	Benign indirect hyperbilirubinemia.
	Indinavir	Kidney stones.
	Nelfinavir	Diarrhea.
	Ritonavir	Potent P-450 inhibitor.
	Saquinavir	Rare side effects.
		All PIs can ↑ lipids, redistribute fat, and cause DM.
Fusion inhibitors	Enfuvirtide (T20)	Injection site reactions.

TABLE 10-8. Prophylaxis in HIV

Disease	Indication	Treatment
PCP	CD4 < 200 or previous PCP or thrush.	TMP-SMX, dapsone, or atovaquone.
Mycobacterium avium–intracellulare (MAI)	CD4 < 50.	Azithromycin weekly.
Toxoplasma gondii	CD4 < 100 and *Toxoplasma* IgG ⊕.	TMP-SMX or dapsone + leucovorin + pyrimethamine.
TB	Recent contact or PPD > 5 mm.	INH for nine months.
Pneumococcal pneumonia	All HIV ⊕.	Vaccine every five years.
Influenza	All HIV ⊕.	Yearly vaccine.
Hepatitis B	Surface antigen/core antibody ⊕.	Hepatitis B vaccine.

Travel Medicine

MALARIA PROPHYLAXIS

- Prophylaxis must be tailored to reflect the prevalence of resistant *Plasmodium falciparum* (high mortality) in the area of proposed travel. Most regimens start 1–2 weeks prior to travel and continue for a month after return.
- Weekly chloroquine is the mainstay of therapy in chloroquine-sensitive areas.
- Mefloquine is active against chloroquine-resistant *P falciparum* and is also given weekly. Mefloquine resistance is emerging in Southeast Asia.
- Daily doxycycline or daily Malarone (atovaquone and proguanil) can be used in those who are unable to take mefloquine or who are traveling to chloroquine-resistant areas. Malarone can be used for short trips.
- **Precautions:**
  - Mefloquine has the potential for neuropsychiatric side effects. Caution should thus be exercised in prescribing it to people with recent or active depression, psychosis, schizophrenia, or anxiety disorders.
  - Other effects include sinus bradycardia and QT-interval prolongation; avoid in patients on β-blockers or in those with known conduction disorders.

TRAVELER'S DIARRHEA (TD)

- Roughly 40–60% of people traveling to developing countries develop TD (see Table 10-9).

TABLE 10-9. Common Pathogens Causing Traveler's Diarrhea

Bacteria	Viruses	Parasites
ETEC (enterotoxic *E coli*)	Rotavirus	*Giardia*
Campylobacter	Enteric adenovirus	*Cryptosporidium*
Salmonella		*Cyclospora*
Shigella		Microsporidia
Vibrio		*Isospora belli*
Yersinia		*Entamoeba histolytica*

- **Sx/Exam:** Patients with uncomplicated TD have watery, unformed stools without systemic symptoms. Those with complicated TD can have bloody diarrhea along with systemic symptoms such as nausea, vomiting, abdominal pain, and fever.
- **Dx:** Since uncomplicated TD is self-limited (48–72 hours), studies are usually not warranted, and treatment is symptomatic. Exceptions are as follows:
  - A stool culture should be considered in those with blood in the stool, fever, and symptoms of colitis.
  - Stool examination for *Giardia* should be done in patients with predominantly upper GI symptoms—eg, nausea, bloating, gas, and persistent nonbloody diarrhea.
- **Tx:**
  - Fluid replacement should be initiated in all cases; oral rehydration should be started in children with cholera.
  - Antimicrobials are indicated for moderate to severe disease. A **fluoroquinolone** or **azithromycin** is the first choice. Antimotility agents should not be used in severe TD.

Tick-Borne Diseases

LYME DISEASE

A systemic disease caused by *Borrelia burgdorferi*, a spirochete carried by the deer tick (*Ixodes* genus). Patients may reside in the Northeast or Midwest.

Symptoms/Exam

- **Stage 1:** Presents with erythema migrans (target or bull's-eye lesion; see Figure 10-10) as well as with fever, arthralgias, myalgias, and lymphadenopathy.
- **Stage 2:** Characterized by myocarditis, possibly accompanied by varying degrees of AV block, Bell's palsy (unilateral or bilateral), peripheral neuropathy, and meningitis.
- **Stage 3:** Marked by arthritis and possibly by chronic neurologic symptoms.

Differential

Erythema migrans is pathognomonic for Lyme disease. The differential for other nonspecific symptoms is broad.

Defined as two systemic inflammatory response syndrome (SIRS) criteria **with evidence of infection.** Divided into three levels of severity (see Table 10-10). SIRS criteria are as follows:

- **Temperature:** < 36°C (< 97°F) or > 38°C (> 100°F).
- **Heart rate:** > 90 bpm.
- **Respiratory rate:** > 24 breaths/min or a Pco_2 of < 32 mm Hg.
- **Leukocytes:** > 12,000 cells/mm^3, < 4000 cells/mm^3, or > 10% bands on peripheral blood smear.

SYMPTOMS/EXAM

- Presents with nonspecific infectious symptoms such as fever, chills, and fatigue.
- Symptoms and signs suggestive of cellulitis, necrotizing fasciitis, meningitis, sinusitis, pneumonia, endocarditis, UTI, or GI infection are seen.
- Vital signs are abnormal (see the SIRS criteria above).
- Evidence of hypoperfusion includes cool, pale extremities, ↓ pulses, altered mental status, and ↓ urine output.

DIFFERENTIAL

MI, PE, cardiac tamponade, acute pancreatitis, acute hemorrhage, transfusion reactions, drug reactions, anaphylaxis, acute adrenal insufficiency, myxedema coma.

DIAGNOSIS

- Find the focus of infection.
- If no clear infectious focus can be found, obtain a CXR, a UA, and a urine Gram stain and culture. Consider obtaining sputum, CSF, pleural fluid, and peritoneal fluid samples; a transesophageal echocardiogram (TEE); and an ultrasound of preexisting catheters or other foreign bodies (eg, pacemakers).
- Always obtain blood cultures and sensitivities.
- Obtain a CBC, electrolytes, glucose, lactate, AST, ALT, aPTT, and PT, and consider an ABG if respiratory failure is a concern.

TREATMENT

- Treat hypotension with **rapid fluid resuscitation.**
- Consider central line access for cardiovascular and pulmonary monitoring as well as administration of high-volume fluid resuscitation, blood products, and/or pressors/inotropes.
- Consider an arterial line for continuous monitoring of BP.
- If an infectious focus is identified, **appropriately tailor antimicrobial treatment.** If the source cannot be identified, start broad-spectrum antimi-

TABLE 10-10. Severity of Sepsis

SEVERITY	CRITERIA
Sepsis	Meets at least two of the SIRS criteria with evidence of infection.
Severe sepsis	Meets the criteria for sepsis with evidence of end-organ damage.
Septic shock	Meets the criteria for sepsis with BP not responding to fluid resuscitation and necessitating the initiation of pressors and/or inotropes.

crobials in accordance with patient risk factors (eg, immune compromise, nursing home residency, recent hospitalization).
- If the patient meets the criteria for severe sepsis or septic shock and has multiorgan failure or ARDS, consider starting activated protein C.

COMPLICATIONS

Can lead to ARDS, DIC, multiorgan failure, and death.

KEY FACT

Early initiation of appropriate antimicrobials is critical in the management of sepsis.

Fungal Infections

Typically affect immunocompromised patients and should always be considered in this population.

CRYPTOCOCCOSIS

- Affects patients with **depressed T-cell immunity.**
- **Sx/Exam:** Presents as a disseminated infection, frequently causing meningoencephalitis. In healthy patients, it typically causes pneumonia that is often self-limited.
- **Dx:**
  - Diagnose with a fungal culture and antigen testing (eg, CSF, blood, sputum). Silver stains of biopsies can aid in diagnosis.
  - Although largely replaced by the antigen test, an India ink test may show a halo 2° to the capsule (see Figure 10-11).
- **Tx:**
  - Treat mild to moderate disease with fluconazole × 6–12 months.
  - Patients with severe disease, immunocompromised hosts, and those with CNS infections should be treated with amphotericin (+/– flucytosine) followed by long-term fluconazole.

HISTOPLASMOSIS

- Affects both healthy and immunocompromised patients.
- **Sx/Exam:**
  - Usually manifests as a respiratory illness, but can present as disseminated disease in the immunocompromised.

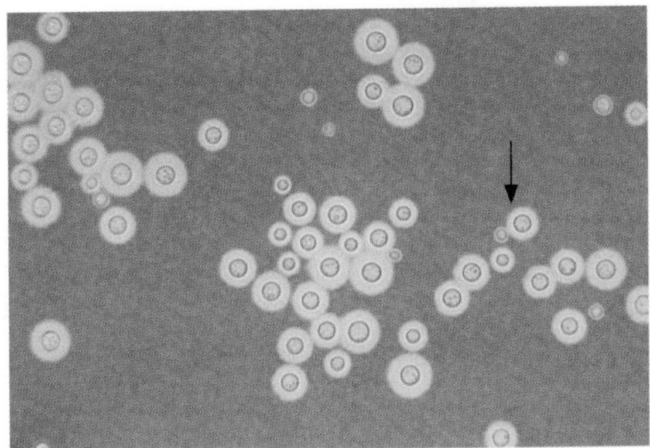

FIGURE 10-11. ***Cryptococcus neoformans.*** India ink preparation demonstrating budding yeast (arrow) and thick, translucent polysaccharide capsules outlined by the dark India ink particles. (Courtesy of Dr. L. Haley, Public Health Image Library, Centers for Disease Control and Prevention, Atlanta, GA, as published in Levinson W. *Review of Medical Microbiology and Immunology,* 10th ed. New York: McGraw-Hill, 2008, Color Plate 38.)

- Disseminated disease can present with palatal ulcerations, fever, weight loss, splenomegaly, anemia, and an elevated ESR.
- Patients have commonly visited the **Ohio/Mississippi river valleys** or have a **history of exposure to bird excrement, bat guano, or construction sites.**

- **Dx:** Diagnosis is best made with silver staining and culture of biopsied infected tissue, but *Histoplasma* antigen tests of urine and serum are available.
- **Tx:** Mild cases in healthy patients do not require treatment. Amphotericin should be used in severe cases, and itraconazole can be given if there is no CNS involvement.

COCCIDIOIDOMYCOSIS

- Typically affects immunocompromised individuals, but not exclusively.
- **Sx/Exam:**
  - 1° disease is usually a self-limited pneumonitis with dry cough and fever; however, disseminated disease affects the CNS (meningitis), skin (erythema nodosum), bones, and joints.
  - Patients have **commonly visited the southwestern United States, particularly Arizona or the San Joaquin Valley in California.**
- **Dx:** Diagnose with silver stains of culture or biopsy, serologic studies, or antibody detection in CSF if meningitis is present.
- **Tx:** Treat with fluconazole and amphotericin if the disease is progressive or disseminated or if the patient is immunocompromised.

Antimicrobial Selection

When a pathogen has been definitively identified, it is important to choose an antimicrobial with narrow coverage. Table 10-11 illustrates common antimicrobials and their spectra of coverage.

TABLE 10-11. Common Antimicrobials and Their Coverage

Antimicrobial Group	Common Examples	Organisms Covered
First-generation or natural penicillins	Penicillin G, penicillin V.	*Treponema pallidum, Enterococcus,* streptococci, and rare penicillin-sensitive staphylococci.
Second-generation or β-lactamase-resistant penicillins	Dicloxacillin, methicillin (no longer used clinically, but important because of methicillin-resistant staphylococci), nafcillin, oxacillin.	Used primarily for methicillin-sensitive staphylococci, but do cover some streptococci.
Third-generation or aminopenicillins	Amoxicillin, amoxicillin/clavulanic acid, ampicillin, ampicillin/sulbactam.	Natural penicillin coverage and *E coli, Proteus, H influenzae,* and *Enterococcus.* β-lactamase inhibitors add coverage for enteric gram-⊖ organisms and anaerobes.
Fourth-generation or extended-spectrum penicillins	Piperacillin/tazobactam, ticarcillin/clavulanic acid.	Aminopenicillin/β-lactamase inhibitor coverage in addition to resistant gram-⊖ organisms and *Pseudomonas.*

TABLE 10-11. Common Antimicrobials and Their Coverage *(continued)*

ANTIMICROBIAL GROUP	COMMON EXAMPLES	ORGANISMS COVERED
First-generation cephalosporins	Cefazolin, cephalexin.	Staphylococci, streptococci, ***Proteus, E** coli,* and ***K**lebsiella* **(PEcK).** Cephalosporins do not cover any enterococci.
Second-generation cephalosporins	Cefaclor, cefuroxime.	First-generation cephalosporin coverage and ***H** influenzae,* **E**nterobacteriaceae, ***N**eisseria* **(HEN PEcK).**
Cephamycins	Cefotetan, cefoxitin.	Second-generation cephalosporin coverage and gram-⊕/gram-⊖ anaerobes.
Third-generation cephalosporins	Cefotaxime, ceftazidime, ceftriaxone.	Most gram-⊖ aerobes. Ceftriaxone adds streptococcal coverage and ceftazidime adds *Pseudomonas* coverage.
Fourth-generation cephalosporins	Cefepime.	Gram-⊖ aerobes, streptococci, and *Pseudomonas.*
Second-generation quinolones	Ciprofloxacin.	Gram-⊖ aerobes and atypicals such as *Legionella, Mycoplasma,* and *Chlamydia.* Best *Pseudomonas* coverage of all quinolones.
Third-generation quninolones	Levofloxacin.	Gram-⊖ aerobes, streptococci, and atypicals.
Fourth-generation quinolones	Gatifloxacin, moxifloxacin.	Gram-⊕ organisms, some anaerobes, weak gram-⊖ coverage, and atypicals.
Carbapenems	Ertapenem, imipenem, meropenem.	Gram-⊕ organisms (except resistant *Staphylococcus* and *Enterococcus*); gram-⊖ organisms, including *Pseudomonas* and anaerobes. Ertapenem has no *Pseudomonas* or *Enterococcus* coverage.
Macrolides	Azithromycin, erythromycin, clarithromycin.	Gram-⊕ organisms and atypicals.
Aminoglycosides	Gentamicin, tobramycin.	Gram-⊖ aerobes.
Others	Aztreonam. Clindamycin. Dalfopristin/quinupristin. Linezolid. Metronidazole. TMP-SMX. Vancomycin. Tetracyclines (doxycycline, minocycline, tigecycline).	Gram-⊖ aerobes, including *Pseudomonas.* Gram-⊕ anaerobes. MRSA and vancomycin-resistant enterococci (VRE). MRSA; VRE. Anaerobes (*Clostridium difficile*). Gram-⊖ organisms, gram-⊕ organisms, PCP. MRSA and *C difficile.* *Rickettsia* and atypicals.

NOTES

CHAPTER 11

MUSCULOSKELETAL

Gout

A 47-year-old man with hypertension and hypercholesterolemia celebrates his birthday by going out for steak and beer. The next morning, his first MTP joint is red and painful even to light touch. He is on lovastatin, ASA, chlorthalidone, and niacin. Which of his medications likely contributed to his gout?

Chlorthalidone.

KEY FACT

Monoarthritis? Think:
- Gout
- Septic arthritis
- Lyme disease
- Pseudogout
- Trauma

A metabolic condition resulting from the intra-articular deposition of monosodium urate crystals. Complications include nephrolithiasis and chronic urate nephropathy.

Symptoms/Exam

- Typically presents in **middle-aged, obese men** (90%) from the Pacific Islands. Incidence in women ↑ after menopause.
- Acute gout attacks often occur at night between periods of remission.
- Patients initially present with severe pain, redness, and swelling in a single lower extremity joint (typically the first MTP joint); subsequent attacks may present in additive fashion with multiple joints.
- Differentiate from pseudogout, in which symptoms may be severe and often affect the knee (> 50%) or shoulder.
- Common precipitants of attacks include a high-purine diet (eg, meats, alcohol), dehydration or diuretic use, high-fructose corn syrup, stress, severe illness, trauma, and tumor lysis syndrome.
- Patients with long-standing disease may develop tophi that lead to joint deformation.

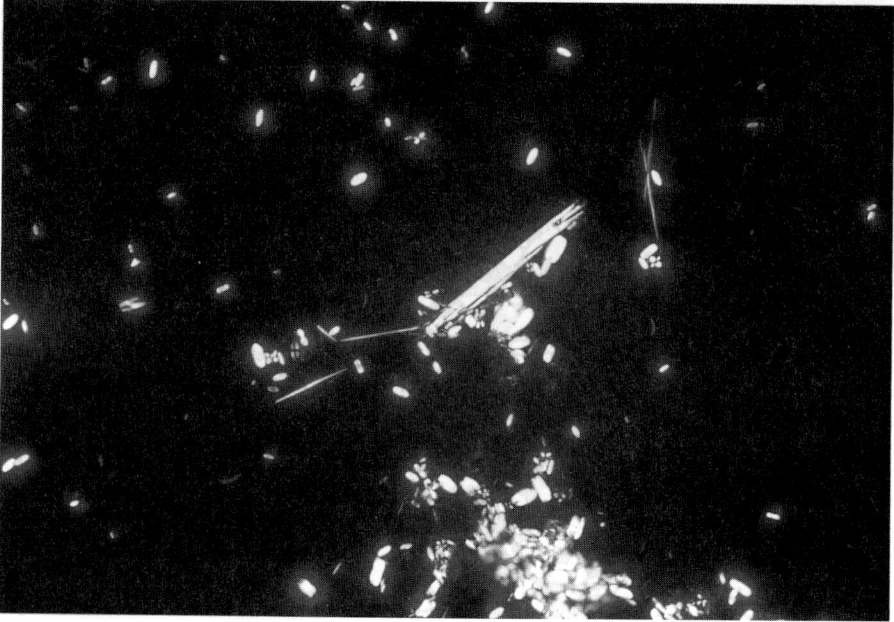

FIGURE 11-3. Gout crystals. Note the needle-shaped, negatively birefringent crystals. (Reproduced with permission from Milikowski C. *Color Atlas of Basic Histopathology.* Stamford, CT: Appleton & Lange, 1997: 546.)

TABLE 11-2. Differential Diagnosis of Gout and Pseudogout

	Gout Crystals	Pseudogout Crystals
Composition	Urate	Calcium pyrophosphate dihydrate
Shape	Needle shaped	Rhomboid shaped
Refringence	Negatively birefringent	Strongly positively birefringent
Red compensator	Ye**LL**ow when para**LL**el	Blue when parallel
Response to colchicine	Good	Weak

Diagnosis

- Joint aspirate is inflammatory with needle-shaped, negatively birefringent (**yeLLow** when **paraLLel** to the condenser) crystals (see Figure 11-3 and Table 11-2).
- Radiographs are normal in early gout. Characteristic punched-out erosions with overhanging cortical bone ("rat bites") are seen in more advanced disease (see Figure 11-4).
- Most patients have ↑ serum uric acid (which is neither sensitive nor specific). Roughly 90% are underexcreters of uric acid, while the remainder are overproducers.
- If you are thinking about starting probenecid, collect a 24-hour urine sample for uric acid while the patient is **off** hyperuricemia-inducing medications (diuretics, alcohol, cyclosporine) to determine whether the hyperuricemia is due to undersecretion or overproduction of urate (see Table 11-3).

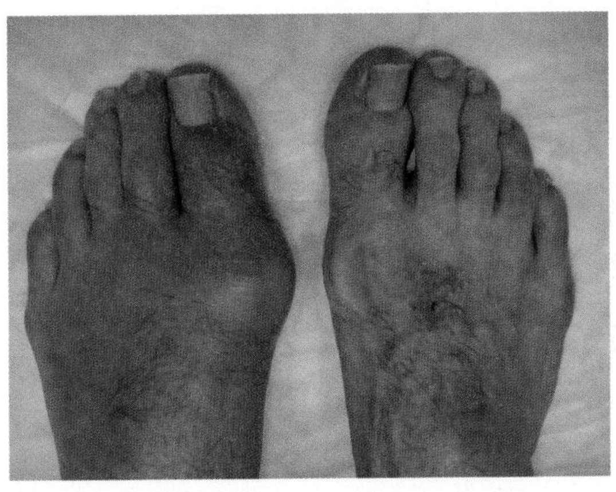

A

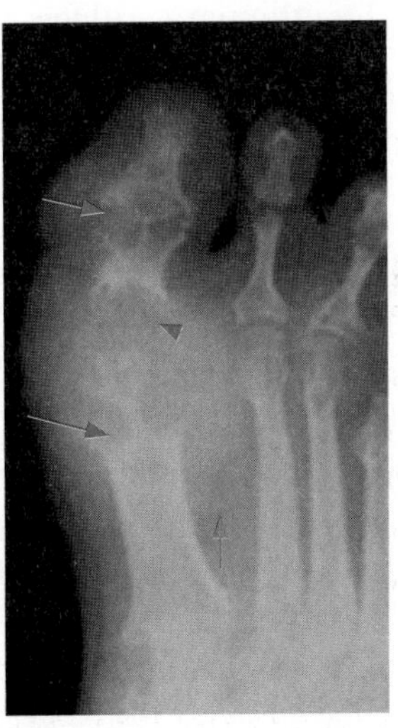

B

FIGURE 11-4. Gout. (**A**) A swollen left first MTP joint with overlying erythema and warmth, characteristic of an acute gout attack (podagra). (**B**) An AP radiograph showing the severe consequences of long-standing gout, including large, nonmarginal erosions with overhanging edges of bone (red arrows), soft tissue swelling, and destruction of the first MTP joint (arrowhead). Note the subtle calcification of a gouty tophus (orange arrow). (Image A reproduced with permission from LeBlond RF et al. *DeGowin's Diagnostic Examination,* 9th ed. New York: McGraw-Hill, 2009, Plate 30. Image B reproduced with permission from USMLERx.com.)

TABLE 11-3. Causes of Hyperuricemia

	Overproduction of Uric Acid	Undersecretion of Uric Acid
24-hour urine collection for uric acid	> 800 mg/day	< 800 mg/day
Etiology	Idiopathic (1°), inherited enzyme defect, myeloproliferative disorders, lymphoproliferative disorders, tumor lysis syndrome, psoriasis	Chronic kidney disease, ASA, diuretics

Treatment

- For acute attacks, administer high-dose NSAIDs (eg, indomethacin) or colchicine. Use oral or intra-articular steroids when first-line therapy fails or is contraindicated.
- Once the acute attack resolves, begin maintenance therapy to ↓ serum uric acid levels (≤ 6 mg/dL). Overproducers are treated with allopurinol; undersecreters are treated with probenecid.
- Patients should avoid precipitants of acute attacks and should consume a low-purine diet (eggs, cheese, fruit, and vegetables). Other key factors in flare prevention are weight loss and BP control.

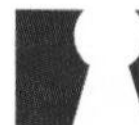

KEY FACT

Remember to **A**void **A**llopurinol in **A**cute gout **A**ttacks.

Osteoarthritis (OA)

A chronic, noninflammatory joint disease characterized by degeneration of the articular cartilage, **hypertrophy** of the bone margins, and changes in the synovial membrane. OA can be 1° or 2° to trauma, chronic arthritis, congenital joint disease, or a systemic metabolic disorder (hemochromatosis, Wilson's disease).

Symptoms/Exam

- Marked by insidious onset of joint pain without inflammatory signs (swelling, warmth, and redness).
- In contrast to the "morning stiffness" of inflammatory arthritis, OA worsens with activity during the day and improves with rest. Crepitus is a common nonspecific finding. There are no systemic manifestations.
- 1° OA usually involves the following joints:
  - **Hands: DIP**, PIP, and first carpometacarpal joints. The classic DIP deformities are also known as Heberden's nodes (see Figure 11-5). Contrast this with the classic MCP lesions of RA.
  - **Feet:** First MTP joint.
  - **Knees, hips.**
  - **Spine:** C5, T9, and L3 are the most common spinal levels.

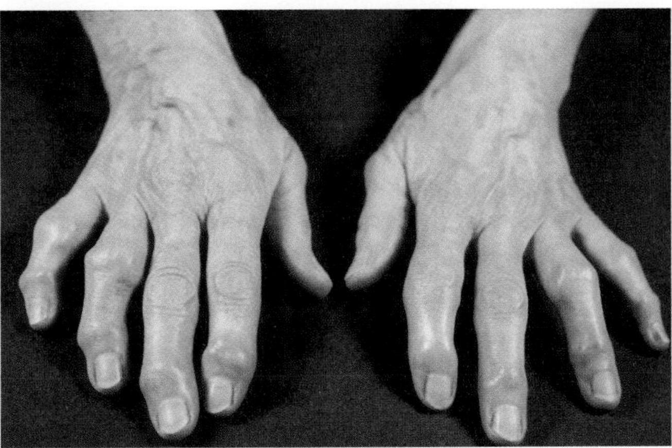

FIGURE 11-5. Osteoarthritis. Severe osteoarthritis of the hands affecting the DIP joints (Heberden's nodes) and the PIP joints (Bouchard's nodes). (Reproduced with permission from Fauci AS et al. *Harrison's Principles of Internal Medicine,* 17th ed. New York: McGraw-Hill, 2008, Fig. 326-2.)

DIAGNOSIS

OA is diagnosed by an overall clinical impression based on the history and physical as well as on radiographic findings (joint space narrowing that is frequently asymmetric [see Figure 11-6], subchondral sclerosis, and osteophytes) and labs (which are normal).

TREATMENT

- 1° treatment consists of nonpharmacologic interventions such as weight loss, physiotherapy, and low-impact exercise.
- If medicating, start with acetaminophen or NSAIDs for mild symptoms. Complementary and alternative treatments include glucosamine and acupuncture. Intra-articular corticosteroid injections may be added for further pain control.
- Joint replacement is used for severe OA in patients who fail medical management and have marked limitation of their daily activities.

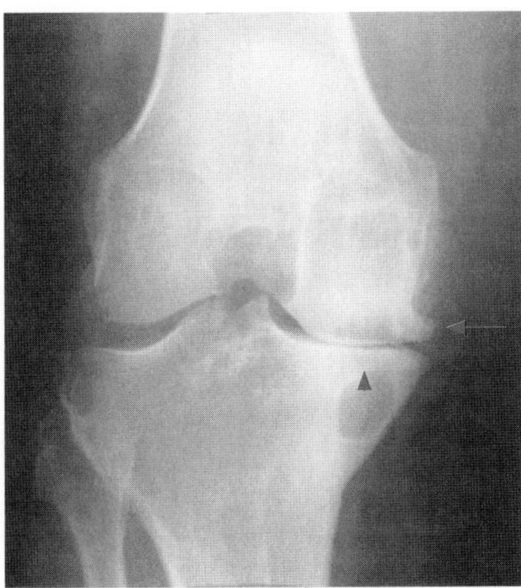

FIGURE 11-6. Radiographic changes in knee osteoarthritis. AP knee radiograph shows a narrowed joint space on the medial side of the joint only; subchondral sclerosis (arrowhead) and a cyst (lucency below the arrowhead); and osteophytes (arrow). (Reproduced with permission from Chen MY et al. *Basic Radiology.* New York: McGraw-Hill, 2004, Fig. 7-40.)

Low Back Pain (LBP)

A 69-year-old man presents with back pain of > 1 year's duration that radiates down his legs. He reports that the pain worsens when he walks downhill but is relieved with he walks uphill or bends over. You diagnose presumed spinal stenosis and order an MRI. You should ask about changes in bowel and bladder function to rule out what complication?

Cauda equina syndrome.

The leading cause of missed workdays in the United States. Table 11-4 outlines the common causes of LBP.

Diagnosis

- Order a stat MRI if you suspect cauda equina syndrome. Assess the range of motion of the lower back. Localize the lower back tenderness to the spine or the paraspinal area.
- Conduct a neurologic exam to determine if the spinal nerves are affected (see Table 11-5).
- Suspect spinal cord involvement if the Babinski reflex is upgoing or if there is sphincter laxity. Remember, an **UP**going toe is an **UP**per motor neuron sign.
- A ⊕ **straight leg raise test** (in which a supine patient experiences leg, buttock, or back pain in the affected leg at < 30° of elevation of the affected leg) is sensitive for spinal nerve irritation or radiculopathy. A ⊕ **crossed straight leg raise test** (in which a supine patient experiences leg, buttock, or back pain in the affected leg at < 30° of elevation of the **unaffected** leg) is specific for spinal nerve irritation.
- Order a **lumbar spine x-ray** for patients in whom osteomyelitis, cancer, fractures, or ankylosing spondylitis is suspected or for those who fail to improve after 2–4 weeks of conservative therapy. Consider screening for osteoporosis if fractures are seen on x-ray.
- An MRI should be ordered if the patient has neurologic deficits for which surgery is being considered.

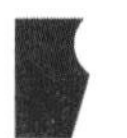

KEY FACT

Order x-rays in geriatric patients with new-onset back pain or if the history and physical are suggestive of malignancy, infection, or inflammatory arthropathy.

Treatment

- Patients with cauda equina syndrome, spinal stenosis, or spinal nerve involvement require surgical evaluation. Degenerative LBP is treated with NSAIDs and physiotherapy. Heavy lifting should be avoided. Ankylosing spondylitis is treated with TNF inhibitors and physiotherapy.
- Most LBP from disk herniation will improve within six weeks; surgery should be considered in cases of progressive neurologic deficits.

TABLE 11-4. Causes of Lower Back Pain

	Symptoms/Exam	Tests
Cauda equina syndrome	Bowel and bladder incontinence or retention, saddle anesthesia. **A medical emergency.**	Order a stat MRI if cauda equina is suspected.
Degenerative processes	Chronic and progressive. **Degeneration of disks** leads to localized pain that can also refer to adjacent spinal nerves (eg, pain that radiates down the thigh). Severe disk disease can lead to **spinal stenosis** in which LBP worsens with standing and walking but improves with sitting or stooping forward (patients typically find it easier to walk uphill than downhill).	Order a lumbar spine x-ray to rule out other causes of LBP.
Neoplastic	1° or metastatic to bone. Suspect in elderly patients with unintentional weight loss or a history of cancer.	A tumor mass may be seen on lumbar spine x-ray. Bone scan or MRI can detect disease not seen on plain film.
Traumatic	Acute onset of LBP is temporally associated with a traumatic event. Look for local spinal tenderness 2° to a **fracture** or a **herniated disk** (pain worsens with cough; L4 or L5 nerve root compression). Perispinal tenderness indicates **myofascial strain.**	CT may be necessary to confirm a fracture and to assess the spinal columns for stability. Myofascial strain and disk herniations cannot be seen.
Osteomyelitis	Fever, chills, or IV drug use. **ESR** will often be ↑↑.	X-ray may show disk narrowing and endplate destruction. MRI may be needed to aid in diagnosis and to assess for epidural abscess.
Ankylosing spondylitis	The typical patient is a young adult male presenting with chronic LBP that is worse in the morning and with sacroiliitis/arthritis of the hip, knee, or shoulder. Acute anterior uveitis, restriction of chest wall expansion, dactylitis, Achilles tendinitis, plantar fasciitis. Reduced spinal mobility.	AP pelvic x-ray shows pseudo-widening, erosions, and sclerosis of the sacroiliac joint. The classic "bamboo spine" on lumbar x-ray is from ossification of spinal ligaments. HLA-B27 is 90% sensitive in Caucasians.
Referred	Can be 2° to disease from the aorta, kidneys, ureter, or pancreas.	Conduct a thorough abdominal exam.

TABLE 11-5. Spinal Nerve Damage and Associated Sensorimotor Deficits

Spinal Nerve	Motor Deficits	Sensory Deficit	Reflexes
L3, L4	Problems rising from a chair and heel walking.	Over the anterior knee or the medial calf.	↓ knee jerk.
L5	Problems heel walking, extending the big toe, or dorsiflexing the ankle.	Over the medial aspect of the foot.	
S1	Problems toe walking or plantar flexing the ankle.	Over the lateral aspect of the foot.	↓ ankle jerk.

Common Orthopedic Injuries

Tables 11-6 and 11-7 outline common adult and childhood orthopedic injuries.

TABLE 11-6. Common Adult Orthopedic Injuries

Injury	Mechanics	Treatment
Shoulder dislocation	Most commonly an anterior dislocation with the **axillary artery and nerve** at risk. Posterior dislocations are associated with seizures and electrocutions and can injure the **radial artery.** Patients with anterior injuries hold the arm in external rotation; those with posterior injuries hold the arm in internal rotation.	Closed reduction followed by a sling and swath. Recurrent dislocations may need surgical repair.
Hip dislocation	Most often a posterior dislocation via a posteriorly directed force on **an internally rotated, flexed,** adducted hip **("dashboard injury").** Anterior dislocations can injure the obturator nerve; posterior dislocations can injure the sciatic nerve and cause avascular necrosis (AVN).	Closed reduction followed by abduction pillow/bracing. Evaluate with CT scan after reduction.
Colles' fracture	**The most common wrist fracture.** Involves the distal radius and commonly results from a **fall onto an outstretched hand,** resulting in a dorsally displaced, dorsally angulated fracture. Commonly seen in the **elderly** (osteoporosis) and in children.	Closed reduction followed by application of a long-arm cast. Open reduction may be needed if the fracture is intra-articular.
Boxer's fracture	Fracture of the fifth metacarpal neck. Often results from forward trauma of a **closed fist** (eg, punching a wall, an individual's jaw, or another fixed object).	Closed reduction and ulnar gutter splint; percutaneous pinning if the fracture is excessively angulated. If skin is broken, assume infection by human oral pathogens **("fight bite")** and treat with surgical irrigation, debridement, and IV antibiotics to cover ***Eikenella.***
Humerus fracture	Results from direct trauma and puts the **radial nerve** at risk (the nerve travels in the spiral groove of the humerus). Signs of radial nerve palsy include **wrist drop** and loss of thumb abduction.	Hanging arm cast vs. coaptation splint and sling. Functional bracing.
Hip fracture	**Most common in osteoporotic women** who sustain a fall. Patients present with a **shortened and externally rotated leg.** Displaced femoral neck fractures are associated with a high risk of AVN and fracture nonunion. Patients are at risk for subsequent DVTs.	Open or percutaneous reduction with internal fixation with parallel pinning of the femoral neck. Displaced fractures in elderly patients (those > 80 years of age) may require a hip hemiarthroplasty. **Anticoagulation** is necessary for DVT prevention.
Achilles tendon rupture	Most commonly seen in unfit men who rupture while participating in sports and hear a sudden **"pop" like a rifle shot.** Exam shows **limited plantar flexion** and a ⊕ **Thompson test** (squeezing the gastrocnemius does not result in foot plantar flexion).	Treatment is with a long-leg cast for six weeks or surgical repair.

TABLE 11-6. Common Adult Orthopedic Injuries *(continued)*

INJURY	MECHANICS	TREATMENT
Knee injuries	Present with knee instability and possibly edema and hematoma. ■ **ACL:** Results from forced hyperflexion; anterior drawer and Lachman's tests are ⊕. Rule out a meniscal or MCL injury. ■ **PCL:** Results from forced hyperextension; posterior drawer test is ⊕. ■ **Meniscal tears: Clicking or locking** may be present. Exam shows **joint line tenderness** and a ⊕ McMurray's test.	Treatment of MCL/LCL and meniscal tears is conservative unless tears are associated with symptoms or concurrent ligamentous injuries. Treatment of ACL injuries is generally surgical reconstruction with graft from the patellar or hamstring tendons. Operative PCL repairs are reserved for highly competitive athletes. Bucket-handle meniscal tears are generally treated arthroscopically. Other tears are treated conservatively.

(Adapted with permission from Le T et al. *First Aid for the USMLE Step 2 CK,* 7th ed. New York: McGraw-Hill, 2010: 257–258.)

TABLE 11-7. Common Pediatric Orthopedic Injuries

INJURY	CHARACTERISTICS	TREATMENT
Clavicular fracture	**The most commonly fractured long bone in children.** May be birth related (especially in large infants), and can be associated with **brachial nerve palsies.** Usually involve the **middle third of the clavicle,** with the proximal fracture end displaced superiorly due to the pull of the sternocleidomastoid muscle.	Figure-of-eight sling vs. arm sling. The need for surgical repair depends on the amount of displacement and the patient's level of function.
Greenstick fracture	Incomplete fracture involving the cortex of only one side of the bone.	Reduction with casting. Order films at 7–10 days.
Nursemaid's elbow	**Radial head subluxation** that typically occurs as a result of being **pulled or lifted by the hand.** The child complains of pain and **will not bend the elbow.**	Manual reduction by gentle supination of the elbow at 90° of flexion. No immobilization is necessary.
Osgood-Schlatter disease	Overuse apophysitis of the tibial tubercle. Causes localized pain, especially with quadriceps contraction, in active young boys.	↓ activity for 1–2 years. A neoprene brace may provide symptomatic relief.
Salter-Harris fractures	Fractures of the growth plate in children. Classified by fracture location (see also Figure 11-7): ■ **I:** Physis (growth plate). ■ **II:** Metaphysis and physis. ■ **III:** Epiphysis and physis. ■ **IV:** Epiphysis, metaphysis, and physis. ■ **V:** Crush injury of physis. **SALTeR-Harris: S**lipped, **A**bove, **L**ower (be**L**ow), **T**hrough, **R**uined (c**R**ushed).	Types I and II can generally be treated nonoperatively. Others, including unstable fractures, must be treated operatively to prevent complications such as leg length inequality.

(Adapted with permission from Le T et al. *First Aid for the USMLE Step 2 CK,* 7th ed. New York: McGraw-Hill, 2010: 273.)

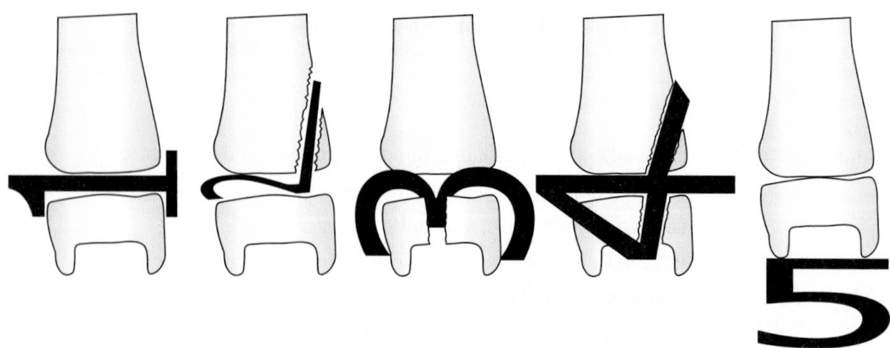

FIGURE 11-7. Mnemonic for Salter-Harris fractures. Imagine the number of the type drawn through the epiphyseal plate. Type 1 is a fracture of the growth plate (physis). Type 2 is a metaphyseal fracture. Type 3 is an epiphyseal fracture. Type 4 goes through both. This mnemonic doesn't work well for type 5, so you just have to remember it is a crush injury of the physis.

Temporal Arteritis (Giant Cell Arteritis)

A 73-year-old woman comes to your office, a small rural clinic with no vascular surgeon. She complains of a headache that has developed over the past month and is now accompanied by severe jaw pain when she chews her food. She has a palpable tender chord on her right temple, and you strongly suspect temporal arteritis. Should you wait to start systemic corticosteroids until she can get a temporal artery biopsy?

No. It may be possible to get an accurate diagnostic biopsy weeks to months after starting treatment, but blindness resulting from temporal arteritis is permanent.

Affects older women more often than men by a ratio of 2:1. Can cause **blindness** 2° to occlusion of the **central retinal artery** (a branch of the internal carotid artery). Half of patients also have polymyalgia rheumatica.

Symptoms/Exam

- Classic symptoms consist of a new headache and scalp tenderness (eg, pain combing hair), **temporal tenderness, jaw claudication,** and visual symptoms such as **monocular blindness.**
- Temporal arteritis is also associated with weight loss, myalgias/arthralgias, and fever.

Diagnosis

Obtain an **ESR** (often > 100 mm/hr), a prompt ophthalmologic evaluation, and a **temporal artery biopsy.** Biopsy will reveal thrombosis; necrosis of the media; and lymphocytes, plasma cells, and giant cells.

Treatment

- Treat immediately with **high-dose prednisone** (40–60 mg/day) and continue for 1–2 months before tapering. Do not delay treatment, as blindness is permanent.
- Conduct serial eye exams for improvements or changes. Complications other than blindness can include angina, stroke, and aortic aneurysm.

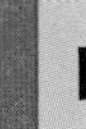

Polymyalgia Rheumatica

An inflammatory disease that causes severe pain and stiffness in proximal muscle groups without weakness or atrophy. Risk factors include female gender and age > 50. PMR is associated with giant cell arteritis, which may precede, coincide with, or follow polymyalgia symptoms.

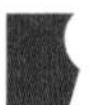

KEY FACT

Polymyalgia causes **P**ain but not weakness.

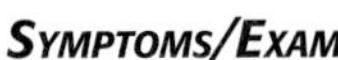

Symptoms/Exam

- Typical symptoms include **pain and stiffness of the shoulder and pelvic girdle** areas with **fever,** malaise, weight loss, and minimal joint swelling.
- Patients classically have difficulty getting out of a chair or lifting their arms above their heads but have **no objective weakness.**

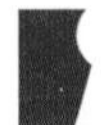

KEY FACT

Long-term steroid use can cause osteoporosis. Screen for bone loss with DEXA scans. Prevent and treat osteoporosis with calcium, vitamin D, weight-bearing exercise, and, when necessary, bisphosphonates.

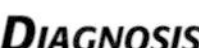

Diagnosis

Look for concurrent **anemia** and an ↑↑ **ESR.**

Treatment

Treat with **low-dose prednisone** (20 mg/day) followed by a long taper. Pain due to polymyalgia responds rapidly to corticosteroids (in 2–4 days).

Fibromyalgia

A chronic pain disorder characterized by soft tissue and axial skeletal pain in the absence of joint pain or inflammation. It is thought to be a central amplification of pain sensory signals. It is typically a diagnosis of exclusion and can be frustrating to manage.

Symptoms/Exam

- Presents as a syndrome of myalgias, insomnia, weakness, and fatigue in the absence of inflammation; laboratory testing is ⊖.
- Associated with depression, anxiety, and irritable bowel syndrome; affects **women** more than men, and prevalence ↑ with age.

Diagnosis

The research criteria used for diagnosis require 11 of 18 tender **trigger points** (see Figure 11-8) that reproduce pain with palpation.

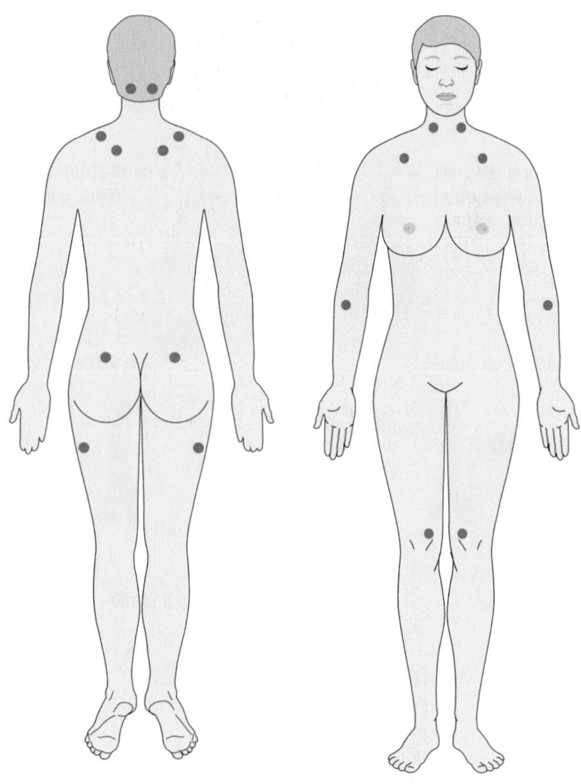

FIGURE 11-8. Trigger points in fibromyalgia. (Reproduced with permission from Le T et al. *First Aid for the USMLE Step 2 CK*, 7th ed. New York: McGraw-Hill, 2010: 265.)

Treatment

- Treatment includes pregabalin (Lyrica), progressive physical reconditioning, improving restorative sleep, and supportive measures such as heat application.
- Consider hydrotherapy, transcutaneous electrical nerve stimulation (TENS), stress reduction, psychotherapy, or low-dose antidepressants.

Polymyositis

A progressive, systemic connective tissue disease characterized by striated muscle inflammation. One-third of patients have **dermatomyositis** with coexisting cutaneous involvement. Patients may also develop myocarditis, pulmonary fibrosis, cardiac conduction deficits, or malignancy. More commonly seen in **older women** (50–70 years of age).

Symptoms/Exam

- **Symmetric**, progressive proximal muscle weakness sometimes accompanied by pain results in the classic complaint of difficulty rising from a chair. Patients may have trouble swallowing and difficulty with phonation, and they may eventually have difficulty breathing. Dyspnea may also be a sign of associated pulmonary fibrosis.

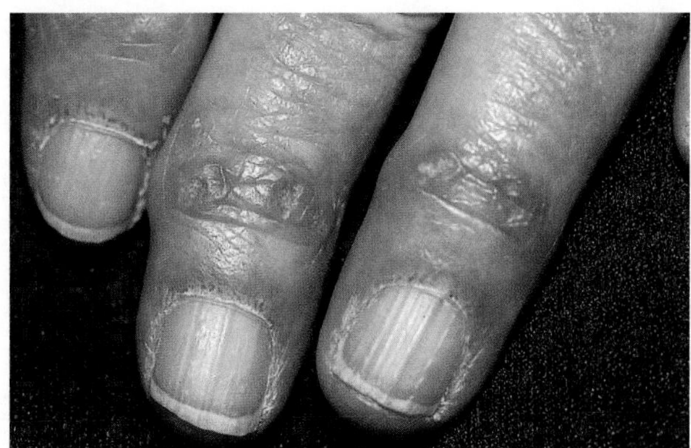

FIGURE 11-9. Gottron's papules in dermatomyositis. Fingers of an elderly woman with classic dermatomyositis. Note the fully formed Gottron's papules over the DIP joints, a hallmark cutaneous feature of dermatomyositis, along with the prominent nail-fold telangiectasias and dystrophic cuticles. The combination of Gottron's papules and nail-fold changes is pathognomonic for dermatomyositis. (Reproduced with permission from Wolff K et al. *Fitzpatrick's Dermatology in General Medicine,* 7th ed. New York: McGraw-Hill, 2008, Fig. 157-5.)

- Dermatomyositis may present with a **heliotrope rash** (a violaceous periorbital rash) and **Gottron's papules** (papules located on the dorsum of the hands over bony prominences; see Figure 11-9).

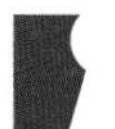

KEY FACT

Evaluate patients with dermatomyositis (more so than with polymyositis) for possible malignancy.

Diagnosis

- Look for ↑ **serum creatinine, aldolase,** and **CK.**
- EMG demonstrates fibrillations. Muscle biopsy, which is necessary for definitive diagnosis, shows inflammatory cells and muscle degeneration.

Treatment

- High-dose **corticosteroids** generally result in improved muscle strength in 4–6 weeks and are then tapered to the lowest effective dose for maintenance.
- Disease-modifying agents such as methotrexate may be used as steroid-sparing therapy or for refractory symptoms.

Scleroderma

A 64-year-old woman with diffuse scleroderma and stable angina underwent an echocardiogram and was found to have pulmonary hypertension. What medication, although typically prescribed for other purposes, is a possible treatment for pulmonary hypertension?

Sildenafil. Remember, however, that nitrates such as sublingual nitroglycerin are strongly contraindicated for 24 hours after the use of sildenafil or other PDE-5 inhibitors.

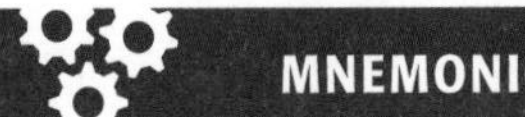

CREST syndrome:

Calcinosis
Raynaud's phenomenon
Esophageal dysmotility
Sclerodactyly
Telangiectasias

A multisystem disease with **symmetric thickening** of the skin on the face and extremities. It typically affects **women** 30–65 years of age. Diagnosis is clinical, supported by immunology and biopsy. There are two subtypes: limited and systemic (see Table 11-8).

TABLE 11-8. Limited vs. Diffuse Scleroderma

	LIMITED (CREST)	DIFFUSE
Skin involvement	Distal, face only	Generalized
Progression	Slow	Rapid
Immunologic finding	Anticentromere antibody	Anti-Scl-70 antibody
Prognosis	Fair	Poor
Calcinosis	+++	+
Telangiectasia	+++	+
Renal failure	0	++
Pulmonary interstitial fibrosis	+	+++

CHAPTER 12

NEPHROLOGY

Electrolytes

SODIUM

Hyponatremia

A 65-year-old man is brought to the ER because his family insists that he is "just not himself." His wife thinks that he has been excessively thirsty lately, and she also notes a worsening cough but no fever. The man has a past medical history of smoking and CAD. A basic metabolic panel shows a serum sodium level of 115 mEq/L. What are the next steps in diagnosis?

Basic steps in evaluating hyponatremia include assessing volume status and checking serum osmolality, urine osmolality, and urine sodium. Given this patient's worsening cough, you might also consider a CXR, as this may be relevant in the setting of SIADH.

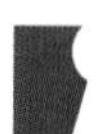

KEY FACT

In pseudohyponatremia, measured serum sodium may be falsely ↓ by hyperlipidemia or hyperproteinemia.

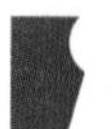

KEY FACT

No, you're **not** an outstanding intern if you ↑ the patient's sodium from 115 mEq/L to 135 mEq/L by the postcall morning. You may be able to bump hyponatremia to the bottom of your problem list, but central pontine myelinolysis will go to spot number one!

Defined as a serum sodium level of < 135 mEq/L.

SYMPTOMS

- Often asymptomatic, but may present with **confusion, lethargy,** muscle cramps, and nausea.
- When serum sodium is low or rapidly decreasing, hyponatremia may lead to cerebral edema that may result in seizures, status epilepticus, coma, or even death.

DIAGNOSIS

Assess volume status, and check serum osmolality, urine osmolality, and urine sodium (see Figure 12-1).

TREATMENT

- **Hypovolemic hyponatremia:** Treat with NS or hypertonic (3%) NS.
- **Euvolemic hyponatremia:** If the patient is symptomatic, give hypertonic NS with furosemide. If asymptomatic, fluid restrict to 1 L/day.
- Note that overly rapid correction may result in central pontine myelinolysis (flaccid paralysis, dysarthria, dysphagia, and gait abnormalities). Maximum target correction should not exceed 8–10 mEq/L/day.

Hypernatremia

Defined as a serum sodium level of > 147 mEq/L.

SYMPTOMS

Hyperpnea, weakness, restlessness, insomnia, altered mental status, coma.

DIAGNOSIS

- Assess volume status, urine output, urine osmolality, and urine sodium.
- Hypernatremia from **hypovolemia** usually presents in the setting of dehydration, when the patient has **limited access to free water.** U_{osm} is usually > 700 mOsm/kg. Causes include ↑ insensible losses (burns, sweating, endotracheal intubation) and diarrhea.

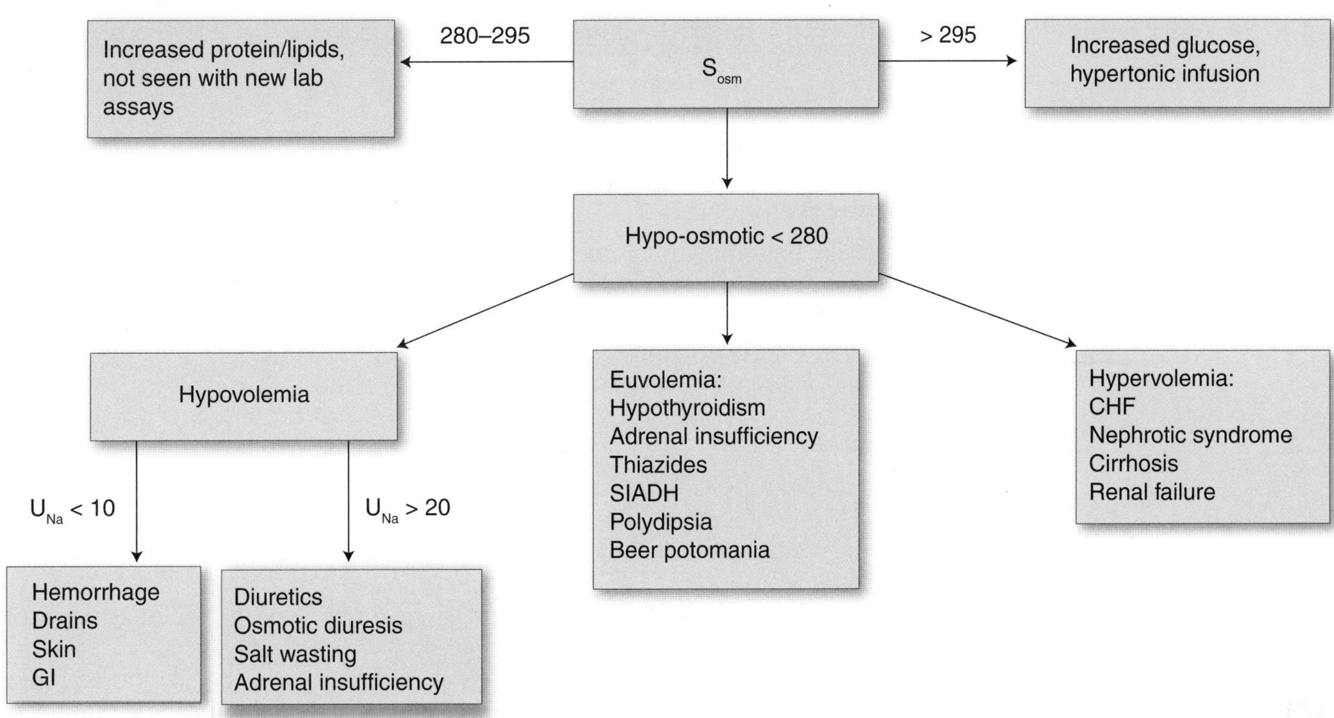

FIGURE 12-1. Evaluation of hyponatremia.

- Hypernatremia from ↑ **total body sodium** generally does **not** present with hypovolemia. Causes include excessive hydration with hypertonic fluids, dysfunction of central regulation, and mineralocorticoid excess (consider if the patient has hypokalemia and hypertension).
- Hypernatremia from **renal losses** (see Table 12-3) usually occurs in the setting of hypovolemia and a U_{osm} < 700 mOsm/kg. Consider the clinical context in the setting of the U_{osm}/P_{osm} ratio to help determine the cause.

KEY FACT

Hypernatremia often occurs with dehydration when a patient has no access to free water. Envision a salty desert.

Treatment

- Always treat underlying causes (eg, DDAVP for central DI; a low-salt diet and thiazides for nephrogenic DI).
- Correct the free-water deficit with hypotonic saline, D_5W, or oral water depending on the patient's volume status.
- To prevent cerebral edema, do not correct hypernatremia at rate of > 12 mEq/L/day.

TABLE 12-3. Causes of Hypernatremia 2° to Renal Losses

	Etiology	Comments
Osmotic diuresis	**Causes:** Mannitol, hyperglycemia, high-protein feeds, postobstructive diuresis.	U_{osm}/P_{osm} > 0.7.
Central DI	The pituitary does not make ADH. **Causes:** Tumor, trauma, neurosurgery, infection.	U_{osm}/P_{osm} < 0.7. U_{osm} should ↑ by 50% in response to DDAVP.
Nephrogenic DI	The kidneys are unresponsive to ADH. **Causes:** Renal failure, hypercalcemia, demeclocycline, lithium, sickle cell anemia.	U_{osm}/P_{osm} < 0.7. U_{osm} should not respond to DDAVP challenge.

POTASSIUM

Hypokalemia

Defined as a serum potassium level of < 3.5 mEq/L.

Symptoms

- May present with fatigue, muscle weakness or cramps, ileus, hyporeflexia, paresthesias, and flaccid paralysis if severe.
- ECG may show T-wave flattening, U waves (an additional wave after the T wave), ST-segment depression, and QT prolongation followed by AV block and subsequent cardiac arrest.

Diagnosis

- Order an ECG and check urine potassium.
- **Urine potassium > 20 mEq/L:** Usually indicates that the kidneys are wasting potassium. Acid-base status must be examined to further stratify the etiology.
  - **Metabolic acidosis:** Type I RTA (eg, amphotericin), lactic acidosis, or ketoacidosis.
  - **Metabolic alkalosis:** 1° or 2° hyperaldosteronism (check plasma renin activity and plasma aldosterone concentration), Cushing's syndrome (check 24-hour urine cortisol), diuretics (loop or thiazide), vomiting, NG suction.
  - **Variable pH:** Gentamicin, platinum-containing chemotherapeutic agents, hypomagnesemia.
- **Urine potassium < 20 mEq/L:** Usually indicates a nonrenal source of hypokalemia. This could be from **transcellular shift** (eg, insulin, β_2-agonists, alkalosis, periodic paralysis) or from **GI losses** (eg, diarrhea, chronic laxative abuse).

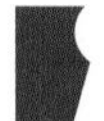

KEY FACT

The main determinant of urinary potassium wasting is urinary flow rate. The greater the urine volume production, the more potassium is wasted.

Treatment

- Treat the underlying disorder.
- Provide oral and/or IV **potassium repletion.** Replete cautiously in patients with renal insufficiency
- Replace **magnesium,** as this deficiency makes potassium repletion more difficult.

Hyperkalemia

A 55-year-old woman with a history of chronic renal insufficiency, likely 2° to hypertension and DM, is in the hospital receiving IV antibiotics for pyelonephritis. On admission, her baseline serum creatinine ↑ from 2.5 to 3.0 mg/dL. She is on her second day of antibiotics and has been afebrile with stable vital signs for the past 24 hours. She is feeling well. A basic metabolic panel this morning shows a serum potassium level of 5.8 mEq/L. You call the laboratory, and they state that the specimen was not hemolyzed. What do you do next?

Get an ECG, as this may show serious signs of hyperkalemia. Next, follow the mnemonic **C BIG K Drop**. Start by administering calcium to stabilize the heart. Then give bicarbonate, insulin, and glucose for a fast-acting but short-lived response. Finally, you can give Kayexalate and furosemide to dispose of the excess potassium. Also make sure you remove any extra potassium from the patient's diet and/or IV fluids.

Defined as a serum potassium level of ≥ 5 mEq/L. Etiologies include the following:

- **Spurious:** Hemolysis (can also ↑ with high platelets or WBCs).
- **Excessive intake:** Ingestion, iatrogenic.
- **Renal:** Renal failure, type IV RTA (see below), adrenal insufficiency (low mineralocorticoid state), drugs (spironolactone, ACEIs, TMP-SMX, digoxin overdose).
- **Cellular release:** Hyperkalemia during acidosis, cell lysis, retroperitoneal hemorrhage.

MNEMONIC

Treatment of hyperkalemia–

C BIG K Drop

Calcium gluconate
Bicarbonate
Insulin
Glucose
Kayexalate
Diuretic/**D**ialysis

Symptoms

- Usually asymptomatic, but may present with muscle weakness and abdominal distention.
- ECG may show tall, peaked T waves and PR prolongation followed by loss of P waves and QRS widening that progress to sine waves, ventricular fibrillation, and cardiac arrest (see Figure 12-2).

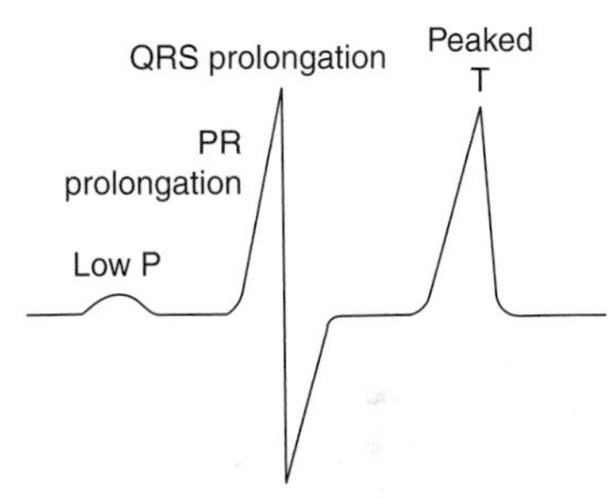

FIGURE 12-2. Effects of hyperkalemia as seen on ECG.

Diagnosis

- Order a repeat blood draw unless suspicion is high.
- Obtain an ECG.
- Urine potassium levels can help determine the etiology of the hyperkalemia.
  - **Urine potassium < 40 mEq/L:** Usually indicates that the hyperkalemia is caused by ↓ potassium excretion by the kidneys. Causes include renal insufficiency, drugs (eg, spironolactone, triamterene, amiloride, ACEIs, TMP, NSAIDs), and mineralocorticoid deficiency (type IV RTA). A plasma renin activity and plasma aldosterone concentration should be ordered if a mineralocorticoid deficiency is suspected.
  - **Urine potassium > 40 mEq/L:** Usually points to a nonrenal etiology. Causes include **cellular shifts** resulting from tissue injury, tumor lysis, insulin deficiency, drugs (eg, succinylcholine, digitalis, arginine, α-blockers), and **iatrogenic** factors.

Treatment

- Values > 6.5 mEq/L or ECG changes (especially PR prolongation or wide QRS) require emergent treatment.
  - **Calcium gluconate** (for cardiac cell membrane stabilization) should be given immediately to prevent arrhythmias,
  - Temporary treatment includes β_2-agonists, insulin and glucose, and sodium bicarbonate.
  - Long-lasting elimination requires Kayexalate and a loop diuretic.
- **Restrict dietary potassium** and discontinue any medications that may be contributing to the hyperkalemia.
- Severe or symptomatic hyperkalemia, hyperkalemia refractory to the above management, or patients on **chronic** hemodialysis may require acute **hemodialysis.**

CALCIUM

Hypocalcemia

- Defined as a serum ionized calcium level of < 8.4 mg/dL.
- **Correct for hypoalbuminemia.** For every 1-mg/dL ↓ in albumin, ↑ the calcium level by 0.8 mg/dL. Alkalosis ↑ calcium binding to albumin.

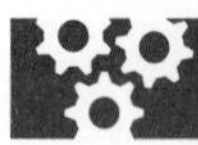

MNEMONIC

Causes of hypocalcemia–

HIPOCAL

Hypoparathyroidism/hypomagnesemia
Infection
Pancreatitis
Overload (rapid volume expansion)
Chronic kidney disease
Absorption abnormalities
Loop diuretics

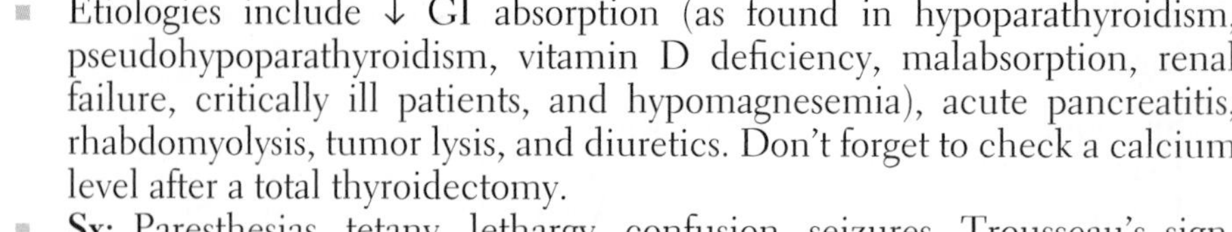

- Etiologies include ↓ GI absorption (as found in hypoparathyroidism, pseudohypoparathyroidism, vitamin D deficiency, malabsorption, renal failure, critically ill patients, and hypomagnesemia), acute pancreatitis, rhabdomyolysis, tumor lysis, and diuretics. Don't forget to check a calcium level after a total thyroidectomy.
- **Sx:** Paresthesias, tetany, lethargy, confusion, seizures, Trousseau's sign, Chvostek's sign, QT prolongation.
- **Tx:** Replace with calcium carbonate orally or with IV calcium gluconate.

Hypercalcemia

Defined as a serum calcium level of > 10.2 mg/dL.

SYMPTOMS

May present with **bones** (fractures), **stones** (kidney stones), abdominal **groans** (anorexia, nausea, constipation), and **psychiatric overtones** (weakness, fatigue, altered mental status). Consider in patients with pancreatitis, refractory peptic ulcer disease, a personal or family history of kidney stones, or bone pain.

DIAGNOSIS

- Inquire about diet and vitamin supplementation.
- Check calcium, phosphate, albumin, ionized calcium, and alkaline phosphatase. Also consider vitamin D levels, SPEP, TSH, and imaging.
- Hyperparathyroidism is a common cause of hypercalcemia, so check PTH and parathyroid hormone–related peptide (PTHrP) levels. To ensure the patient's safety, order an ECG (may show a **short QT interval**).
  - **Elevated PTH:** Indicates that 1° hyperparathyroidism (eg, from adenoma, hyperplasia, carcinoma, or MEN 1/2) is the likely cause (see Chapter 5 for more details). Consider an ectopic PTH-producing tumor as well.
  - **Normal or low PTH:**
    - Indicates that the cause could be excessive calcium or vitamin D intake, granulomatous disease, sarcoidosis, malignancy (eg, hematologic, lymphoproliferative, multiple myeloma, bone metastases), milk-alkali syndrome, or Paget's disease.
    - PTHrP secretion from cancer cells (often squamous cell carcinoma) can cause a paraneoplastic hypercalcemia. The elevated calcium suppresses the normal parathyroid gland, resulting in low PTH levels.
    - Testing options include phosphate, vitamin D, TSH, serum immunoelectrophoresis (for MGUS), alkaline phosphatase (for Paget's), GGT (to determine the origin of the elevated alkaline phosphatase), spot urine calcium, spot urine creatinine, BUN/creatinine, and x-rays/bone scan (to look for lytic lesions).

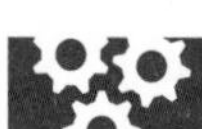

MNEMONIC

Causes of hypercalcemia–

CHIMPANZEES

Calcium supplementation
Hyperparathyroidism
Iatrogenic/**I**mmobility
Milk-alkali syndrome
Paget's disease
Addison's disease/**A**cromegaly
Neoplasm
Zollinger-Ellison syndrome
Excess vitamin A
Excess vitamin D
Sarcoidosis

TREATMENT

- Identify and treat the underlying cause.
- For 1° hyperparathyroidism, parathyroidectomy is needed. In all other cases, additional treatment measures depend on the severity of the hypercalcemia. Possible interventions include the following:
  - Discontinue all drugs that can cause hypercalcemia (eg, thiazides).
  - Place the patient on a low-calcium diet.
  - **Hydrate** and use **furosemide** to ↑ calcium excretion and, if necessary, to prevent volume overload.
- Patients with symptomatic hypercalcemia or a serum calcium level > 14 mg/dL require **IV bisphosphonates** (eg, pamidronate) or **calcitonin.** However, each takes 12–24 hours to have an effect, and the therapeutic benefits of both may be short-lived.
- **Hemodialysis** is a last resort.

Syndrome of Inappropriate Secretion of ADH (SIADH)

A major cause of hyponatremia due to ↑ ADH release without osmolality-dependent or volume-dependent physiologic stimuli. Causes include the following:

- **Pulmonary:** Small cell carcinoma, TB, pneumonia, pulmonary abscess. Consider ordering a CXR.
- **CNS:** Meningitis, brain abscess, head trauma. Consider ordering a head CT.
- **Drugs:** Clofibrate, chlorpropamide, phenothiazine, carbamazepine.
- **Ectopic ADH production:** Lymphoma, sarcoma, duodenal/pancreatic cancer.

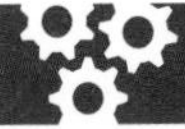

MNEMONIC

Causes of SIADH–

BCDE

Breathing (pulmonary)
CNS
Drugs
Ectopic

DIFFERENTIAL

Hypothyroidism; consumption of too much water with not enough salt (psychogenic polydipsia, beer potomania).

DIAGNOSIS

- Asymptomatic unless serum sodium becomes very low (< 120 mEq/L).
- Check plasma and urine osmolalities and sodium. Findings include P_{osm} < 270 mOsm/kg; U_{osm} > 100 mOsm/kg; euvolemia; and normal renal, adrenal, and thyroid function. **SIADH cannot be diagnosed in a hypovolemic patient regardless of plasma or urine osmolalities.**

TREATMENT

- Fluid restriction (free-water consumption < 1 L/day). If response is inadequate, add demeclocycline to antagonize ADH.
- Treat symptomatic hyponatremia with hypertonic saline (see the discussion of hyponatremia). Do not give patients with SIADH NS, as this can paradoxically worsen the hyponatremia.

Acute Renal Failure (ARF)

A 65-year-old man who is otherwise healthy comes to your primary care clinic for a routine checkup after getting a set of labs. The patient's serum creatinine is 1.8 mg/dL, up from 1.1 mg/dL three months ago. The patient states that he has been producing plenty of urine, maintaining that he goes to the bathroom every 20 minutes. He adds that his urine "mostly just dribbles out" and that he's not sure if he is completely emptying his bladder, as he feels some fullness in his suprapubic region. On exam, you feel a suprapubic mass. What should you do next?

Evaluate the patient for urinary retention, as this is likely the cause of his renal failure. Consider ordering a bladder scan, a straight catheterization, or placement of a Foley catheter. If the patient has a large postvoid residual, he should keep his Foley in place and be referred to urology. As this condition is most commonly 2° to BPH, consider starting α-blockers and 5α-reductase inhibitors.

A ↓ in GFR (usually corresponding to an ↑ in creatinine of 0.5 mg/dL or > 50% over the baseline value) occurring over a period of hours to days. Results in failure of the kidneys to excrete nitrogenous waste and to maintain fluid and electrolyte balance. Oliguria (defined as < 500 mL/day) is not required for ARF but should prompt one to test for it.

SYMPTOMS/EXAM

- Patients are often asymptomatic but may present with dyspnea, **uremic symptoms** (eg, anorexia, nausea, malaise, hyperpigmented skin, asterixis, pericarditis [listen for a friction rub]), and anemia.
- Examination should include checking BP, daily weights, and assessment of volume status. Other findings are specific to the etiology of the renal failure.

DIAGNOSIS

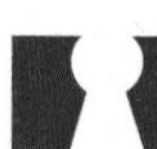

KEY FACT

An Fe_{Na} < 1% suggests prerenal failure.

ARF is categorized as prerenal, intrinsic, or postrenal (see Table 12-4). To determine the etiology, order electrolytes, BUN/creatinine, and a UA with micro and urine eosinophils, and calculate Fe_{Na} (see the discussion of renal basics).

- **Prerenal failure:** Caused by ↓ renal perfusion. Fe_{Na} is usually **< 1%** and the **BUN/creatinine ratio > 20.** Can be due to anything that causes the kidneys to "see" less volume.
  - Listen for a renal artery bruit characteristic of renal artery stenosis.
  - If a bolus of isotonic fluids improves the BUN/creatinine ratio, prerenal failure due to shock is the likely cause, but make sure the patient is not in CHF before giving the bolus!
- **Intrinsic failure:** Can be vascular, glomerular, tubular (most common), or interstitial. Usually presents with **hematuria, proteinuria, and/or casts on UA.**
  - Glomerulonephritis presents with a nephritic syndrome (RBCs/RBC casts).

TABLE 12-4. Causes of Acute Renal Failure

Prerenal	Intrinsic	Postrenal
Dehydration (anorexia, burns, GI losses) ACEIs, NSAIDs Renal artery stenosis All causes of shock (eg, cardiogenic, hypovolemic) Hepatorenal syndrome Cardiomyopathies	**Interstitial:** Acute interstitial nephritis (eg, penicillins, systemic infections) **Glomerular:** Nephritides **Tubular:** ATN (often drug induced, eg, aminoglycosides, radiocontrast) **Vascular:** Emboli, occlusion, vasculitis, renal vein thrombosis	**Ureteral stenosis:** Papillary necrosis, stones, blood clot, retroperitoneal fibrosis **Bladder neck:** Anticholinergics, tumor **Prostate:** BPH, cancer, prostatitis

  - Acute interstitial nephritis yields a UA with eosinophils, WBCs, and WBC casts.
  - ATN presents with an $Fe_{Na} > 1\%$ and a urine sediment with pigmented granular ("muddy brown") casts and renal tubular epithelial cells.
  - Suspect a vascular cause in predisposed patients (eg, those with a hypercoagulable state) presenting with abdominal pain.
- **Postrenal failure:** Caused by urinary outflow obstructions in one or both ureters, the bladder neck, the urethra, or the prostate. Patients can present in fluid overload from urinary retention.
  - Determine a **postvoid residual**—ie, have the patient urinate, and then insert a Foley catheter to measure the urine remaining in the bladder. A postvoid residual of > 75 mL points to bladder outlet obstruction (from a large prostate, a high bladder neck, or a urethral stricture) or indicates that the bladder is unable to contract fully.
  - **Renal ultrasound** or CT scan can detect hydronephrosis.
  - Men should have a prostate exam in cases of postrenal failure.

Treatment

Treat the underlying cause **and** the sequelae. Protect the kidneys with the following interventions:

- Discontinue nephrotoxic medications, and ↓ any renally excreted medications in proportion to the GFR.
- Avoid contrast studies unless they are essential.
- To keep patients euvolemic, give IV fluids and, if absolutely necessary, furosemide (be careful to prevent further damage!). Volume expansion, however, may not shorten the duration of ATN.
- Initiate a low-potassium diet.
- Monitor and correct calcium, PO_4, and potassium.
- If the pH is < 7.2, bicarbonate may be used to treat a nongap acidosis or to temporize an anion-gap metabolic acidosis (until dialysis).
- Dialyze if indicated (see the mnemonic **AEIOU**).

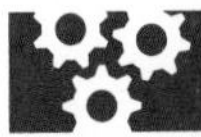

MNEMONIC

Indications for emergent dialysis—

AEIOU

Acidosis
Electrolytes (hyperkalemia)
Ingestion (of toxins)
Overload (volume)
Uremic symptoms (encephalopathy, pericarditis)

Acute Glomerulonephritis

- Relatively acute onset of hypertension, hematuria, edema, and oliguria.
- **Dx:**
  - UA shows microscopic hematuria with RBC casts and dysmorphic red cells. Proteinuria is usually present in subnephrotic ranges.

    - Renal biopsy is the gold standard for diagnosis.
    - Evaluation may also include checking complement levels, ANCA, ANA, anti-dsDNA, cryoglobulin, hepatitis B and C, anti-GBM antibodies, ASO, and blood cultures.
- **Tx:** Treat inflammatory disorders with steroids and cytotoxic agents. In cases 2° to systemic disease, treat the underlying disorder.

Acute Tubular Necrosis (ATN)

The most common form of intrinsic ARF. Usually caused by toxic or ischemic damage. Causes include the following:

- **Exogenous nephrotoxins:** Chemotherapeutic agents (cisplatin, methotrexate) and other immunosuppressants (cyclosporine, tacrolimus), aminoglycosides, amphotericin B, cephalosporins, heavy metals, and radiocontrast dyes (effects can be minimized by hydration and oral N-acetylcysteine).
- **Endogenous nephrotoxins:** Hyperuricemia, rhabdomyolysis, massive intravascular hemolysis, Bence Jones proteins (from multiple myeloma).
- **Ischemia:** All causes of shock. ATN can therefore be a complication of prerenal ARF.

Diagnosis

Check the same labs/studies as one would with other forms of ARF plus a serum CK and uric acid level. Fe_{Na} is usually > 1%, and routine UA shows a sediment with pigmented granular ("muddy brown") casts and renal tubular epithelial cells.

Treatment

- Treat as per ARF. If the patient is ischemic, treat the underlying cause. If toxic, remove or minimize the toxin.
- With rhabdomyolysis, aggressively hydrate to keep urine output > 300 mL/hr; the use of mannitol for diuresis and bicarbonate to alkalinize urine remains controversial.

Contrast Nephropathy

- Characterized by an acute decline in GFR that occurs 24–48 hours after a patient receives IV radiocontrast.
- Risk factors include preexisting renal insufficiency, diabetes, ↓ effective arterial volume, a high volume of contrast, and concomitant nephrotoxic medications.
- Patients with an ↑ risk of developing contrast nephropathy should receive prophylaxis with IV fluids, sodium bicarbonate, and acetylcysteine.
- **Tx:** Treatment is supportive. Contrast nephropathy usually resolves in one week.

Chronic Kidney Disease (CKD)

An irreversible or only partially reversible state in which the kidneys have lost the ability to regulate some combination of the body's fluid state, electrolyte levels, and acid-base status. Erythropoiesis and vitamin D metabolism are often compromised as well.

SYMPTOMS/EXAM

- May be asymptomatic, or may present with a clinical picture that appears inconsistent with the severity of the disease. If mild or gradual, other organ systems may compensate (eg, hyperventilation to blow off CO_2).
- As CKD worsens—ie, as GFR approaches zero—uremic and anemic symptoms worsen, and patients appear progressively more ill.
- Urine volume may remain normal despite marked changes in serum (elevation) or urine (reduction) electrolytes, urea nitrogen levels, and creatinine. Urine output will ↓ as CKD reaches a terminal stage.

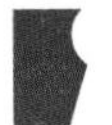

KEY FACT

Urine volume may be completely normal in acute and chronic renal failure.

DIAGNOSIS

- A serum creatinine that is persistently > 1.4 mg/dL is generally considered diagnostic. Lower cutoffs are applied to patients with less muscle mass (often shorter or older patients), particularly women, and higher cutoffs to large, muscular patients (remember to examine the labs **and** the patient).
- Etiologies vary, and appropriate identification of the cause is critical to preventing disease progression. Most causes are similar to those of ARF and include the following:
  - **ARF:** Persistent ARF can lead to CKD. Identifying what caused the ARF remains important (see the earlier discussion).
  - **Prerenal causes:** Addison's disease, CHF, cirrhosis.
  - **Intrinsic renal disease:** Diabetes, hypertension, drugs, glomerulonephritis, malignancy, hereditary renal disease, renal vascular disease. Diabetes and hypertension are the most common causes of CKD.
  - **Postrenal causes:** Includes anything that causes postrenal obstruction, such as kidney stones, compression of the ureters (eg, masses, scarring), neurogenic bladder, and an enlarged prostate.
- Note that high-protein diets, rhabdomyolysis, and certain medications (eg, cimetidine, TMP) can ↓ creatinine excretion, in which case serum creatinine may be high without renal impairment.

TREATMENT

- Detect and treat any reversible causes. Follow the indications for dialysis as laid out in the discussion of ARF.
- For intrinsic renal disease, it is important to optimize the kidney in other respects—ie, to control hypertension, avoid nephrotoxic drugs, control blood glucose level, restrict protein intake, and control lipids. Patients should be placed on a renal diet to prevent a high potassium load.
- Long-term treatment often involves erythropoietin (if the patient is anemic), vitamin D, phosphate binders, and calcium. Bicarbonate may be used for severe acidosis.
- Prepare the patient for dialysis. Avoid IVs in the arm that will be used for AV shunts.
- The only definitive treatment for irreversible end-stage renal disease is transplantation.

Hematuria

Defined as three or more RBCs/hpf on urine microscopy. Gross hematuria is present when blood is visible to the naked eye.

DIFFERENTIAL

Pseudohematuria is defined as urine that gives the false impression of hematuria either grossly or by laboratory testing. It may result from certain drugs,

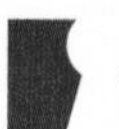

KEY FACT

Remember—true hematuria must have RBCs.

foods, or dyes that cause myoglobinuria, hemoglobinuria, or simple discoloration of urine.

DIAGNOSIS

- Patients with gross hematuria should have a UA to rule out UTI, nephrolithiasis (indicated by crystals on urine microscopy), and tubulointerstitial nephritis (indicated by urine WBCs, WBC casts, and/or eosinophils, though less common). If the UA shows RBC casts or the daily urinary protein is > 1 g, suspect a glomerular cause for the hematuria (see the discussion of nephritic syndrome below).
- First repeat the UA, as there are benign causes for isolated hematuria, such as vigorous exercise. If an infection is evident, treat the infection and then repeat the UA to confirm resolution of the hematuria with elimination of the infection.
- In all patients with confirmed hematuria, check PTT, PT, and platelets to determine if any coagulopathy is present. Male patients should undergo a prostate exam to look for BPH or prostatitis as a cause of the hematuria. Urine cytology can be sent if there is reason to suspect bladder cancer (eg, smoking, exposure to organic compounds). If the initial workup is ⊖ or hematuria persists despite treatment, proceed as follows:
  - Look for **upper tract** (renal and ureteral) causes of hematuria by ordering an IVP, a CT urogram, or a renal ultrasound to look for renal masses, polycystic kidneys, or hydronephrosis/hydroureter that may be 2° to nephrolithiasis.
  - If no upper tract cause can be found, cystoscopy can look for **lower tract** causes of hematuria, such as interstitial cystitis, or bladder cancer.
  - If the workup is still ⊖ and suspicion is high, a **renal angiogram** may be ordered to look for vascular causes (eg, renal vein thrombosis, varices, aneurysms, AVMs).

Proteinuria

Urinary protein excretion of > 150 mg/24 hrs. **Nephrotic syndrome** consists of severe proteinuria that is defined as a daily urinary protein excretion of > 3.5 g (see the following section). Microalbuminuria is defined as a **persistent** daily urinary protein excretion of 30–300 mg in a patient with diabetes. Transient microalbuminuria can occur with infection, stress, and illness.

SYMPTOMS/EXAM

Presentation is generally unremarkable unless the patient has nephrotic-range proteinuria. In such instances, patients usually present with generalized edema and/or frothy urine.

DIAGNOSIS

To ascertain the cause of proteinuria, it is important to know the quantity and type of protein involved. To determine this, proceed as follows (see also Table 12-5):

- Obtain a 24-hour urine collection to quantify daily urinary protein excretion. If this is not possible, check a urine protein/creatinine ratio (normal is < 0.2; nephrotic syndrome is > 3.0).
- Check a UA, electrolytes, BUN/creatinine, urine protein electrophoresis, and serum total protein.
- Examine urine sediment. A benign appearance suggests benign causes, while red cells and casts suggest acute nephritic syndrome, and fat bodies

TABLE 12-5. Location of Renal Disease in Proteinuria

Location	Urine Protein	Lab Findings	Etiologies
Interstitial nephritis	< 2 g/24 hrs	Routine UA shows WBCs, WBC casts, and eosinophils.	Infection, medications (NSAIDs, quinolones, sulfonamides, rifampin), connective tissue diseases (SLE, sarcoidosis, Sjögren's syndrome).
Glomerular disease	> 2 g/24 hrs	Routine UA shows RBCs or RBC casts.	See the discussion of nephritic and nephrotic syndromes.
Overflow proteinuria	< 2 g/24 hrs; mostly light-chain or low-molecular-weight proteins.	↑ serum protein.	Amyloid, multiple myeloma, lymphoproliferative disease, hemoglobin, myoglobin.

point to nephrotic syndrome. (Note the difference between nephritic and nephrotic syndromes.)

- A UA significant only for protein in the absence of other signs of renal disease suggests **benign proteinuria.** Causes include pulmonary edema, CHF, fever, exercise, head injury, CVA, stress, orthostatic proteinuria, and idiopathic factors.

Treatment

- Treat any underlying causes:
  - **Hyponatremia:** Free water restriction.
  - **Peripheral edema:** Furosemide.
  - **Diabetes with microalbuminuria or proteinuria:** Treat diabetes and use ACEIs.
- Proteinuria itself does not require treatment. Patients in whom proteinuria persists for many years are at ↑ risk for renal failure. In these cases, consider a low-salt and low-saturated-fat diet, and limit protein intake to 1 g/kg/day.

Nephrotic Syndrome

A mother brings her two-year-old boy to the clinic because his face seems swollen and he is heavier overall. The child recently had a URI, and you were able to reassure the parents over the phone. Although the child's upper respiratory symptoms have improved, he has grown more fatigued. On exam, you note dependent edema, and you send some labs and a UA, which reveals 3+ protein. Light microscopy shows normal-appearing glomeruli, and biopsy reveals podocyte effacement. What is your diagnosis?

Minimal change disease. The mother is only minimally impressed.

A syndrome of edema, hypoalbuminemia, and severe proteinuria that is defined as > 3.5 g of urinary protein/24 hrs. Patients may also have hyperlipidemia and hypercoagulability. Causes are summarized in Table 12-6.

NOTES

CHAPTER 13

NEUROLOGY

Localization

Localization involves determining **where** a lesion exists in the nervous system. It is the first step in the neurological thought process derived from the history and physical exam. You do not need to know detailed neuroanatomy in order to localize. The following is a list of the major locations for lesions and their associated patterns of findings. See Table 13-1 for a definition of upper motor neuron (UMN) and lower motor neuron (LMN) signs.

- **Muscle:** Proximal limb weakness (eg, hip girdle muscles) in a symmetric pattern; no sensory loss; muscles may be tender.
- **Neuromuscular junction:** Fatigable weakness (ie, weakness that is exacerbated by repetition of movement); the face and proximal limbs are affected; symmetric pattern; no sensory loss.
- **Peripheral nerve:** Distal asymmetric or symmetric pattern; LMN signs; ↓ sensation in a patch innervated by nerve.
- **Root:** Shooting pain in a proximal or distal asymmetric pattern; weakness in movement corresponding to the root; LMN signs; dermatomal sensory change without spinal cord signs.
- **Spinal cord:** Sensory level ("band" with ↓ sensation below); bladder or bowel incontinence or retention; symmetric pattern; UMN signs below the level affected.
- **Brain stem:** Cranial nerve deficits; hemibody UMN signs; hemibody sensory changes; possible stupor or coma; crossed motor and sensory signs (eg, right face and left body).
- **Cerebellum:** Ipsilateral ataxia (distal limbs = cerebellar hemispheres; core body = vermis); nystagmus; dysmetria; breakdown of rapid alternating movements.

TABLE 13-1. UMN vs. LMN Lesions

	UMN Lesions	LMN Lesions
Anatomy	Motor cortex → internal capsule → pons → medulla (pyramidal decussation) → corticospinal tract ("CNS lesions").	Anterior horn cell → plexus → peripheral nerve ("PNS lesions").
Paresis (muscle weakness)	Affects the upper extremity extensors more than the flexors, and the lower extremity flexors more than the extensors.	Affects the distribution of the anterior horn cell, plexus, or peripheral nerve.
Tone	Spasticity.	Flaccidity.
Wasting	Absent.	Present.
DTRs	Hyperactive.	Hypoactive or absent.
Plantar reflexes	Upgoing (⊕ Babinski's).	Downgoing (normal).
Fasciculations	Absent.	Present.
Examples	Strokes, TIA, brain tumors, head trauma, MS, epidural abscess.	Guillain-Barré syndrome, neuropathies, **Bell's palsy,** herpes zoster, Lyme disease, cauda equina syndrome.

- **Subcortical brain:** Hemibody UMN signs; hemibody sensory changes; extrapyramidal signs (rigidity, bradykinesia, tremor); visual field cuts.
- **Cortical brain:** Cortical signs (aphasia → left hemisphere; neglect → right hemisphere, gaze deviation); UMN weakness that is not fully hemibody (eg, face and arm > leg); sensory changes that are not fully hemibody.

For practice in localization, www.lesionlocalizer.com is a useful preparation tool.

KEY FACT

Bell's palsy involves damage to the facial nerve that leads to hemifacial weakness, diminished taste, hyperacusis, ↑ tearing, and variable hyperesthesia of the face.

Stroke

An 81-year-old woman with a history of hypertension presents with sudden onset of left-sided weakness. On exam, she displays left-sided neglect and left facial and arm paralysis with relative sparing of the left leg. Is this likely a large-vessel or a small-vessel stroke? Which vessel territory is affected?

The woman is likely experiencing a large-vessel stroke involving the right MCA territory. This is supported by the neglect (a cortical sign) and sparing of the left leg, indicating preservation of the ACA territory and the MCA perforators to the internal capsule.

An acute onset of neurologic deficit referable to a cerebrovascular territory. Stroke is a clinical diagnosis that can be divided into two categories, **ischemic** and **hemorrhagic,** each of which consists of pathologic diagnoses facilitated by imaging.

- **Ischemic:**
  - **Ischemic stroke:** An infarction of CNS tissue that accounts for 85% of all strokes. It results from vessel obstruction caused by cerebral thrombosis (clot development at the site of obstruction) or cerebral embolism (clot development, usually in the heart or neck vessels, that migrates to the site of obstruction). Risk factors include untreated hypertension, atrial fibrillation (AF), diabetes, cigarette smoking, recent MI, valvular heart disease, carotid artery disease, TIA, OCP use, illicit drug use (eg, cocaine, amphetamines), and hyperlipidemia (see Figure 13-1).
  - **Transient ischemic attack (TIA):** A transient episode of neurologic dysfunction caused by focal brain, spinal cord, or retinal ischemia without acute infarction. Typically lasts 10–60 minutes. The etiologies of TIA are the same as those of ischemic stroke, and therefore the same workup is required.
- **Hemorrhagic:**
  - **Intracerebral hemorrhage (ICH):** Focal bleeding from a blood vessel in the brain parenchyma. This usually results from rupture of an atherosclerotic small artery weakened by chronic hypertension (see Figure 13-2).
  - **Subarachnoid hemorrhage (SAH):** Sudden bleeding into the subarachnoid space. The most common cause is head trauma, although spontaneous bleeding is usually the result of a ruptured aneurysm (see Figure 13-3).

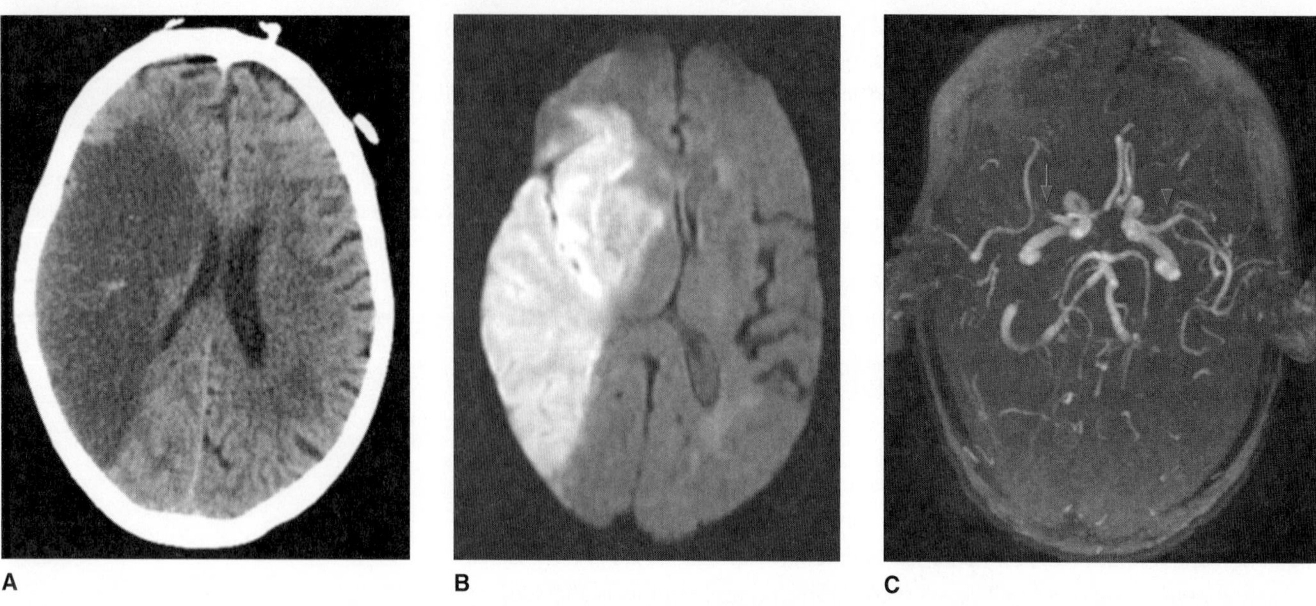

FIGURE 13-1. Acute ischemic stroke. Acute left hemiparesis in a 62-year-old woman. (**A**) Noncontrast transaxial head CT with loss of gray and white matter differentiation and asymmetrically decreased size of the right lateral ventricle in a right MCA distribution (indicating mass effect). (**B**) Transaxial diffusion-weighted MRI with reduced diffusion in the same distribution, consistent with an acute infarct. (**C**) Maximum-intensity projection of a transaxial time-of-flight MRA shows the cause: an abrupt occlusion of the proximal right MCA (arrow). Compare with the normal left MCA (arrowhead). (Reproduced with permission from USMLERx.com.)

Symptoms/Exam

- **Ischemic strokes** have an abrupt, dramatic onset of focal neurologic symptoms.
- By contrast, **intracranial hemorrhagic strokes** usually involve headache, vomiting, hypertension, and impaired consciousness, although a CT scan is needed to truly differentiate them from ischemic strokes.

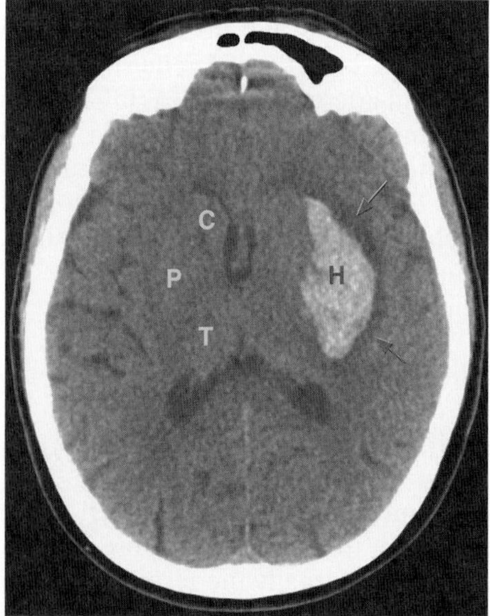

FIGURE 13-2. Intracerebral hemorrhage. Transaxial image from a noncontrast head CT shows an intraparenchymal hemorrhage (H) and surrounding edema (arrows) centered in the left putamen, a common location for hypertensive hemorrhage. C, P, and T denote the normal contralateral caudate, putamen, and thalamus. (Reproduced with permission from Fauci AS et al. *Harrison's Principles of Internal Medicine,* 17th ed. New York: McGraw-Hill, 2008, Fig. 364-17.)

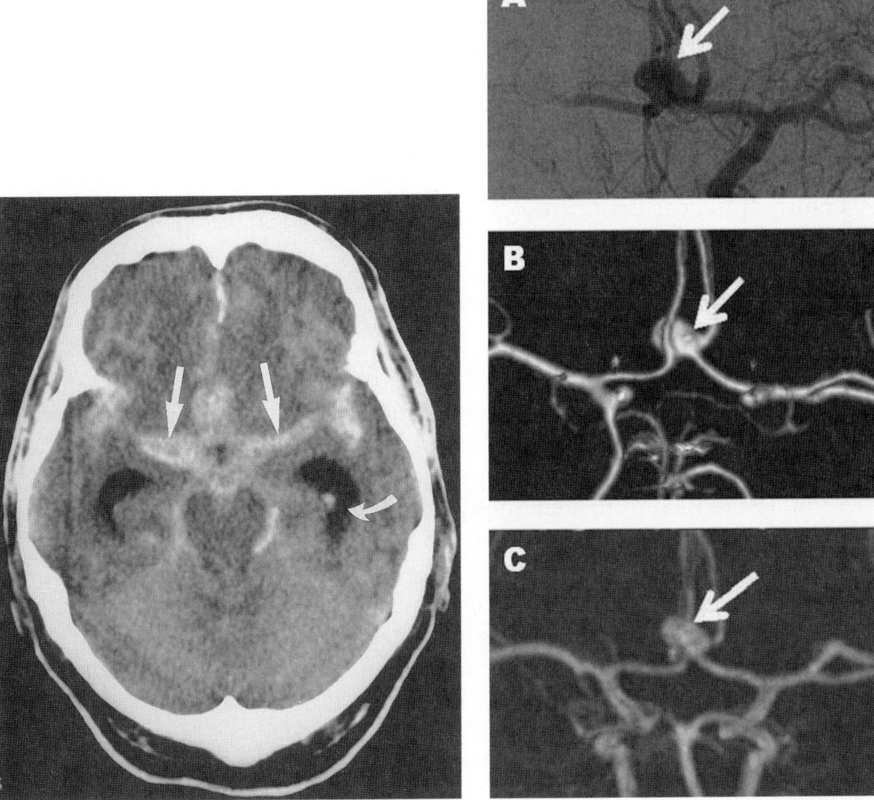

FIGURE 13-3. Subarachnoid hemorrhage. Transaxial noncontrast CT (left) showing SAH filling the basilar cisterns and sylvian fissures (straight arrows). The curved arrow shows the dilated temporal horns of the lateral ventricles/hydrocephalus. Coned-down images (right) from a catheter angiogram (**A**), a CT angiogram (**B**), and an MRA (**C**) show a saccular aneurysm arising from the anterior communicating artery (arrow). (Left image reproduced with permission from Tintinalli JE et al. *Tintinalli's Emergency Medicine: A Comprehensive Study Guide,* 6th ed. New York: McGraw-Hill, 2004, Fig. 237-4. Right image reproduced with permission from Doherty GM. *Current Diagnosis & Treatment: Surgery,* 13th ed. New York: McGraw-Hill, 2010, Fig. 36-6.)

- Specific symptoms are as follows:
  - **Superior division MCA stroke:** Contralateral hemiparesis that affects the face, hand, and arm; contralateral hemisensory deficit in the same distribution; ipsilateral gaze preference; facial droop. If the dominant hemisphere is affected, **Broca's aphasia** results.
  - **Inferior division MCA stroke:** Contralateral homonymous hemianopia; neglect of the contralateral limbs; apraxia. If the dominant hemisphere is affected, **Wernicke's aphasia** results.
  - **ACA stroke:** Leg paresis.
  - **PCA stroke:** Homonymous hemianopia with macular sparing; prosopagnosia (inability to recognize familiar faces).
  - **Basilar artery stroke:** Coma, cranial nerve palsies, "locked-in" syndrome.
  - **Lacunar stroke:** Pure motor or sensory deficit; dysarthria–clumsy hand syndrome; hemiparesis involving the face, arm, and leg.

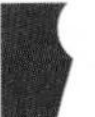

KEY FACT

Broca's (expressive) aphasia involves nonfluent speech; good auditory comprehension; and poor repetition and naming.

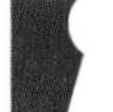

KEY FACT

Wernicke's (receptive) aphasia involves fluent speech and poor auditory comprehension, repetition, and naming.

DIFFERENTIAL

Seizure, brain tumor or abscess, subdural or epidural hematoma, hypo- or hyperglycemia, migraine, TIA.

Diagnosis

- **Head CT without contrast** to rule out bleed.
- **MRI with diffusion-weighted imaging (DWI) and perfusion-weighted imaging (PWI) or CT perfusion:** DWI shows dying tissue; PWI shows penumbra, or tissue at risk of dying.
- **MRA or CT angiography:** To evaluate vessels, including the carotids and circle of Willis.
- **Transesophageal echocardiography (TEE):** To evaluate for cardiac emboli and patent foramen ovale.
- **Labs:** CBC, electrolytes, coagulation studies, HbA_{1c}, fasting lipids.
- **Telemetry or ECG:** To evaluate for AF.

Treatment

- Check airway, breathing, and circulation **(ABCs);** order a stat glucose. **Keep NPO** until intracranial hemorrhage has been ruled out and the patient has been assessed for dysphagia (aspiration risk).
- Admit to the ICU or to a telemetry-monitored bed.
- For ischemic stroke patients who are tPA candidates, proceed by keeping BP < 185/110. For patients with ischemic stroke who are not tPA candidates, allow permissive hypertension (> 160/> 80). For hemorrhagic stroke, lower systolic BP to < 160 unless intracranial pressure is very high.
- In hemorrhagic stroke, **obtain an urgent neurosurgical evaluation** for possible posterior craniotomy for cerebellar ICHs of > 3 cm or aneurysm clipping/coiling in SAH.
- If the head CT shows a normal or hypodense area consistent with **acute ischemic stroke,** consider the following:
  - **Antiplatelet agents:** ASA ↓ the incidence of a second event. Patients already on ASA may be given clopidogrel, ticlopidine, or dipyridamole.
  - **Thrombolytics:** IV recombinant tPA has strict inclusion and exclusion criteria.
    - **Inclusion criteria** include a symptom duration of < **4.5 hours,** age > 18 years, a CT scan without hemorrhage, a diagnosis of ischemic stroke, and a measurable neurologic deficit.
    - **Exclusion criteria** include stroke or head trauma within the prior three months; a history of intracranial hemorrhage; major surgery within two weeks; acute MI within the past three months; LP within seven days; uncontrolled hypertension requiring aggressive therapy; pregnancy or lactation; and evidence of cerebral hemorrhage.
  - Patients with **basilar artery thrombosis** may receive intra-arterial tPA up to **six hours after symptom onset.**

Prevention

- **Antiplatelet therapy:** ASA, ASA/dipyridamole (Aggrenox), or clopidogrel (Plavix).
- **BP goals:** Treat most patients to < 130/80.
- **Lipid goals:** Treat patients to an LDL of < 100 mg/dL.
- **Other:**
  - The HbA_{1c} goal is < 7%.
  - Discontinue smoking.
  - Encourage physical activity.
  - If > 50% carotid stenosis is seen on angiography, consider carotid endarterectomy.
  - If AF is present or if the LVEF is ≤ 25%, consider warfarin.

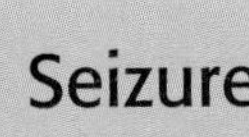

Seizures

Paroxysmal events due to neuronal discharges that are inappropriately excessive and hypersynchronous.

Symptoms

- **Partial seizures:** Involve only part of the brain. There are two subtypes, both of which can progress to a **generalized tonic-clonic (GTC) seizure.**
  - **Simple partial seizures:** Acute onset of motor, sensory, autonomic, or psychiatric symptoms **without** alteration of consciousness.
  - **Complex partial seizures:** Acute onset of motor, sensory, autonomic, or psychiatric symptoms **with** transient alteration of consciousness. These seizures frequently begin with an aura.
- **Generalized seizures:** Arise at once from both cerebral hemispheres. There are four major subtypes:
  - **GTC ("grand mal") seizures:** Acute onset of loss of consciousness accompanied by tonic contraction of the jaw, larynx, and extremity muscles for 10–20 seconds, followed by a clonic phase marked by periods of muscle relaxation for no more than one minute. Incontinence and confusion may occur in the postictal period. EEG shows generalized low-voltage activity followed by high-amplitude, polyspike discharges and then a spike-and-wave pattern. Generally there is also a postictal acidosis with a low HCO_3, elevated serum **CK,** and elevated serum **prolactin.**
  - **Absence ("petit mal") seizures:** Acute onset of brief lapses of consciousness with no loss of postural control and no postictal confusion. These seizures usually begin in childhood (4–8 years). EEG shows generalized **spike-and-wave discharges at 3 Hz.**
  - **Atonic seizures:** Acute onset of loss of postural muscle tone lasting 1–2 seconds with brief impairment of consciousness and no postictal confusion.
  - **Myoclonic seizures:** Acute onset of shocklike contraction of muscle groups.
- **Status epilepticus:** Continuous seizures or repetitive, discrete seizures with impaired consciousness in the interictal period. A medical emergency with up to a 20% mortality rate.

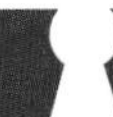

KEY FACT

Jacksonian march seizure activity presents as progressive jerking that spreads from one limb to the next.

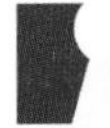

KEY FACT

Postictally, seizure patients may have a focal neurologic deficit that mimics a stroke (eg, Todd's paralysis) and resolves within minutes to days.

Exam

- **Fever** suggests CNS infection or status epilepticus.
- Look for **tongue biting, urinary incontinence,** and **meningeal signs** (nuchal rigidity, ⊕ Brudzinski's, ⊕ Kernig's).

Differential

- ICH, acute or **old stroke (particularly cortical),** SAH, meningitis, head injury, subdural or epidural hematoma, migraines.
- **Hyponatremia** (or changes in magnesium, calcium, or glucose), **EtOH withdrawal,** cocaine or amphetamine intoxication.
- Medications associated with seizures include imipramine, meperidine, INH, metronidazole, bupropion, and **fluoroquinolones.**
- 1° **CNS tumor** or brain metastases.

TABLE 13-2. First-Line Drugs for the Prevention of Seizure

Partial Onset[a]	Primary Generalized	Absence	Myoclonic, Atonic
Carbamazepine	Valproate	Ethosuximide	Valproate
Lamotrigine	Lamotrigine	Valproate	
Phenytoin			
Valproate			

[a]Includes simple partial, complex partial, and secondarily generalized.

KEY FACT

Signs and symptoms of elevated ICP include headache on awakening, nausea/vomiting, drowsiness, diplopia, blurry vision, papilledema, and CN VI palsies.

Diagnosis

- **Labs:** Order a CBC, electrolytes, glucose, magnesium, calcium, ammonia, an EtOH level, a toxicology screen, and an antiepileptic drug level if appropriate.
- **EEG:** To establish a baseline, localize the focus and confirm the diagnosis. If a focal deficit is present, get a **CT** or **MRI** of the brain.
- **If CNS infection is suspected, get an LP**—but only if there is **no evidence of ↑ ICP.**

Treatment

- **Acute:**
  - Check **ABCs; intubation may be required to protect the airway.**
  - Gently turn the patient onto his left side to prevent aspiration. Unless the patient is being intubated, do not put anything into his mouth (eg, tongue blade, fingers)!
  - Always check a **glucose level,** as hypoglycemia is a common cause of convulsions. If the patient is hypoglycemic, give IV thiamine and then glucose. If the glucose level is normal, give lorazepam 0.1 mg/kg in 2-mg increments each over 2–3 minutes up to 8 mg.
  - If the seizure continues, give fosphenytoin 15–20 mg/kg at a rate no faster than 150 mg/min. If the seizure persists, consider induction of coma with anesthetic (propofol, midazolam, phenobarbital).
- **Chronic:** Table 13-2 outlines pharmacotherapeutic options for the long-term prevention of seizures.

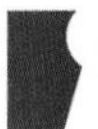

KEY FACT

Most antiepileptic drugs are teratogenic. Rule out pregnancy before starting treatment.

Brain Death

A state characterized by the absence of cerebral or brain stem function with maintenance of other organs through artificial means. Clinical criteria for the determination of brain death include the following:

- A comatose state (unresponsiveness to verbal, tactile, or painful stimuli).
- Absent pupillary light, corneal, oculovestibular (tested by cold calorics), and gag reflexes.
- Absent motor responses to painful stimuli.
- Complete apnea denoted by no respirations at a $PaCO_2$ of 60 mm Hg, or 20 mm Hg above normal values.
- Exclusion of sedative medications, hypothermia, hypotension, or metabolic derangements.

KEY FACT

Common causes of coma include ischemic brain injury, traumatic brain injury, and metabolic derangements (eg, profound hypoglycemia).

Diagnosis

Auxiliary tests include the following:

- Radionuclide brain scanning
- EEG
- Cerebral angiography
- Transcranial Doppler measurements

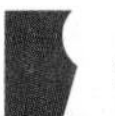

KEY FACT

For comatose patients, always rule out nonconvulsive status epilepticus with an EEG.

Epidural Hematoma

- An accumulation of blood between the skull and the dura. It typically results from tearing of the **middle meningeal artery** 2° to head trauma. A true **neurologic emergency.**
- **Sx/Exam:**
  - The patient is initially unconscious from concussion resulting from head trauma.
  - The patient awakens and has a "lucid interval" in which the hematoma subclinically expands.
  - Lethargy and rapid neurologic deterioration follow, including evidence of herniation (hemiparesis and a fixed, dilated pupil).
- **Dx:** Head CT without contrast shows a **biconvex, lens-shaped hyperdensity** that respects cranial suture lines (see Figure 13-4A).
- **Tx:** Open craniotomy and evacuation of blood.

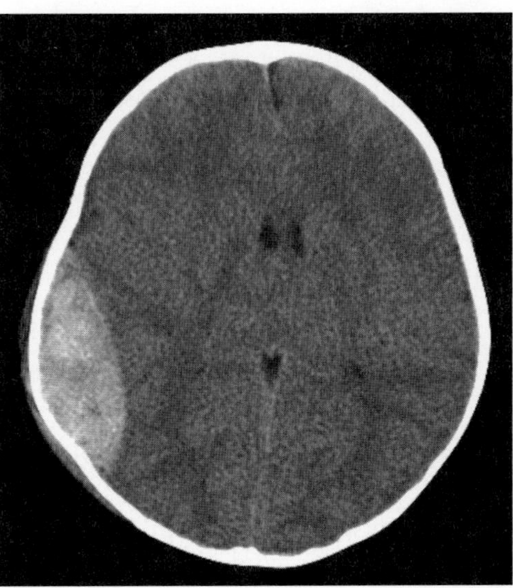

A

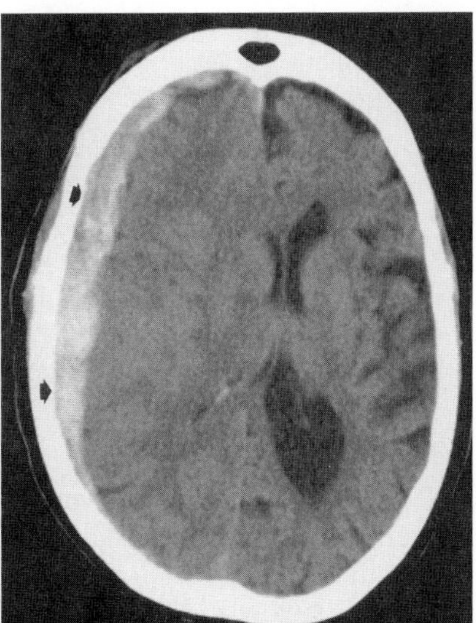

B

FIGURE 13-4. Acute epidural and acute subdural hematoma. (**A**) Noncontrast transaxial CT showing a right temporal acute epidural hematoma. Note the characteristic biconvex shape. (**B**) Noncontrast transaxial CT demonstrating a right acute holohemispheric subdural hematoma. Note the characteristic crescentic shape. (Image A reproduced with permission from Doherty GM. *Current Diagnosis & Treatment: Surgery,* 13th ed. New York: McGraw-Hill, 2010, Fig. 36-8. Image B reproduced with permission from Chen MY et al. *Basic Radiology.* New York: McGraw-Hill, 2004, Fig. 12-32.)

Subdural Hematoma

- An accumulation of blood between the arachnoid membrane and the dura. This typically results from blunt head trauma (commonly a fall) that leads to rupture of the **bridging veins** (common in the **elderly** and in **alcoholics**).
- **Sx/Exam:** Presents with headache, altered mental status, and possible hemiparesis.
- **Dx:** Head CT shows a **crescent-shaped,** concave hyperdensity that may have a less distinct border and does not cross the midline (see Figure 13-4B).
- **Tx: Surgical evacuation** of blood if symptoms are present or if the lesion is increasing in size.

Spinal Cord Compression

A 58-year-old male-to-female transgender patient who has been treated with estrogen presents with an inability to walk or to urinate. Exam shows a distended bladder, ↓ rectal tone, weakness in the bilateral lower extremities, and bilateral ankle clonus. Where is the lesion, and what are the most likely etiologies?

Given this patient's bilateral weakness, spasticity, and bowel and bladder involvement, the lesion is likely in the spinal cord at the lumbar level or higher. The most likely etiologies are neoplastic, infectious, inflammatory, vascular, or structural (disk herniation). In this rare case, the etiology was a metastatic lesion at the thoracic level from a 1° breast cancer 2° to estrogen treatment.

KEY FACT

Loss of anal reflex ("anal wink") indicates a lesion in S2–S4.

KEY FACT

Always look for a sensory level when considering a spinal cord process. The pinprick test is precise and reproducible.

A neurologic emergency! The approach is to evaluate for trauma (immobilize the neck if necessary), localize the lesion, image the spine, and call neurosurgery (see Figure 13-5).

Symptoms/Exam

- Symptoms include back pain, bilateral weakness, paresthesias, and bladder/bowel incontinence or retention.
- Exam includes bilateral weakness, sensory level (by pinprick), hyperreflexia below the sensory level, saddle anesthesia, and loss of anal wink. These last two findings are common with conus medullaris and cauda equina involvement.
- Abrupt onset of radicular pain, flaccid weakness, sphincter dysfunction, and a sensory level could indicate **cord infarction.**
- Trauma to the neck should be suspected if there is trauma to the face and body. Signs of skull fracture include the following:
  - **Battle's sign** (ecchymosis over the mastoid process).
  - **Raccoon eyes** (periorbital ecchymosis).
  - Hemotympanum and CSF rhinorrhea/otorrhea.

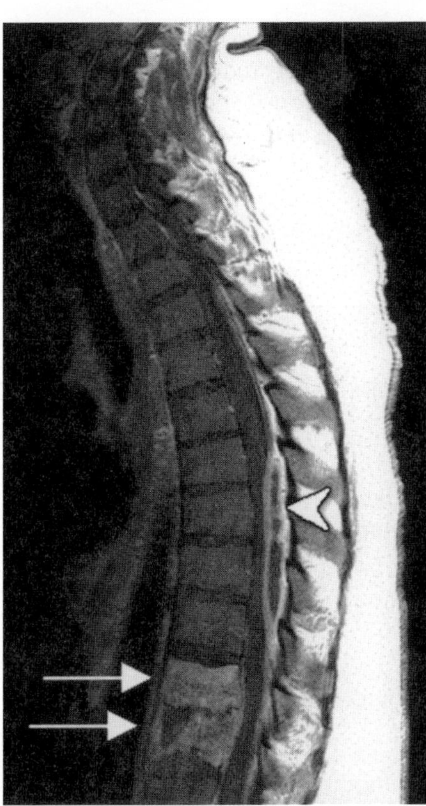

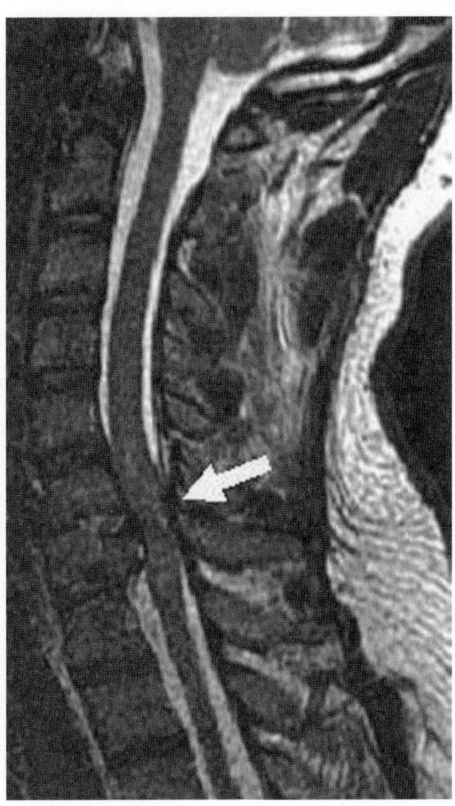

FIGURE 13-5. Spinal cord compression. (**A**) Sagittal postcontrast MRI shows diskitis/osteomyelitis (arrows) and a rim-enhancing epidural abscess (arrowhead) compressing the spinal cord. (**B**) Sagittal T2-weighted MRI in another patient shows a traumatic fracture at C6–C7 compressing the spinal cord. Note the abnormally high signal within the spinal cord (arrow). (Image A reproduced with permission from Tintinalli JE et al. *Tintinalli's Emergency Medicine: A Comprehensive Study Guide,* 6th ed. New York: McGraw-Hill, 2004, Fig. 305-5. Image B reproduced with permission from Doherty GM. *Current Diagnosis & Treatment: Surgery,* 13th ed. New York: McGraw-Hill, 2010, Fig. 36-12.)

DIFFERENTIAL

The etiologies of spinal cord compression include the following:

- **Trauma:** Motor vehicle accidents; sports-related injuries.
- **Infection:** Epidural abscess in IV drug users; spinal TB (Pott's disease) in immunocompromised patients; vertebral osteomyelitis.
- **Neoplasms:** Metastases are most common.
- **Degenerative disease:** Cervical and lumbar disk herniations.
- **Vascular:** Infarction, epidural and subdural hematomas, and AVMs are rare.

DIAGNOSIS

Spinal MRI; CT or CT myelography for patients in whom MRI is contraindicated (eg, those with pacemakers).

TREATMENT

- **Acute spinal cord injury:** Methylprednisolone 30 mg/kg IV bolus. Wait 45 minutes; then give methylprednisolone in a 5.4-mg/kg/hr continuous infusion over the next 24 hours.

- **Spinal tumor:** Dexamethasone 100 mg IV bolus.
- **Fractures, subluxations, and dislocations:** Surgical reduction.
- **Epidural abscess:** Neurosurgical drainage and broad-spectrum antibiotics (a third-generation cephalosporin, vancomycin, and metronidazole).

Headache

TENSION HEADACHE

A chronic syndrome characterized by tight, bandlike pain bilaterally.

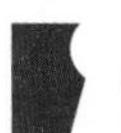

KEY FACT

Headache danger signs include a change in frequency or severity, fever, neurologic signs, and new-onset headaches.

KEY FACT

Severe, sudden-onset headache should raise concern for a subarachnoid/ aneurysm rupture.

KEY FACT

Even if the head CT is ⊖, get an LP if there is a high suspicion for SAH. Fifteen percent of patients with an aneurysmal SAH have a ⊖ CT scan. LP will show high RBCs in all tubes and xanthochromia (yellow CSF).

SYMPTOMS/EXAM

Presents with nonthrobbing, bilateral occipital head pain that is generally not associated with nausea, vomiting, photophobia, phonophobia, or aggravation with movement. Exam is usually normal.

DIFFERENTIAL

- **Sinus tenderness:** May point to sinusitis.
- **Temporal artery tenderness:** Associated with temporal arteritis.
- **Cranial bruit:** Rule out AVM.

DIAGNOSIS

Obtain a CT scan under the following conditions:

- If the headache is acute and extremely severe (**"thunderclap headache"**).
- If the headache is progressive over days to weeks, particularly if it is not similar to previous headaches.
- In the presence of focal neurologic signs.
- In the setting of papilledema.
- If the headache has a morning onset or awakens the patient from sleep.

TREATMENT

Treat with **NSAIDs** or acetaminophen. Relaxation techniques may be of benefit.

MIGRAINE

An episodic headache syndrome that is associated with sensitivity to light, sound, and movement and is often accompanied by nausea and vomiting. Its prevalence in the United States is 15% in women and 6% in men. Migraine has a familial predisposition, with > 50% of patients having an affected family member.

SYMPTOMS/EXAM

- **Migraine without aura ("common migraine"):** Recurrent headaches of 4–72 hours' duration that are characterized by at least two of the following—unilateral, throbbing, severe enough in intensity to limit daily activity, and aggravated by movement—plus nausea/vomiting or photophobia/ phonophobia.
- **Migraine with aura ("classic migraine"):** Common migraine that also includes a preceding homonymous visual disturbance (eg, scintillations, blind spots), unilateral paresthesias, and, rarely, weakness.

TREATMENT

- Identify and **eliminate triggers.**
- Treat according to severity:
  - **Mild:** NSAIDs plus an antiemetic such as metoclopramide.
  - **Moderate:** Abortive (**triptans** as soon as headache begins).
  - **Severe:** IV hydration, metoclopramide, dexamethasone, prochlorperazine, or ergotamine.
- **Preventive therapy:** TCAs, α-blockers, valproate, β-blockers.

CLUSTER HEADACHE

- A brief, severe, **unilateral, periorbital, stabbing** headache, with attacks occurring at the same hour each day and with periods of remission during the year.
- Affects men more than women; onset is at 20–30 years of age.
- **Sx/Exam:** Exam reveals ipsilateral lacrimation, **conjunctival injection,** Horner's syndrome, and nasal congestion.
- **Tx:** Responds to 100% O_2 or low-dose prednisone.

KEY FACT

Horner's syndrome presents with ipsilateral miosis (pupillary constriction), ipsilateral ptosis (eyelid droop), and ipsilateral anhidrosis (lack of sweating) of the face.

Guillain-Barré Syndrome (GBS)

An acute polyradiculoneuropathy (**root** and **peripheral nerve** process) that usually has an autoimmune basis. It typically presents as an ascending motor paralysis with areflexia, autonomic involvement (eg, postural hypotension), and possible sensory symptoms. Seventy percent of patients have a recent history of respiratory or GI infection (particularly *Campylobacter jejuni*).

SYMPTOMS/EXAM

Exam shows leg > arm weakness, facial weakness with difficulty handling secretions, **absent reflexes,** proprioception > pain/temperature sensation, postural hypotension, and respiratory failure.

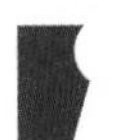

KEY FACT

Absence of reflexes, ascending weakness, and recent infection—think GBS.

DIAGNOSIS

- GBS is a clinical diagnosis; it is supported by ancillary tests that are most effective at excluding mimics (eg, acute myelopathies, botulism, diphtheria, Lyme disease).
- **LP:** Typically shows ↑ protein with normal WBC levels ("**albuminocytologic dissociation**"), but often normal in the first 48 hours.
- **CBC:** May show an ↑ WBC count. Obtain an ESR and a Lyme titer.
- **Nerve conduction study (NCS):** May show evidence of demyelination.

TREATMENT

- Give **IVIG** or **plasmapheresis** as soon as possible.
- Measure **vital capacity** and **maximum inspiratory force** to monitor for respiratory compromise.
- Watch for **autonomic instability,** including hypotension, temperature dysregulation, and cardiac arrhythmias.

Myasthenia Gravis (MG)

A 31-year-old man complains that when he looks up to catch a baseball, he sees two balls and cannot make the catch. On exam, he displays ptosis and weakness in all extraocular muscles. Where is the lesion, and what is the likely diagnosis? How should the diagnosis be confirmed, and how should he be treated?

The lesion is in the neuromuscular junction isolated to the eyes, and the likely diagnosis is ocular myasthenia gravis. Confirmatory tests include edrophonium (Tensilon) injection and an acetylcholine receptor antibody blood test. The patient should be treated with pyridostigmine 60 mg TID.

An autoimmune disorder in which antibodies attack the acetylcholine (ACh) receptor proteins at the neuromuscular junction. This causes weakness and fatigability of skeletal muscles. There is a bimodal distribution, with an earlier peak in the 30s–40s (women) and a late peak in the 70s–90s (men).

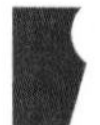

KEY FACT

Neuromuscular blocking agents used during anesthesia can unmask or worsen MG, leading to prolonged postoperative weakness and ventilator dependence.

Symptoms/Exam

The main features are **weakness** and **fatigability** of muscles. The weakness may be worse at the end of the day or after exercise and may improve with rest. There is an ↑ in weakness with repeated use of the skeletal muscles (fatigability). Categorized as follows:

- **Ocular MG:** Muscle weakness limited to the eyelids and extraocular muscles, with ptosis and/or diplopia. Fifty percent of patients go on to develop generalized MG.
- **Generalized MG:** Weakness may be seen in ocular, bulbar (dysarthria, dysphagia, fatigable chewing), facial (expressionless), limb, and respiratory muscles. Worsening respiratory muscle strength can lead to respiratory failure, or a **"myasthenic crisis."**

Differential

Lambert-Eaton myasthenic syndrome, botulism, drug-induced myasthenia, motor neuron diseases (eg, ALS), generalized fatigue, intracranial mass lesion, hyperthyroidism.

Diagnosis

- **Bedside tests:**
  - **Edrophonium chloride (Tensilon)** is an acetylcholinesterase inhibitor that prolongs the presence of ACh at the neuromuscular junction. A ⊕ test results in an immediate ↑ in the strength of affected muscles.
  - The **ice pack test** is the use of ice that improves ptosis in patients with MG.
- Immunologic assays for **ACh receptor antibody;** if seronegative, **muscle-specific kinase (MuSK) antibodies.**
- **Repetitive nerve stimulation:** The nerve is stimulated and action potentials are measured in muscles. In MG, there is a rapid ↓ in the amplitude of action potentials.
- **Single-fiber electromyography:** This test measures single-muscle-fiber discharges. It is the most sensitive diagnostic test for MG.

TREATMENT

- **Symptomatic treatment:** First-line treatment is an acetylcholinesterase inhibitor (pyridostigmine).
- **Chronic immunomodulating agents:** Corticosteroids, azathioprine, cyclosporine, mycophenolate mofetil.
- **For myasthenic crisis:** Plasmapheresis and/or IVIG.
- **Surgery:** Thymectomy.

Vertigo

An illusion of movement of either the patient or his/her surroundings. Mimickers of vertigo include orthostatic hypotension, cardiac arrhythmia, and presyncope/syncope. Once a diagnosis of vertigo has been established, one must determine whether it is peripheral or central.

PERIPHERAL VERTIGO

A lesion of the vestibular apparatus of the inner ear or CN VIII. It is often intermittently severe, positional, and associated with auditory sensations (tinnitus, hearing loss) and postural unsteadiness.

SYMPTOMS/EXAM

Nystagmus is rotary, unidirectional, and fatigable. Examine the external auditory canal for vesicles (herpes zoster or **Ramsay Hunt** syndrome). Use Dix-Hallpike and head thrust maneuvers to evaluate for positional effects. Rule out cerebellar signs (ataxia, wide-based gait) and cranial neuropathies.

DIFFERENTIAL

- **Medication side effects: Furosemide, aminoglycosides, salicylates.**
- **Benign paroxysmal positional vertigo (BPPV):** Episodic attacks of severe vertigo. Self-limited; probably caused by crystals floating inside the semicircular canals brushing against the sensory cilia.
- **Labyrinthitis/neuronitis:** Viral inflammation of CN VIII or the labyrinth; usually self-limited.
- **Ménière's disease:** Overproduction of endolymph in the vestibular canals. Presents with the **triad** of vertigo, tinnitus, and hearing loss.
- **Schwannoma:** A mass compressing CN VIII, causing hearing loss and vertigo.

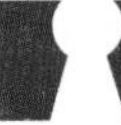

KEY FACT

If there are episodic attacks of severe vertigo associated with head position, think of BPPV.

DIAGNOSIS

The history and exam should reveal the diagnosis. No imaging is needed, although an audiogram is necessary to rule out vestibular schwannoma.

TREATMENT

Canalith repositioning (the Epley maneuver), physical therapy, antihistamines/benzodiazepines/scopolamine, possible surgery for schwannoma.

CENTRAL VERTIGO

A lesion that affects the brain stem vestibular nuclei or their connections. It is usually acute onset, with symptoms independent of head positioning.

SYMPTOMS/EXAM

- Spontaneous nystagmus that cannot be suppressed with visual fixation; nystagmus that changes direction with gaze; purely vertical, horizontal, or torsional nystagmus; saccade dysmetria (overshoot and undershoot of gaze).
- Cranial nerve signs such as facial droop, dysarthria, and loss of corneal reflexes are also seen.

DIFFERENTIAL

- **Brain stem stroke:** Associated neurologic deficits seen include weakness, ataxia, and cranial nerve dysfunction.
- **Cerebellar stroke:** Associated neurologic deficits seen include midline and appendicular ataxia.
- **Demyelination:** MS.
- **Neoplasm:** Brain stem glioma.

DIAGNOSIS

Head CT without contrast; MRI of the brain with DWI.

TREATMENT

In the setting of a posterior circulation stroke, careful monitoring is necessary for 24–48 hours followed by stroke workup.

Multiple Sclerosis (MS)

A disease involving inflammation and destruction of the CNS myelin, likely from an autoimmune process. **Young women** are at higher risk, as are those who reside in **northern latitudes.**

SYMPTOMS

- Initial symptoms are varied. The most common are sensory loss, optic neuritis, weakness, paresthesias, diplopia, and ataxia.
- The four clinical courses of MS are relapsing-remitting, 2° progressive, 1° progressive, and progressive/relapsing.

EXAM

Some of the classic findings include the following:

- Hyperreflexia, **weakness,** and ataxia.
- **Lhermitte's sign:** Radiating/shooting pain up or down the neck on flexion or extension.
- **Optic neuritis:** ↓ visual acuity; pain with eye movements; central scotoma; red desaturation.
- **Afferent pupillary defect (Marcus Gunn pupil):** The pupil paradoxically dilates to a light stimulus owing to delayed conduction.
- **Internuclear ophthalmoplegia (MLF syndrome):** The classic finding is bilateral weakness on adduction of the ipsilateral eye with nystagmus on abduction of the contralateral eye, together with incomplete or slow abduction of the ipsilateral eye on lateral gaze with complete preservation of convergence.

CHAPTER 14

OBSTETRICS

Prenatal Care and Nutrition

All prenatal visits should document weight, BP, extremity edema, urine protein and glucose, fundal height (> 20 weeks), and fetal heart rate. Further recommendations are as follows:

- **Weight gain:** Average-size women should gain 25–35 lbs; obese women should gain less (15–25 lbs) and thin women more.
- **Nutrition:** Requirements for total calories, protein, iron, folate, calcium, and zinc should ↑. All patients should take prenatal vitamins.
  - **Caloric intake:** An additional 300 kcal/day is needed during pregnancy and 500 kcal/day during breast-feeding.
  - **Folate:** Supplement with 400 μg/day to ↓ the risk of neural tube defects (NTDs). **Women with twin gestation or a prior history of a fetus with NTDs should receive 4 mg/day.**
  - **Iron:** Supplement in the latter half of pregnancy to prevent anemia.
  - **Calcium:** Supplement in the later months of pregnancy and during breast-feeding.
- **Smoking and alcohol cessation.**
- **Prenatal labs:** See Table 14-1 for lab work that should be scheduled during pregnancy.

TABLE 14-1. Prenatal Labs During Pregnancy

Gestational Age (GA)	Labs to Be Obtained
Initial visit	CBC, blood type, Rh antibody screen, UA with culture, Pap smear, cervical gonorrhea and chlamydia cultures, rubella antibody titer, hepatitis B surface antigen, syphilis screen, PPD, HIV. Toxoplasmosis and sickle cell screening for at-risk patients. Women with prior gestational diabetes or a family history (in a first-degree relative) should get early glucose testing.
6–11 weeks	**Ultrasound** to determine GA (more accurate than later scans).
15–19 weeks	**Triple-marker screen/quadruple test** (quad screen). Offer amniocentesis for those of advanced maternal age (≥ 35 years of age at delivery).
18–21 weeks	**Screening ultrasound** to survey fetal anatomy, placental location, and amniotic fluid.
26–28 weeks	**One-hour glucose challenge test.** If ≥ 140 mg/dL, follow with a three-hour glucose tolerance test. Repeat hemoglobin/hematocrit.
28 weeks	**RhoGAM** injection for Rh-⊖ patients. Start fetal kick counting (the patient should count 10 fetal movements in < 1 hour).
35–37 weeks	Screen for **group B streptococcus** (GBS) with a rectovaginal swab. Repeat hemoglobin/hematocrit. Cervical gonorrhea and chlamydia cultures, RPR, and HIV (in at-risk patients). Assess fetal position with Leopold maneuvers and ultrasound.

Prenatal Diagnostic Testing

TRIPLE-MARKER SCREEN/QUADRUPLE TEST (QUAD SCREEN)

- Measured between 15 and 20 weeks' gestation.
- Any maternal serum α-fetoprotein (MSAFP) result > 2.5 multiples of the mean (MoM) can signify an open NTD, an abdominal wall defect, multiple gestation, incorrect dating, fetal death, or placental abnormalities.
- The sensitivity for detecting chromosomal abnormalities (trisomies 18 and 21) can be ↑ through the addition of estriol and β-hCG (**triple-marker screen**) to MSAFP. See Table 14-2 for trends in the detection of genetic abnormalities.
- The addition of **inhibin-A** to the three markers above (**quadruple test**) will ↑ the sensitivity for Down syndrome.

AMNIOCENTESIS

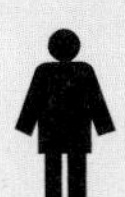

A 32-year-old G4P2 woman at 16 weeks' gestation has an abnormal triple-marker screen that raises concern for trisomy 21. What is the next step?

The next step depends on the patient's desire to confirm the diagnosis. If the patient desires termination of pregnancy with a positive result, amniocentesis would be confirmatory.

- Performed primarily between 15 and 20 weeks' gestation to detect possible genetic diseases or congenital malformations.
- Risks include fetal-maternal hemorrhage (1–2%) and fetal loss (0.5%).
- Amniocentesis is used:
  - In conjunction with an **abnormal triple-marker screen/quadruple test.**
  - In **women > 35 years of age** at the time of delivery.
  - In **Rh-sensitized pregnancy** to ascertain fetal blood type or to detect fetal hemolysis.
  - For the evaluation of **fetal lung maturity** in the third trimester.

CHORIONIC VILLUS SAMPLING

- Performed to evaluate possible genetic diseases at an earlier time than is possible with amniocentesis, with comparable diagnostic accuracy.
- Done at **10–12 weeks' gestation via transabdominal or transvaginal** aspiration of chorionic villus tissue (a precursor of the placenta). Risks include fetal loss (1–5%) and an association with distal limb defects.

TABLE 14-2. Detection of Genetic Abnormalities with the Triple-Marker Test

	NEURAL TUBE DEFECT	TRISOMY 18	TRISOMY 21
MSAFP	↑	↓	↓
Estriol	Not used	↓	↓
β-hCG	Not used	↓	↑

Tests of Fetal Well-Being

NONSTRESS TEST (NST)

- Fetal heart rate is monitored externally by Doppler.
- A **normal response** is an acceleration of ≥ 15 bpm above baseline lasting > 15 seconds.
- A normal or "reactive" test includes two such accelerations in a **20-minute** period.
- An abnormal or "nonreactive" NST warrants a biophysical profile or a contraction stress test (see below).
- A nonreactive NST can be due to fetal sleep cycle, GA < 30 weeks, a fetal CNS anomaly, or maternal sedative or narcotic use.

CONTRACTION STRESS TEST (CST)

- Used to assess uteroplacental dysfunction.
- Fetal heart rate is monitored during spontaneous or induced (nipple stimulation or pitocin) contractions.
- A normal or "negative" CST has no late decelerations and is highly predictive of fetal well-being.
- An abnormal or "positive" CST is defined by late decelerations in conjunction with at least 50% of contractions. A minimum of three contractions within a 10-minute period must be present for an adequate CST.

MNEMONIC

When performing a BPP, remember to—

Test the Baby, MAN!

Fetal **T**one
Fetal **B**reathing
Fetal **M**ovements
Amniotic fluid volume
Nonstress test

BIOPHYSICAL PROFILE (BPP)

- Ultrasound is used to assess five parameters (see the mnemonic **Test the Baby, MAN**).
- A score of 2 (normal) or 0 (abnormal) is given to each of the parameters.
- A normal or "negative" test (a score of 8–10) is reassuring for fetal well-being.
- An abnormal or "positive" test (a score < 6) is worrisome for fetal compromise.

TABLE 14-3. Fetal Heart Rate Patterns

Type of Deceleration	Description	Common Cause
Early	Deceleration begins and ends at approximately the same time as maternal contractions.	Fetal head compression **(no fetal distress).**
Variable	Variable onset of abrupt (< 30-sec) slowing of fetal heart rate in association with contractions. The return is similarly abrupt in most situations.	Umbilical cord compression.
Late	Decelerations begin after onset of maternal contractions and persist until after the contractions are finished. The time from peak to nadir is > 30 sec.	Late decelerations indicate fetal hypoxia **(fetal distress).** If late decelerations are repetitive and severe, immediate delivery is necessary.

FETAL HEART RATE PATTERNS

Table 14-3 outlines different types of heart rate patterns seen in near-term and term fetuses.

Medical Complications of Pregnancy

DIABETES MELLITUS (DM)

The **most common** medical complication of pregnancy. See Table 14-4 for a comparison of pregestational and gestational DM.

> **KEY FACT**
>
> An HbA_{1c} > 6.5 prior to conception or during the first trimester will lead to a higher rate of fetal malformations.

TABLE 14-4. Pregestational vs. Gestational Diabetes Mellitus

	Pregestational	Gestational
Definition	Diagnosed **prior to pregnancy.**	Diagnosed **during pregnancy.**
Risk factors	Family history; autoimmune disorders (type 1), obesity (type 2).	Obesity, family history (in a first-degree relative), prior history of DM in pregnancy.
Diagnosis	See above.	Diagnosed if the one-hour glucose test is **≥ 140 mg/dL and** the follow-up three-hour glucose test has at least two ↑ levels.
Treatment	Strict control of blood glucose levels with diet, exercise, and **insulin:** ▪ **Fasting morning:** < 90 mg/dL. ▪ **Two-hour postprandial:** < 120 mg/dL.	ADA diet and regular exercise. If blood sugars are ↑ after one week, initiate insulin therapy. Glyburide can be considered.
Labor	Fingersticks every 1–2 hours while the patient is in active labor with dextrose infusion +/– an insulin drip to maintain tight glycemic control.	**Diet controlled (A1):** Fingersticks on admission and every four hours in labor. **A2:** Same as pregestational.
Postpartum	Continue glucose monitoring; the body's insulin requirements quickly ↓.	Resume normal diet; no insulin is required.
Complications		
Fetus	Congenital malformations, stillbirth, macrosomia, IUGR, hypoglycemia, birth trauma.	Hypoglycemia from hyperinsulinemia; macrosomia; birth trauma.
Mother	Hypoglycemia, DKA, spontaneous abortion, polyhydramnios, preterm labor, worsening end-organ dysfunction, ↑ risk of preeclampsia.	Perineal trauma from macrosomic infant; ↑ lifetime risk of developing DM.

PREECLAMPSIA/ECLAMPSIA

> A 32-year-old G1P0 at 34 weeks' gestation with a diagnosis of preeclampsia presents with a refractory headache and nausea. She is found to have a BP of 208/112 and 3+ protein on urine dipstick. Her labs are pending. What is the next step?
>
> The patient is presenting with severe preeclampsia that raises concern for the development of eclampsia. You should administer antihypertensives and magnesium for seizure prophylaxis and prepare for emergent delivery.

Preeclampsia is characterized by hypertension and proteinuria and is thought to be due to ↓ organ perfusion 2° to vasospasm and endothelial activation. Risk factors include nulliparity, African American ethnicity, extremes of age, multiple gestations (ie, twins), renal disease, and chronic hypertension. **Eclampsia** is defined as seizures in a patient with preeclampsia. Preeclampsia is further distinguished as follows:

- **Mild:** Systolic BP (SBP) > 140, diastolic BP (DBP) > 90, and 1+ on dipstick or > 300 mg on 24-hour urine.
- **Severe:** SBP > 160, DBP > 110, and 3+ on dipstick or > 5 g on 24-hour urine.

SYMPTOMS/EXAM

Table 14-5 outline differences in the presentation of mild preeclampsia, severe preeclampsia, and eclampsia.

DIAGNOSIS

- Check UA, 24-hour urine for protein and creatinine clearance, CBC, BUN, creatinine, uric acid, LFTs, PT/PTT, fibrinogen, and a toxicology screen.
- Determine the precise GA; consider amniocentesis to assess fetal lung maturity for mild preeclampsia.
- Diagnosis is based on clinical findings as described in Table 14-5.

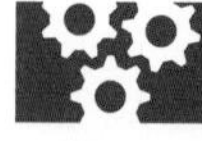

MNEMONIC

HELLP syndrome:

Hemolysis
Elevated **L**iver enzymes
Low **P**latelets

TREATMENT

Definitive treatment is **delivery.** See Table 14-5 for management.

HYPEREMESIS GRAVIDARUM

- Defined as refractory vomiting that leads to **weight loss,** poor weight gain, dehydration, ketosis from starvation, and metabolic alkalosis. Typically persists beyond 14–16 weeks' gestation.
- Risk factors include nulliparity, multiple pregnancies, and trophoblastic disease.
- **DDx:** Rule out molar pregnancy, hepatitis, gallbladder disease, reflux, and gastroenteritis.
- **Dx:** Labs show **hyponatremia** and a hypokalemic, hypochloremic **metabolic alkalosis.** Ketonuria on UA suggests starvation ketosis.
- **Tx:** If there is evidence of weight loss, dehydration, or altered electrolytes, **hospitalize** and give antiemetics, IV hydration, and vitamin and electrolyte replacement. Advance the diet slowly and avoid fatty foods.

TABLE 14-5. Mild and Severe Preeclampsia vs. Eclampsia

	Mild Preeclampsia	Severe Preeclampsia	Eclampsia
Symptoms/exam	**SBP > 140 or DBP > 90** on ≥ 2 occasions. **Proteinuria** (> 300 mg/24 hrs or 1+ on urine dipstick).	**SBP > 160 or DBP > 110** on > 2 occasions. **Proteinuria** (> 5 g/24 hrs or > 3+ on urine dipstick). HELLP syndrome (see mnemonic). Oliguria (< 500 mL/24 hrs). Pulmonary edema.	**Seizures with the diagnosis of preeclampsia.**
Treatment	Deliver if near term, fetal lungs are mature, or preeclampsia worsens. If far from term, treat with bed rest and conservative management. Use of magnesium sulfate for seizure prophylaxis is controversial.	Magnesium sulfate for seizure prophylaxis. Hydralazine +/– labetalol for BP control. When stable, deliver. Postpartum: Continue magnesium sulfate for at least 12–24 hours after delivery. Watch for magnesium toxicity; treat life-threatening toxicity with IV calcium gluconate.	**Magnesium sulfate to control seizures.** Monitor ABCs closely. When stable, deliver. Seizures may occur before delivery, during delivery, and up to six weeks postpartum.
Complications	Fetal distress, stillbirth, placental abruption, DIC, seizures, fetal/maternal death, cerebral hemorrhage.	Same as with mild preeclampsia.	Fetal/maternal death.

GESTATIONAL TROPHOBLASTIC DISEASE

Can range from benign (eg, hydatidiform mole) to malignant (eg, choriocarcinoma). Hydatidiform mole accounts for approximately 80% of cases.

Symptoms/Exam

- Suspect in patients with **first-trimester uterine bleeding** and excessive nausea and vomiting.
- Look for patients with **preeclampsia or eclampsia at < 24 weeks.**
- Other findings include uterine size greater than dates and hyperthyroidism.
- **No fetal heartbeat** is detected.
- Pelvic exam may show enlarged ovaries and possible expulsion of **grape-like molar clusters** into the vagina or blood in the cervical os.

Diagnosis

- β-hCG levels are markedly ↑ (usually > 100,000 mIU/dL).
- Pelvic ultrasound shows a **"snowstorm" appearance** with no gestational sac and no fetus or heart tones present.
- Obtain a CXR to look for metastases.

Treatment

- D&C.
- Carefully monitor β-hCG levels after D&C for possible progression to malignant disease.
- Pregnancy prevention (contraception) is needed for one year to ensure accurate monitoring of β-hCG levels.
- Treat malignant disease with chemotherapy and residual uterine disease with hysterectomy.

Peripartum Complications

KEY FACT

If postpartum uterine bleeding persists after conventional therapy, uterine/internal iliac artery ligation or hysterectomy can be lifesaving.

POSTPARTUM HEMORRHAGE

- Defined as blood loss of > 500 mL during a vaginal delivery or > 1000 mL during a cesarean section occurring before, during, or after delivery of the placenta. Table 14-6 summarizes common causes.
- Complications include **Sheehan's syndrome** (see below).

SHEEHAN'S SYNDROME (POSTPARTUM HYPOPITUITARISM)

- The most common cause of anterior pituitary insufficiency in adult females. It occurs 2° to **pituitary ischemia,** usually as a result of postpartum blood loss and hypotension.
- **Sx/Exam:**
  - The most common presenting symptom is **failure to lactate** as a result of ↓ prolactin levels.
  - Other symptoms include lethargy, anorexia, weight loss, amenorrhea, and loss of sexual hair, but these may not be recognized for many years.
- **Tx: Lifelong hormone replacement therapy** (corticosteroids, levothyroxine, estrogen and progesterone).

TABLE 14-6. Common Causes of Postpartum Hemorrhage

	Uterine Atony	Genital Tract Trauma	Retained Placental Tissue
Risk factors	Uterine overdistention, exhausted myometrium, uterine infection, grand multiparity.	Precipitous delivery, operative vaginal delivery, large infant, laceration.	Placenta accreta/increta/percreta, placenta previa, prior C-section, curettage, accessory placental lobe, retained membranes.
Diagnosis	Palpation of a soft, enlarged, "boggy" uterus.	Inspection of the cervix, vagina, and vulva for lacerations or hematoma.	Inspection of the placenta and uterine cavity. Ultrasound to look for retained placenta.
Treatment	Vigorous bimanual massage. Oxytocin infusion. Methylergonovine if not hypertensive; PGF_{2a} if not asthmatic; misoprostol.	Surgical repair of the defect.	Removal of remaining placental tissue.

INTRAPARTUM AND POSTPARTUM FEVERS

A 31-year-old healthy woman develops fevers (39.1°C/102.4°F) and shaking chills eight hours following a C-section performed for fetal malposition. The baby is doing well, and the amniotic fluid at C-section is clear. What is the likely source of infection?

The uterus (endometritis). This is a rapid postoperative presentation, making the standard causes of postoperative fever less likely.

- Most commonly due to infections (see Table 14-7).
- Remember the mnemonic for the 7 **W's** for the causes of postpartum fever.

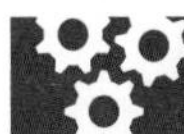

MNEMONIC

The 7 W's of postpartum fever:

Womb—endomyometritis
Wind—atelectasis, pneumonia
Water—UTI
Walk—DVT, pulmonary embolism
Wound—incision, lacerations
Weaning—breast engorgement, mastitis, breast abscess
Wonder drugs—drug fever

MASTITIS

- Cellulitis of the periglandular tissue in breast-feeding mothers, typically due to *S aureus*, occurring at about 2–4 weeks postpartum.
- **Sx/Exam:** Symptoms include breast pain and redness along with a **high fever**, chills, and flulike symptoms. Look for **focal** breast erythema, swelling, and tenderness. **Fluctuance** points to a breast abscess.
- **DDx:** Distinguish from simple breast engorgement, which can present as a swollen, firm, tender breast with low-grade fever and a breast abscess.
- **Dx:** Diagnosis includes breast milk cultures and CBC.
- **Tx:** Treat with **dicloxacillin** or **erythromycin.** Continue nursing or manually expressing milk to prevent milk stasis. Incision and drainage is necessary if an abscess is present.

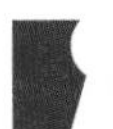

KEY FACT

The treatment of mastitis includes antibiotics and continued breast-feeding.

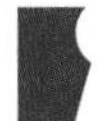

KEY FACT

Contraindications to breast-feeding include HIV infection, active hepatitis, and certain drugs (eg, tetracycline, chloramphenicol, warfarin).

TABLE 14-7. Common Infections During Labor and After Delivery

	Chorioamnionitis	Endometritis
Definition	Infection of the **chorion, amnion,** and **amniotic fluid,** diagnosed **during labor.**	Infection of the **uterus,** diagnosed **after delivery.**
Risk factors	**Prolonged rupture of membranes (ROM);** multiple vaginal exams while being ruptured in labor.	**C-section,** prolonged ROM, multiple vaginal exams while being ruptured in labor.
Symptoms/ exam	Fever with no other obvious source **and** one of the following: ▪ Fetal **or** maternal tachycardia ▪ Abdominal tenderness ▪ Foul-smelling amniotic fluid ▪ Leukocytosis	Fever within 24 hours postpartum without an obvious source.
Diagnosis	Clinical; CBC with differential.	Pelvic exam to rule out hematoma or retained membranes. CBC with differential, UA, urine culture, and blood cultures as indicated.
Treatment	Delivery of the fetus (chorioamnionitis is **not** an indication for cesarean delivery). Antibiotics until the patient is afebrile for 24 hours after delivery. Some practitioners stop antibiotics after delivery.	Antibiotics until the patient is afebrile for 24 hours (vaginal) or 48 hours (cesarean) after delivery

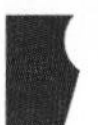

KEY FACT

CT scans of the fetus should be avoided at all trimesters of pregnancy in light of concerns over increasing the risk of childhood cancer.

TABLE 14-8. Radiation Exposure Resulting from Common Radiologic Procedures

Radiologic Film	Exposure (mrad)
Abdominal x-ray (one view)	100
Chest x-ray (two views)	0.02–0.07
CT head/chest	< 1000
CT abdomen/ lumbar spine	3500
MRI	0
Ultrasound	0

Teratogens in Pregnancy

- **Radiation:** Diagnostic and nuclear medicine studies have not been shown to pose any risk of fetal teratogenicity if overall exposure during pregnancy is < 5000 mrads. Table 14-8 outlines radiation exposure levels associated with such procedures.
- **Medications:** See Table 14-9 for safe and teratogenic medications during pregnancy.

TABLE 14-9. Safe vs. Teratogenic/Unsafe Medications During Pregnancy

Indication	Safe to Use	Contraindicated
Acne	Benzoyl peroxide.	Vitamin A and derivatives (eg, isotretinoin, etretinate) → heart and great vessel defects, craniofacial dysmorphism, and deafness.
Antibiotics	Penicillins, cephalosporin, macrolides.	Tetracycline → discoloration of deciduous teeth. Quinolones → cartilage damage. Sulfonamides late in pregnancy → kernicterus. Streptomycin → CN VIII damage/ ototoxicity.
Bipolar disorder	Assess the risks and benefits of medications.	Lithium → congenital heart disease and Ebstein's anomaly (also avoid if the mother is breast-feeding).
Cancer	Alkylating agents can be used in the second and third trimesters.	Folic acid antagonists → abnormalities of the cranium.
Contrast solution	Indigo carmine.	Methylene blue → jejunal and ileal atresia.
Depression	Assess risks vs. benefits; TCAs, SSRIs.	SSRIs may cause persistent pulmonary hypertension of the newborn, poor feeding, and/or jitteriness.
GERD	OTC antacids (calcium carbonate, milk of magnesia), ranitidine, cimetidine, omeprazole.	Alka-Seltzer (has aspirin).
Headache/ migraine	Acetaminophen, codeine, caffeine.	Avoid aspirin in late pregnancy in light of the risk of bleeding to the mother and fetus at birth. Ergotamines have abortifacient potential and a theoretical risk of fetal vasoconstriction.

TABLE 14-9. Safe vs. Teratogenic/Unsafe Medications During Pregnancy *(continued)*

INDICATION	SAFE TO USE	CONTRAINDICATED
Hypertension	Labetalol, hydralazine, nifedipine, methyldopa, clonidine.	ACEIs and angiotensin receptor blockers → fetal renal damage and oligohydramnios.
Hyperthyroidism	PTU.	Methimazole → aplasia cutis.
Hypothyroidism	Levothyroxine.	
Nausea/vomiting	Pyridoxine (B_6), doxylamine, prochlorperazine, metoclopramide, ondansetron, granisetron, promethazine.	Thalidomide → limb reduction and malformation of the ear, kidney, and heart.
Pain	Acetaminophen, menthol, topical patches, morphine, hydrocodone, propoxyphene, meperidine; these medications should not be used continuously.	Avoid NSAIDs in late pregnancy for > 48 hours. When used over a long period, will → premature closure of the ductus arteriosus.
Seizure	Use an anticonvulsant that works best to control maternal seizures. Monotherapy at the lowest dose is preferred. Folate supplementation should be started three months prior to conception.	Phenytoin → dysmorphic facies, microcephaly, mental retardation, hypoplasia of the nails and distal phalanges, and NTDs. Valproic acid → craniofacial defects and NTDs. Carbamazepine → craniofacial defects, mental retardation, and NTDs. Phenobarbital → **cleft palate** and **cardiac defects.** Trimethadione and paramethadione have strong teratogenic potential and → mental retardation, speech difficulty, and abnormal facies.
Thromboembolic disease	Heparin, low-molecular-weight heparin. Warfarin must be used in cases of highly thrombogenic artificial heart valves.	Warfarin → fetal nasal hypoplasia and bony defects (chondrodysplasia).
URI	Guaifenesin (Robitussin), acetaminophen, diphenhydramine, loratadine (Claritin).	

Obstetric Complications of Pregnancy

INTRAUTERINE GROWTH RESTRICTION (IUGR)

- Defined as an estimated fetal weight at or below the 10th percentile for GA. See Table 14-10 for common causes of IUGR.
- **Sx/Exam:** Suspect IUGR clinically if the difference between fundal height and GA is > 2 cm.
- **Tx: Focus on prevention**—eg, smoking cessation, BP control, and dietary changes. Order an ultrasound every 3–4 weeks to assess interval growth. Deliver once the pregnancy reaches term.

KEY FACT

Oligohydramnios almost always indicates the presence of a fetal abnormality.

OLIGOHYDRAMNIOS AND POLYHYDRAMNIOS

Table 14-11 contrasts oligohydramnios with polyhydramnios.

RHESUS (Rh) ISOIMMUNIZATION

When fetal Rh-⊕ RBCs leak into Rh-⊖ maternal circulation, **maternal anti-Rh IgG antibodies** can form. These antibodies can cross the placenta and react with fetal Rh-⊕ RBCs, leading to fetal hemolysis (erythroblastosis fetalis).

TREATMENT

- **Give RhoGAM to Rh-⊖ women:**
  - With prior delivery of an Rh-⊕ baby.
  - If the father is Rh ⊕, Rh status is unknown, or paternity is uncertain.
  - If the baby is Rh ⊕ at delivery.
  - If the woman has had ectopic pregnancies, abortions, amniocentesis or other traumatic procedures during pregnancy, vaginal bleeding, blood transfusions, or placental abruption.
- Sensitized Rh-⊖ women with titers > 1:16 should be closely monitored for evidence of fetal hemolysis with serial ultrasound and amniocentesis or middle cerebral artery Doppler velocimetry.
- In severe cases, intrauterine blood transfusion via the umbilical vein or preterm delivery is indicated.

TABLE 14-10. Causes of IUGR

FETAL	MATERNAL
Chromosomal abnormalities: Trisomy 21 is most common, followed by trisomies 18 and 13. **Infection: CMV is most common;** then toxoplasmosis. Placental abnormalities, uterine abnormalities, multiple gestations.	**Hypertension.** **Drugs: Cigarette** smoking is most common; also alcohol, heroin, methamphetamines, and cocaine. **SLE.** Maternal thrombophilia. Malnutrition, malabsorption (eg, cystic fibrosis). Ethnic/genetic variation.

TABLE 14-11. Oligohydramnios vs. Polyhydramnios

	Oligohydramnios	Polyhydramnios
Definition	Amniotic fluid index (AFI) ≤ 5 cm on ultrasound.	AFI ≥ 25 cm on ultrasound.
Causes	**Fetal urinary tract abnormalities** (renal agenesis, polycystic kidneys, GU obstruction). Chronic uteroplacental insufficiency, ROM.	Normal pregnancy, uncontrolled maternal DM, multiple gestations, pulmonary abnormalities, fetal anomalies (duodenal atresia, tracheoesophageal fistula).
Diagnosis	Ultrasound for anomalies. Rule out ROM with ferning test and Nitrazine paper.	Ultrasound for fetal anomalies; glucose testing for DM.
Treatment	Possible amnioinfusion during labor to prevent cord compression.	Depends on the cause; therapeutic amniocentesis.
Complications	**Cord compression** → fetal hypoxia. Musculoskeletal abnormalities (facial distortion, clubfoot). Pulmonary hypoplasia, IUGR.	Preterm labor, placental abruption, fetal malpresentation, cord prolapse.

THIRD-TRIMESTER BLEEDING

A 32-year-old G3P2 at 35 weeks' gestation is brought to the ER by ambulance with severe abdominal pain following a motor vehicle accident. Her BP is 92/47 and her pulse is 135/min. Her exam is significant for a severely tender, asymmetric gravid uterus. Fetal monitoring is worrisome. What is the cause?

Uterine rupture. The patient needs to go to the OR emergently for an exploratory laparotomy and a C-section.

- Describes any bleeding after 20 weeks' gestation.
- The most common causes are placental abruption and placenta previa (see Table 14-12).
- Other causes of bleeding include bloody show, preterm/early labor, vasa previa, genital tract lesions, and trauma (eg, intercourse).

TABLE 14-12. Common Causes of Third-Trimester Bleeding

	Placental Abruption	Placenta Previa	Uterine Rupture
Pathophysiology	**Placental separation** from the site of uterine implantation before delivery of the fetus.	**Abnormal placental implantation** near or covering the os.	**A complete rupture disrupts the entire thickness of the uterine wall.**
Risk factors	**Hypertension,** abdominal/pelvic trauma, tobacco or **cocaine use,** uterine distention.	**Prior C-section,** grand multiparity, multiple gestations, prior placenta previa.	**Prior uterine scar,** trauma (eg, motor vehicle accident), uterine anomalies, grand multiparity.

(continues)

TABLE 14-12. Common Causes of Third-Trimester Bleeding *(continued)*

	Placental Abruption	Placenta Previa	Uterine Rupture
Symptoms	Abdominal pain; vaginal bleeding that does not spontaneously cease. Prolonged tightening of the abdomen coupled with prolonged contraction. **Fetal distress.**	Painless vaginal bleeding that ceases spontaneously with or without uterine contractions. The first bleeding episode usually occurs in the second or third trimester. **Usually no fetal distress.**	Severe abdominal pain, usually during labor, typically at the scar site. Change in the shape of the abdomen. **Fetal distress.** Loss of fetal station.
Diagnosis	**Primarily clinical.** Ultrasound to look for retroplacental hemorrhage (low sensitivity).	**Ultrasound** for placental position.	**Primarily clinical; based on symptoms and fetal distress.**
Treatment	**Mild abruption or premature infant:** Hospitalization, fetal monitoring, type and cross, bed rest. **Moderate to severe abruption:** ABCs, type and cross, immediate delivery.	**No cervical exams!** Stabilize patients with a premature fetus. Serial ultrasound to assess fetal growth and resolution of previa. C-section for total or partial previa or if the patient/infant is in distress.	**Immediate C-section** with delivery of the infant and repair of the rupture.
Complications	Hemorrhagic shock; DIC; fetal death with severe abruption.	↑ risk of placenta accreta. Persistent hemorrhage requiring hysterectomy.	Fetal and maternal death.

Abnormal Labor and Delivery

PRETERM PREMATURE RUPTURE OF MEMBRANES (PPROM)

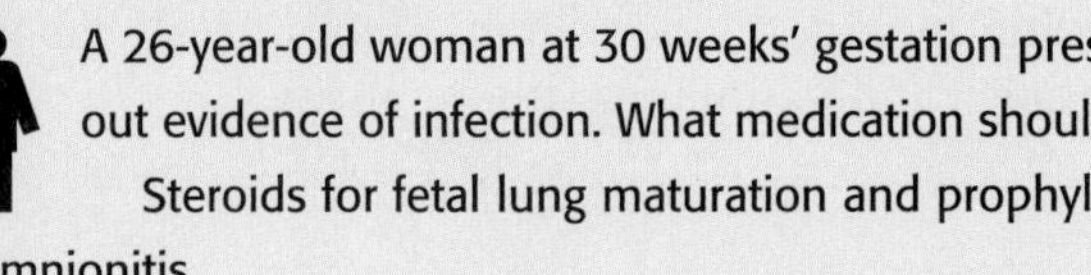

A 26-year-old woman at 30 weeks' gestation presents with PPROM without evidence of infection. What medication should be administered?

Steroids for fetal lung maturation and prophylactic antibiotics for chorioamnionitis.

Defined as spontaneous ROM at < **37 weeks,** prior to the onset of labor. Distinguished from premature rupture of membranes (PROM), which refers to loss of fluid at term prior to the onset of contractions. Risk factors include low socioeconomic status, young maternal age, smoking, and STDs.

Symptoms/Exam

- Sterile speculum exam shows pooling of amniotic fluid in the posterior vaginal vault.
- Look for cervical dilation.

DIAGNOSIS

- **Nitrazine paper test:** Paper turns blue in alkaline amniotic fluid.
- **Fern test:** A ferning pattern is seen under the microscope after amniotic fluid dries on glass slide.
- Determine AFI by ultrasound to assess amniotic fluid volume.

TREATMENT

- Obtain cultures and/or wet mounts to look for infectious causes. If signs of infection are present, assume **amnionitis** (maternal fever, fetal tachycardia, foul-smelling amniotic fluid). Give antibiotics (ampicillin +/– gentamicin) and **induce labor** regardless of GA.
- If no signs of infection are present and GA is **24–32 weeks,** treat with **antibiotics (ampicillin and erythromycin)** to prolong pregnancy and **steroids** for fetal lung maturation +/– **tocolytics.**
- If no signs of infection are present and GA is ≥ **33 weeks,** hospitalize and treat expectantly until labor begins, signs of infection are seen, or 34 weeks' gestation is achieved.

PRETERM LABOR

Labor between 20 and 36 weeks' gestation.

SYMPTOMS/EXAM

- Patients may complain of menstrual-like cramps, uterine contractions, low back pain, pelvic pressure, new vaginal discharge, or bleeding.
- Rule out cervical insufficiency (treated with cerclage if early enough) and **preterm contractions** (no cervical dilation).
- Can lead to fetal respiratory distress syndrome, intraventricular hemorrhage, retinopathy of prematurity, necrotizing enterocolitis, or fetal death.

DIAGNOSIS

- Obtain an **ultrasound** to verify GA, fetal presentation, and AFI.
- Look for **regular** uterine contractions (three or more contractions lasting 30 seconds each over a 30-minute period) coupled with a concurrent cervical change at < 37 weeks' gestation.

TREATMENT

- Begin with **hydration** and **bed rest.**
- Unless contraindicated, **administer steroids (to accelerate fetal lung maturity)** +/– tocolytics.
- Give **penicillin or ampicillin** for GBS prophylaxis if preterm delivery is likely.

FETAL MALPRESENTATION

Defined as any presentation other than cephalic (head down). Breech presentation is the most common fetal malpresentation (affects 3% of all pregnancies).

DIAGNOSIS

- Perform Leopold maneuvers to identify fetal lie.
- Check by ultrasound if there is **any** doubt.

Treatment

- **Follow:** Up to 75% of cases spontaneously change to cephalic presentation by 38 weeks.
- **External cephalic version** can be attempted at 36–37 weeks' gestation in the setting of persistent malpresentation.
  - Involves pressure applied to the maternal abdomen to turn the infant.
  - Risks of the procedure are placental abruption and cord compression; the infant **must** be monitored after the procedure, and consent must be obtained for emergent C-section.

SHOULDER DYSTOCIA

Defined as difficult delivery due to entrapment of the fetal shoulder at the level of the pubic bone. Risk factors include the following:

- A prior history of a shoulder dystocia.
- Fetal macrosomia or inadequate pelvis.

Diagnosis

- A prolonged second stage of labor with retraction of the head ("turtle sign") back into the vaginal canal after pushing.
- After delivery of the head, difficulty delivering the anterior shoulder without performing additional maneuvers.

Treatment

Flex and open the maternal hips (McRoberts maneuver), followed by suprapubic pressure. Most dystocias will be relieved with these two maneuvers:

- Delivery of the posterior fetal arm or internal rotation of the fetal shoulders to lessen the shoulder diameter.
- Replacement of the fetal head into the vaginal canal, followed by cesarean section (Zavanelli maneuver).

INDICATIONS FOR CESAREAN SECTION

Table 14-13 outlines the indications for C-section.

TABLE 14-13. Indications for Cesarean Section

Maternal Factors	Fetal and Maternal Factors	Fetal Factors
Prior C-section Active genital herpes infection Cervical carcinoma Maternal trauma/demise	**Cephalopelvic disproportion** (the most common cause of 1° C-section) Placenta previa/placental abruption Failed vaginal delivery	Fetal malposition Fetal distress Cord prolapse Erythroblastosis fetalis (Rh incompatibility)

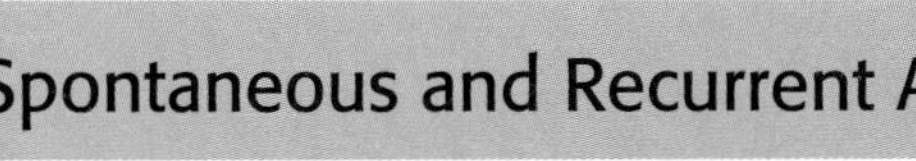

Spontaneous and Recurrent Abortion

SPONTANEOUS ABORTION (SAB)

Defined as **nonelective** termination of pregnancy at < 20 weeks' gestation. Also known as "miscarriage." Occurs in 10–15% of clinically recognizable pregnancies.

Symptoms/Exam

Differentiate types of SABs on the basis of symptoms, cervical exam, and ultrasound (see Table 14-14).

Differential

Common causes of first-trimester bleeding include normal pregnancy (implantation bleeding), postcoital bleeding, ectopic pregnancy, vaginal or cervical lesions, pedunculated myomas or polyps, and extrusion of molar pregnancy.

TABLE 14-14. Types of Spontaneous Abortions

Type	Symptoms	Cervix/Ultrasound	Treatment
Threatened abortion	Minimal bleeding +/− cramping. Most cases are thought to be due to implantation bleed. **No products of conception (POC) are expelled.**	Closed os; ⊕ gestational sac.	Expectant management; consider pelvic rest for several weeks.
Inevitable abortion	Cramping with bleeding. **No POC are expelled.**	Open os; normal ultrasound.	D&C.
Incomplete abortion	Cramping with bleeding. **Some POC are expelled.**	Open os; normal ultrasound.	D&C.
Complete abortion	Slight bleeding; pain has usually ceased. **All POC are expelled.**	Closed os; empty uterus on ultrasound.	None.
Missed abortion	Often no symptoms. **No POC are expelled.**	Closed os; no fetal cardiac activity; retained fetal tissue on ultrasound.	Allow up to four weeks for POC to pass; offer medical management with misoprostol or D&C.
Septic abortion	Constitutional symptoms; malodorous discharge. Patients often have a recent history of therapeutic abortion; maternal mortality is 10–50%.	Cervical motion tenderness.	Monitor ABCs; D&C, IV antibiotics, supportive care.

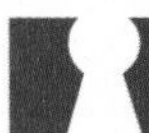

KEY FACT

All women with potential SABs should receive RhoGAM if appropriate.

Treatment

- Hemodynamic monitoring for significant bleeding.
- Check β-hCG to confirm pregnancy and transvaginal ultrasound to establish GA and rule out ectopic pregnancies; assess fetal viability or check for remaining tissue in the setting of a completed abortion.
- Check blood type and antibody screen; give RhoGAM if appropriate.

RECURRENT ABORTION

- Defined as three or more consecutive pregnancy losses before 20 weeks' gestation.
- Usually due to **chromosomal** or **uterine abnormalities,** but can also result from hormonal abnormalities, infection, or systemic disease.
- **Dx:** Based on clinical and lab findings.
  - Perform a pelvic exam (to look for anatomic abnormalities).
  - Check cervical cultures for chlamydia and gonorrhea.
  - Perform a maternal and paternal genetic analysis.
  - Obtain a hysterosalpingogram to look for uterine abnormalities.
  - Obtain TFTs, progesterone, lupus anticoagulant, and anticardiolipin antibody.
- **Tx:** Treatment is based on the diagnosis.

CHAPTER 15

GYNECOLOGY

KEY FACT

Any woman > 35 years of age with unexplained bleeding needs an endometrial biopsy to rule out malignancy.

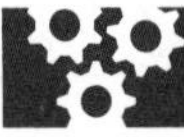

MNEMONIC

Causes of uterine bleeding–

MS. PDA

Malignancy
Systemic
Postmenopausal
Dysfunctional
Anatomic

Abnormal Uterine Bleeding

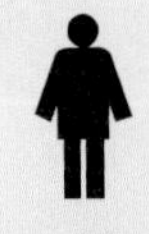

A 38-year-old woman has a history of bilateral tubal ligations five years ago. She presents to her gynecologist with intermittent and painless noncyclic vaginal bleeding of two months' duration. She otherwise feels well and has a normal cervical exam. What is the next step?

You must rule out endometrial cancer by performing an endometrial biopsy or a D&C (the gold standard).

Abnormalities in the frequency, duration, volume, and/or timing of menstrual bleeding. Defined as follows:

- **Menorrhagia:** Heavy or prolonged menstrual flow.
- **Metrorrhagia:** Bleeding between menses.
- **Metromenorrhagia:** Heavy bleeding at irregular intervals.

There are multiple causes of abnormal uterine bleeding (see Table 15-1 and the mnemonic **MS. PDA**).

TABLE 15-1. Types of Abnormal Uterine Bleeding

Category	Etiology	Diagnosis
Malignancy	Endometrial and cervical malignancies are most common, but malignancies may occur anywhere along the genital tract.	Endometrial biopsy, Pap smear/cervical biopsy, D&C (gold standard).
Systemic	1° bleeding disorders (eg, von Willebrand's disease), endocrine abnormalities.	Coagulation profile, bleeding time, endocrine tests (FSH, LH, TSH, and prolactin).
Postmenopausal bleeding	Endometrial cancer, vaginal atrophy, exogenous hormones.	By definition, occurs one or more years after menopause. Malignancy must be ruled out!
Dysfunctional uterine bleeding (DUB)	A **diagnosis of exclusion.** Ninety percent of cases are due to unopposed estrogen in anovulation that leads to proliferative endometrium; 10% of cases are ovulatory.	Other causes must be ruled out.
Anatomic	Leiomyoma, adenomyosis, or polyps.	Pelvic ultrasound, sonohysterogram, hysteroscopy.

Exam/Diagnosis

- Determine if the bleeding is **ovulatory** or **anovulatory.**
  - **Ovulatory:**
    - Characterized by midcycle bleeding or changes in menstrual flow.
    - Can present with premenstrual syndrome symptoms (weight gain, breast tenderness, dysmenorrhea).
  - **Anovulatory:**
    - Unpredictable bleeding patterns.
    - Excessive and prolonged bleeding due to unopposed estrogen on the endometrium.
    - Seen mostly in adolescent and perimenopausal women.
    - Associated with an ↑ risk of endometrial hyperplasia and cancer.
- Look for a cervical lesion on speculum exam or an enlarged uterus on bimanual exam.

Treatment

- Treat the underlying cause.
- Acute, profuse bleeding can be treated with high-dose IV estrogen, D&C, uterine artery embolization, or hysterectomy.
- DUB and anovulatory bleeding are treated with OCPs or NSAIDs.

Amenorrhea

Defined as either 1° or 2° amenorrhea.

- **1° amenorrhea:** Absence of menses and lack of 2° sexual characteristics by age 14 **or** absence of menses by age 16 with or without 2° sexual characteristics. Associated with gonadal failure, congenital abnormalities, and constitutional symptoms (see Figure 15-1).
- **2° amenorrhea:** Absence of menses for three cycles or for six months with prior normal menses. Etiologies include pregnancy, anorexia nervosa, stress, strenuous exercise, intrauterine adhesions, chronic anovulation, hypothyroidism, and hyperprolactinemia (see Figure 15-2).

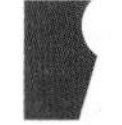

KEY FACT

Always rule out pregnancy in a patient with amenorrhea.

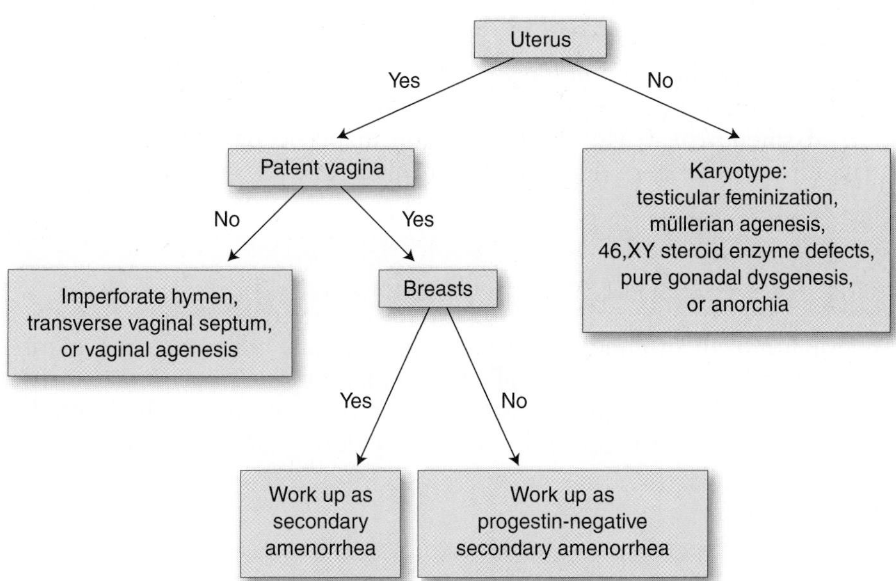

FIGURE 15-1. Workup for patients with 1° amenorrhea. (Modified with permission from DeCherney AH, Nathan L. *Current Diagnosis & Treatment: Obstetrics & Gynecology,* 10th ed. New York: McGraw-Hill, 2007, Fig. 56-2.)

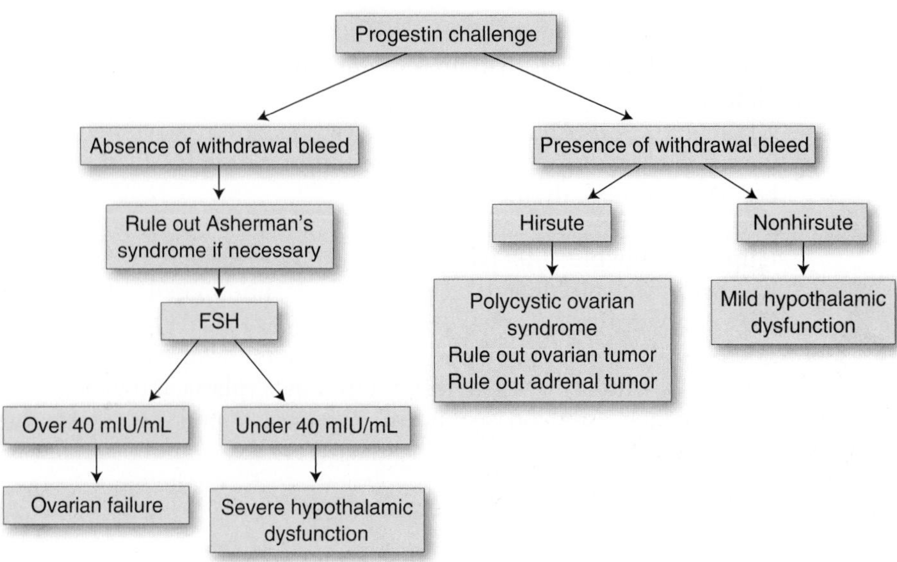

FIGURE 15-2. Workup for patients with 2° amenorrhea. (Modified with permission from DeCherney AH, Nathan L. *Current Diagnosis & Treatment: Obstetrics & Gynecology,* 10th ed. New York: McGraw-Hill, 2007, Fig. 56-4.)

KEY FACT

Amenorrhea is a symptom, not a diagnosis.

Diagnosis

- **Check β-hCG** to make sure the patient is not pregnant.
- **1° amenorrhea:** See Figure 15-1.
- **2° amenorrhea:** See Figure 15-2.

Treatment

Depends on the etiology; may include surgery or hormonal therapy +/– drug therapy.

Dysmenorrhea

Defined as pain with menstrual periods that requires medication and prevents normal activity. It is divided into 1° and 2° dysmenorrhea.

- **1° dysmenorrhea:** No clinically detectable pelvic pathology. Most likely due to ↑ uterine prostaglandin production.
- **2° dysmenorrhea:** Menstrual pain due to pelvic pathology, most commonly endometriosis, adenomyosis, myomas, or PID.

Endometriosis

Abnormal growth of endometrial tissue in locations other than the uterine lining, usually in the ovaries (called endometriomas or "chocolate cysts"), cul-de-sac, and broad ligament. Associated with premenstrual pelvic pain due to stimulation from estrogen and progesterone during the menstrual cycle.

Symptoms/Exam

- Presents with pelvic pain, dysmenorrhea, dyspareunia, and infertility.
- On pelvic exam, patients may have tender nodularity along the uterosacral ligament +/– a fixed, retroflexed uterus or enlarged ovaries.

DIAGNOSIS

Diagnosis can be made by the history and physical, but the gold standard is direct visualization during laparoscopy with biopsy showing endometrial glands.

TREATMENT

Treatment depends on the patient's symptoms, age, desire for future fertility, and disease stage.

- If the patient's main complaint is **infertility,** operative laparoscopy should be performed to excise the endometriomas.
- If the patient's main complaint is **pain,** the objective is to induce a state of anovulation:
  - For mild pain, first-line treatment is NSAIDs and/or continuous OCPs.
  - For moderate to severe pain, options include medical treatment to induce anovulation (GnRH agonists) or **excision.**
- Hysterectomy with bilateral oophorectomy is curative.

Polycystic Ovarian Syndrome (PCOS)

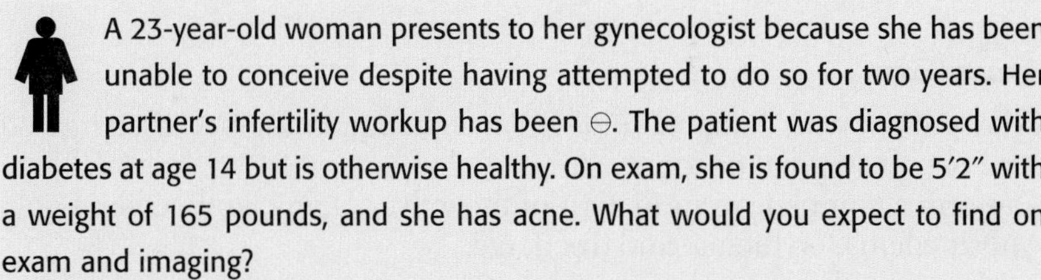

A 23-year-old woman presents to her gynecologist because she has been unable to conceive despite having attempted to do so for two years. Her partner's infertility workup has been ⊖. The patient was diagnosed with diabetes at age 14 but is otherwise healthy. On exam, she is found to be 5′2″ with a weight of 165 pounds, and she has acne. What would you expect to find on exam and imaging?

The patient probably has PCOS. You would expect to find enlarged ovaries on bimanual exam and polycystic ovaries on ultrasound/CT scan.

The most common cause of female hirsutism (male-pattern hair growth). Typically affects adolescent women. The cause is unknown.

SYMPTOMS

Look for an obese woman with hirsutism, oligo- or amenorrhea, infertility, acne, and diabetes or insulin resistance.

EXAM

- Exam may reveal hirsutism with no evidence of cortisol or adrenal androgen excess.
- Pelvic exam may reveal palpably enlarged ovaries.

DIAGNOSIS

- Two out of three of the following clinical signs must be present to diagnose PCOS:
  - Oligo- or anovulation.
  - Hyperandrogenism (acne, hirsutism, or elevated testosterone).
  - Polycystic ovaries.
- An ↑ LH/FSH ratio (> 2) is also characteristic.
- Perform a glucose tolerance test to evaluate for **diabetes/hyperglycemia.**

TREATMENT

Treat the specific symptoms:

- **Infertility:** Induce ovulation with clomiphene and/or metformin.
- **Hirsutism:** Start combination OCPs to suppress ovarian steroidogenesis.
- **Hyperglycemia/diabetes:** Weight loss; hypoglycemic agents.

Vulvovaginitis

A 19-year-old woman who is sexually active with multiple partners presents to your clinic with vaginal pruritus and ↑ discharge. A wet mount and KOH prep reveal no organisms. What organism is likely contributing to her vulvovaginitis?

Chlamydia.

The most common outpatient gynecologic problem. Vulvovaginitis can be bacterial (bacterial vaginosis), fungal (*Candida*), or protozoal (*Trichomonas vaginalis*). Figure 15-3 depicts the histologic appearance of two common causes of vulvovaginitis.

KEY FACT

Sexual abuse must be considered in any child with vulvovaginitis.

SYMPTOMS/EXAM

- May present with ↑ vaginal discharge, a change in vaginal discharge odor, and/or vulvovaginal pruritus.
- Perform a complete examination of the vulva, vagina, and cervix. Look for vulvar edema, erythema, and discharge.

DIAGNOSIS/TREATMENT

Obtain swabs from the vagina to perform a wet mount and cultures for gonorrhea and chlamydia (see Table 15-2).

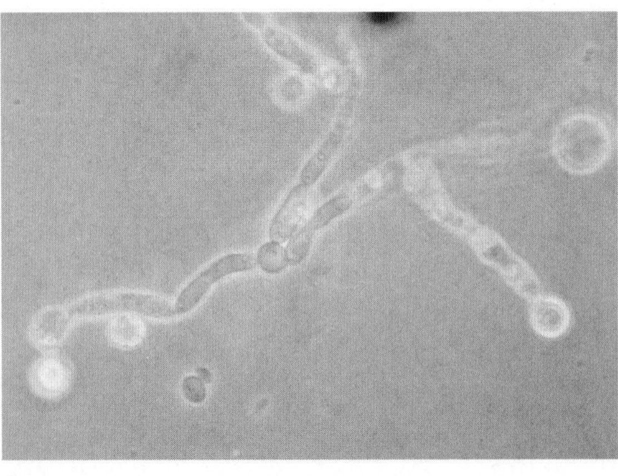

A

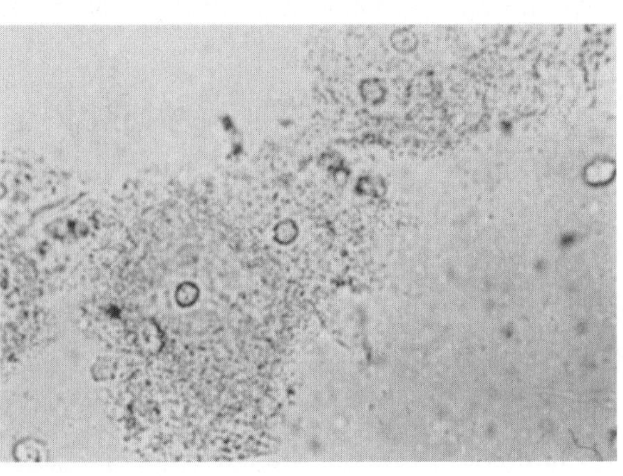

B

FIGURE 15-3. Causes of vaginitis. (**A**) Candidal vaginitis. *Candida albicans* organisms are evident on KOH wet mount. (**B**) *Gardnerella vaginalis.* Note the granular epithelial cells ("clue cells") and indistinct cell margins. (Image A reproduced with permission from Wolff K, Johnson RA. *Fitzpatrick's Color Atlas & Synopsis of Clinical Dermatology,* 6th ed. New York: McGraw-Hill, 2009: 720. Image B reproduced with permission from Kasper DL et al. *Harrison's Principles of Internal Medicine,* 16th ed. New York: McGraw-Hill, 2005: 767.)

TABLE 15-2. Common Causes of Vulvovaginitis

	Bacterial Vaginosis	Yeast (usually *Candida*)	*Trichomonas vaginalis*
Exam	Can be unremarkable except for discharge.	Erythema and irritation.	The vagina and cervix may be swollen and red.
Discharge	Grayish or white, having a **fishy odor;** pronounced after intercourse.	White, curdlike.	Yellow-green, malodorous.
Wet mount	Reveals > 20% of epithelial cells with indistinct cell margins ("clue cells"; see Figure 15-3).	Nothing.	Motile, flagellated protozoans.
KOH prep	⊕ **"whiff test"** (KOH placed on a slide leads to a fishy odor).	Pseudohyphae and spores (see Figure 15-3).	**Nothing.**
pH	Elevated (ie, > 7).	Normal or < 7.	Elevated or > 7.
Treatment			
Nonpregnant	Metronidazole.	Topical antifungal × 3–7 days or oral fluconazole × 1 dose.	Metronidazole.
Pregnant	Metronidazole.	Use only topical antifungals × 7 days.	Metronidazole.

Ectopic Pregnancy

A 28-year-old woman who found out that she was pregnant one week ago presents to the ER complaining of fevers and RLQ abdominal pain. Her exam is significant for RLQ tenderness and no cervical motion tenderness. What should be the next step?

Abdominal ultrasound to look for an adnexal mass. It is too early to visualize an intrauterine gestational sac. Also, trend the patient's β-hCG, as levels tend to rise less in ectopic as opposed to intrauterine pregnancies. It is also important to consider nongynecologic causes.

Defined as any pregnancy that is implanted outside the uterine cavity. The most common location is the fallopian tube (95%). Risk factors include a history of PID, prior ectopic pregnancy, tubal/pelvic surgery, DES exposure in utero leading to abnormal tubal development, and IUD use.

Symptoms/Exam

- Patients may complain of lower abdominal or pelvic pain as well as abnormal vaginal spotting or bleeding and amenorrhea.
- The abdomen may be tender to palpation. Bimanual exam may also reveal cervical motion tenderness and an adnexal mass.
- A ruptured ectopic may present with unstable vital signs, diffuse abdominal pain, rebound tenderness, and shock.

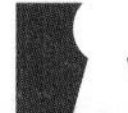

KEY FACT

Any woman with abdominal pain needs a urine pregnancy test.

DIFFERENTIAL

Spontaneous abortion, molar pregnancy, ruptured corpus luteum cyst, PID, ovarian torsion, appendicitis, pyelonephritis, diverticulitis, regional ileitis, ulcerative colitis.

DIAGNOSIS

- **An ↑ β-hCG in the absence of an intrauterine pregnancy on ultrasound is highly suspicious for an ectopic pregnancy.**
- Do an ultrasound to look for an intrauterine pregnancy, an adnexal mass, or free fluid (see Figure 15-4).
- The gestational sac may be visualized on:
  - **Transvaginal** ultrasound when β-hCG is approximately 1000–2000 mIU/mL, or at approximately 4–5 weeks' GA.
  - **Transabdominal** ultrasound when β-hCG is > 1800–3600 mIU/mL.
- Fetal heart motion of the embryo can be seen after 5–6 weeks' GA.
- Definitive diagnosis is made by laparoscopy, laparotomy, or ultrasound visualization of a pregnancy outside the uterus.

KEY FACT

↑ β-hCG in the absence of an intrauterine pregnancy on ultrasound is suspicious for an ectopic pregnancy.

TREATMENT

- For **hemodynamically unstable** patients, immediate surgery is required.
- For **hemodynamically stable** patients:
  - Follow serial β-hCG levels closely with or without ultrasound studies.
  - **Methotrexate** is used for small (< 3.5-cm), unruptured ectopic pregnancies in asymptomatic women until levels are undetectable.
  - **Laparoscopy or laparotomy for removal of ectopic pregnancy.**
- Expectant management is appropriate for stable, compliant patients with decreasing β-hCG levels or β-hCG < 200 mIU/mL, and if the risk of rupture is low.
- Prevention of ectopic pregnancies includes prevention and thorough **treatment of STDs.**

KEY FACT

All women with ectopic pregnancies should be typed and screened and given RhoGAM if Rh is ⊖.

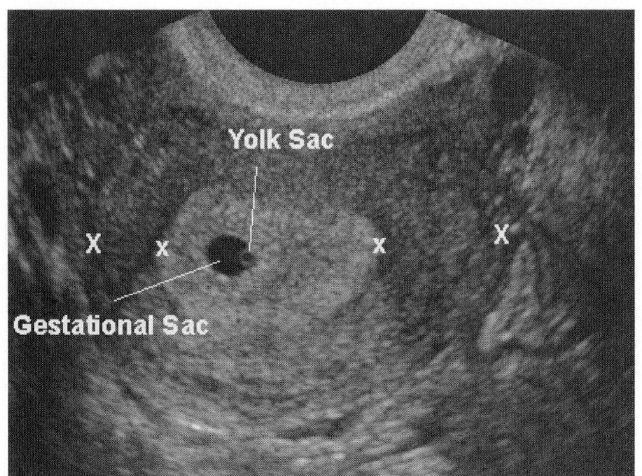

A

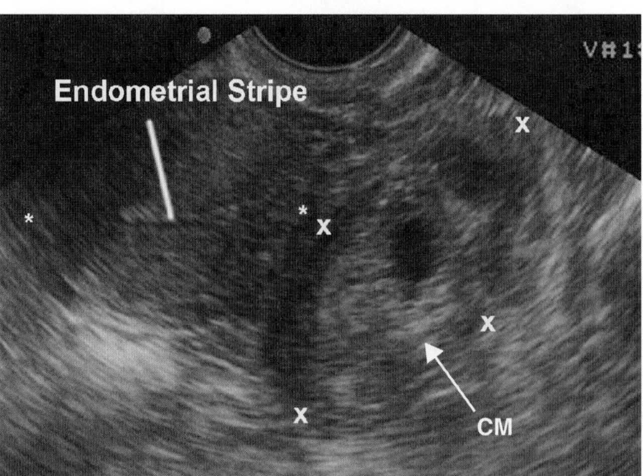

B

FIGURE 15-4. Normal intrauterine pregnancy and ectopic pregnancy. Transvaginal ultrasound showing (**A**) a normal intrauterine pregnancy with a gestational sac containing a yolk sac within the uterine cavity, and (**B**) a complex mass (CM)/ectopic pregnancy adjacent to an empty uterus. (Reproduced with permission from Tintinalli JE et al. *Tintinalli's Emergency Medicine: A Comprehensive Study Guide,* 6th ed. New York: McGraw-Hill, 2004, Figs. 113-15 and 113-22.)

Contraception

ORAL CONTRACEPTIVES (OCPs)

The long-term consequences of OCP use include a ↓ in ovarian and endometrial cancers, a ↓ incidence of breast disease (but not breast cancer), ↓ menstrual flow, and ↓ dysmenorrhea. OCP use also ↑ the risk of hypertension and stroke. Contraindications to OCP use include the following:

- Pregnancy.
- Previous or active thromboembolic disease.
- Smoking in patients > 35 years of age.
- Undiagnosed genital bleeding.
- Estrogen-dependent neoplasms.
- Hepatocellular carcinoma.
- Acute liver dysfunction.

OTHER HORMONAL CONTRACEPTIVES

Have fewer compliance issues than OCPs. Include the following:

- **Injectable (Depo-Provera):** Administered intramuscularly every three months.
- **Transdermal (Ortho Evra):** A patch that is changed weekly for three weeks followed by a one-week holiday.
- **Vaginal (NuvaRing):** A vaginal ring that is removed after three weeks followed by a one-week holiday.
- **Intrauterine (Mirena):** See the discussion of IUDs below.

INTRAUTERINE DEVICES (IUDs)

A 36-year-old mother with a history of breast cancer presents to her gynecologist seeking a reliable, "hassle-free" birth control option. She has been in a long-term relationship with her husband. What method would you recommend?

A copper IUD would be optimal for this patient, since she has a contraindication to using hormonal contraceptives and is not at high risk for contracting STDs.

Two types of IUDs are approved for use in the United States. Both are highly effective, with > 99% efficacy during the first year of use.

- **Levonorgestrel IUD** (trade name Mirena):
  - Lasts 5 years.
  - ↓ the amount of menstrual bleeding and dysmenorrhea; thus, a good choice for the treatment of menorrhagia.
  - **Side effects:** Irregular menstrual bleeding or amenorrhea.
- **Copper IUD** (trade name ParaGard):
  - Lasts 10 years.
  - Nonhormonal; a good choice for women who have contraindications to hormone treatment.
  - **Side effects:** Dysmenorrhea and ↑ menstrual bleeding.

EMERGENCY CONTRACEPTION

- Should be taken immediately after intercourse; can be taken up to five days afterward, but with decreasing effectiveness.
- Options include levonorgestrel +/– estradiol.

Infertility

Defined as the inability of a couple to conceive after one year of unprotected intercourse. It affects 10–15% of couples. Causes include the following:

- **Male dysfunction (35%):** Defects in spermatogenesis (male factor); varicoceles.
- **Female dysfunction (50%):**
  - **Uterine/tubal factors: Endometriosis** or myomas that distort the endometrium or fallopian tubes, PID, congenital genital tract abnormalities.
  - **Ovulatory dysfunction:** Ovarian failure, prolactinoma.
  - **Endocrine dysfunction:** Thyroid/adrenal disease, PCOS.
- **Unexplained infertility and rare problems (15%).**

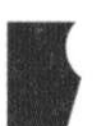

KEY FACT

Endometriosis is the leading cause of female infertility, followed by PID.

DIAGNOSIS

- Semen analysis to rule out male factors.
- Serum FSH/LH/TSH/prolactin to rule out endocrine dysfunction.
- Hysterosalpingography to rule out tubal and uterine cavity abnormalities.
- Basal body temperatures or ovulation kits to rule out ovulatory dysfunction.

TREATMENT

- Treat the underlying cause.
- Fertility rates in endometriosis can be improved through laparoscopic removal of implants outside the uterine cavity.
- Ovulation can be induced with **clomiphene,** but this can lead to ovarian hyperstimulation and multiple gestations.
- For refractory cases, assisted reproductive technologies such as in vitro fertilization can be used.

Menopause

Cessation of menstruation for > 12 months. Average age of onset is 51. Surgical menopause occurs following removal or irradiation of the ovaries. Postmenopausal women are at ↑ risk for developing **osteoporosis** and **heart disease.**

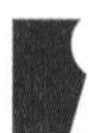

KEY FACT

Premature menopause occurs before age 40 and is often due to idiopathic premature ovarian failure.

SYMPTOMS/EXAM

- Patients may complain of menstrual irregularities, hot flashes, sweating, sleep disturbances, mood changes, ↓ libido, and vaginal dryness.
- Exam may reveal vaginal dryness, ↓ breast size, and genital tract atrophy.

DIAGNOSIS

- Requires **one year** without menses with no other known cause.
- ↑↑ **serum FSH** (> **30 IU/L**) is suggestive.

TREATMENT

- Hormone therapy with estrogen (in woman without a uterus) or combined estrogen and progesterone (in woman with an intact uterus) can be used for short-term symptomatic relief.
- Absolute contraindications to hormone therapy include undiagnosed vaginal bleeding, active liver disease, recent MI, recent or active vascular thrombosis, and a history of endometrial or breast cancer.
- Alternatives to hormone therapy include the following:
  - **Vasomotor instability:** Venlafaxine and some SSRIs.
  - **Vaginal atrophy:** Vaginal lubricants or topical estrogens.
  - **Osteoporosis:** Calcium, vitamin D, calcitonin, bisphosphonates (alendronate), and selective estrogen receptor modulators (raloxifene).
- Unopposed estrogen (without progesterone therapy) can lead to endometrial hyperplasia and/or carcinoma.

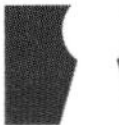

KEY FACT

Use the lowest possible dose of hormone therapy for the shortest duration to treat symptoms.

Urinary Incontinence

A 43-year-old mother of four presents to her primary care physician complaining of urinary leakage that has occurred during her aerobics classes and when she coughs or lifts heavy objects. These symptoms started after the birth of her last child. She wants to avoid surgery if at all possible. What do you recommend?

This patient has stress incontinence from a weakened pelvic floor. Kegel exercises can strengthen the pelvic floor and improve symptoms. Pessaries can also be used to prevent embarrassing leakage.

Involuntary loss of urine that is a social or hygienic problem. See Table 15-3 for an outline of stress, urge, and mixed incontinence.

EXAM/DIAGNOSIS

- Voiding diaries can help quantify the frequency and volume of urine lost, the circumstances of leakage (to diagnose stress or urge types of incontinence), voiding patterns, and the amount and type of fluid taken in.
- Patients with incontinence should have a screening neurologic exam to rule out neurologic causes.
- A standing cough stress test can be used to diagnose stress incontinence; cystometry can be used to diagnose urge incontinence.
- Urinary retention with overflow can be a cause of urinary incontinence and can be diagnosed with an elevated postvoid residual.

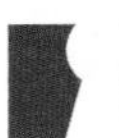

KEY FACT

UTI must be ruled out in all women complaining of urinary incontinence.

TREATMENT

Table 15-3 outlines treatment measures for urinary incontinence.

TABLE 15-3. Types of Urinary Incontinence

	Stress Incontinence	Urge Incontinence (Detrusor Instability)	Mixed Incontinence
History	Loss of urine with exertion (running) or straining (coughing, laughing).	Loss of urine with strong desire to void. Often associated with urinary frequency and urgency.	Stress and urge incontinence present simultaneously.
Mechanism	Poor support or poor function of the urethral sphincter.	Involuntary detrusor muscle contractions.	A combination of both mechanisms.
Etiology	Urethral hypermobility; weakened urethral closing mechanisms.	Idiopathic, neurologic (Alzheimer's, diabetes, MS).	As for both conditions.
Diagnosis	Patient history. Demonstrable leakage with stress (cough).	Patient history. Cystometry reveals involuntary detrusor muscle contraction associated with urinary leakage.	As for both conditions.
Treatment	Pelvic floor strengthening exercises (Kegel) +/– biofeedback, pessaries, weight loss, surgery to restore bladder neck support.	Behavior modification (eg, limiting fluid intake; avoiding caffeinated or alcoholic beverages). Bladder training. Medical therapy (anticholinergic). Surgical therapy (sacral neurostimulators, intravesical Botox injections).	Based on the patient's worst symptom; some treatments overlap (eg, Kegel exercises).

Benign Breast Disorders

Include **fibrocystic change** (the most common), fibroadenoma, intraductal papilloma (a common cause of bloody nipple discharge), duct ectasia, fat necrosis, mastitis, and breast abscess. See Table 15-4 for a list of common examples.

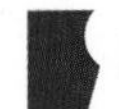

KEY FACT

Always rule out a breast malignancy with a biopsy in anyone who is high risk.

TABLE 15-4. Benign Breast Disease

Disease Type	Symptoms/Exam	Treatment	Associated with Carcinoma
Fibrocystic changes	Mild to moderate pain in the breasts +/– lumps premenstrually; multifocal, bilateral nodularity. Most common in women 20–50 years of age.	OCPs.	Patients are at ↑ risk of breast cancer only in the presence of cellular atypia. Cancer must be excluded in high-risk groups.
Fibroadenoma	**The most common tumor in menstruating women** < 25 years of age. Presents as a small, firm, unilateral, nontender mass that is freely movable and slow growing. Ultrasound can be used to differentiate from a cyst.	Thirty percent will spontaneously disappear. Removal is not necessary, but surgical excision is both diagnostic and curative. Biopsy if the patient is in a high-risk group. Recurrence is common.	Risk is twice as high as that of control patients.
Intraductal papilloma	Clear, bloody, or discolored fluid from a single duct opening. Milking of the breast shows drainage from one duct opening.	Drainage and surgical exploration of the duct. **A malignant process must always be excluded.**	Risk is twice as high as that of control patients.
Mastitis	Seen in breast-feeding women; presents as a hard, red, tender, swollen area of breast accompanied by fever, myalgias, and general malaise.	Continued breast-feeding; NSAIDs and antibiotics to cover common etiologies (staph, strep, *E coli*).	None.
Abscess	Can develop if mastitis is inadequately treated. Exam reveals a fluctuant mass accompanied by systemic symptoms similar to those seen in mastitis.	Needle aspiration or surgical drainage in addition to antibiotics.	None.
Fat necrosis	Firm, tender, and ill defined with surrounding erythema; related to trauma/ischemia.	Analgesia. An excisional biopsy may be done to rule out malignancy.	None.

Well-Child Care/Routine Health Screening

Routine health screening includes the monitoring of growth and development, the prevention of illness, safety, and anticipatory guidance to help parents prepare for their child's next steps. Routine screening should be conducted at the following intervals:

- **Metabolic/genetic diseases:** At one day of life, a state newborn screen is drawn. The exact tests conducted vary by state but typically include testing for disorders for which early identification and treatment would significantly improve morbidity and mortality for affected infants.
- **Growth parameters/development/behavior:** Screen at each visit—ie, at 2–4 weeks, 2 months, 4 months, 6 months, 9 months, 12 months, 15 months, 18 months, and 2 years. Then screen annually.
- **Lead/anemia:** Screen at 9–15 months in communities where more than one-third of the houses were built before 1950; where > 12% of one- and two-year-old children have been found to have elevated serum lead levels; or where limited information is available about the lead levels of the children in the community. Lead screening should be repeated at age two, especially in high-risk communities. Consider repeating anemia screening in menstruating adolescents and screening for anemia at six months in premature infants.
- **BP:** Screen with every medical exam starting at age three. Norms are based on sex, age, and height percentile.
- **Vision and hearing screening:** Conduct subjective testing at each visit; red-reflex testing at all infant visits; and objective hearing and vision screening at birth and annually starting at age three.
- **TB:** Conduct a risk assessment at each well-child check. PPD placement is appropriate for high-risk children.
- **High-risk behaviors/STD screening:** Screen at each adolescent visit (beginning at approximately 10–11 years of age).

KEY FACT

Commonly tested disorders on newborn screens:

- Phenylketonuria
- Congenital hypothyroidism
- Galactosemia
- Sickle cell disease
- Biotinidase deficiency
- Congenital adrenal hyperplasia
- Maple syrup urine disease
- Tyrosinemia
- Cystic fibrosis (CF)
- Medium-chain acyl-CoA dehydrogenase deficiency
- Toxoplasmosis

GROWTH AND DEVELOPMENT

A concerned parent brings his 11-month-old son to see you because the child is smaller than his cousins, who are approximately the same age. The boy has been meeting his developmental milestones, and when you plot his height and weight, you find that his weight is in the 10th percentile and height in the 25th percentile. His physical exam is unremarkable. According to his past records, his height has been in the 25th percentile since birth, and his weight has been in the 10th to 25th percentile. What further evaluation should you consider?

None; the boy's growth is appropriate.

Failure to Thrive (FTT)

Although there is no consensus for the definition of FTT, criteria that are often used include the following:

- Weight less than the third to fifth percentile for gestation-corrected age and sex on growth charts on more than one occasion.
- Weight for height less than the 10th percentile.
- ↓ weight velocity with crossing of two major percentiles (90th, 75th, 50th, 25th, 10th, 5th) on the growth chart.

- Daily weight gain less than expected for age.
- **Failure to grow:** Growth that is significantly slower than that of children of the same age. Height and weight are both slow (eg, growth hormone deficiency, genetic disease).
- **Failure to gain weight:** The child is or was previously able to maintain normal height velocity, but weight is disproportionately low or has "fallen off" the growth curve. Height velocity may subsequently slow if the child has been underweight for a prolonged period of time. Head circumference is the last to fall off the curve.
- **Short stature:**
  - Height less than the third percentile for age, with weight in the normal range.
  - ↓ height velocity with crossing of two major percentiles on the growth chart, with normal or ↑ weight gain for age.

SYMPTOMS/EXAM

- Obtain a thorough feeding/nutrition history, and if possible, observe the parent or caretaker feeding the child.
- Ask about malabsorption, quality and frequency of stools, and/or systemic symptoms.
- Obtain a detailed social history (family stressors) and family history (CF, genetic diseases, HIV).
- Conduct formal development and behavioral testing.
- Plot height, weight, and head circumference since birth.
- Conduct a complete physical exam.

DIFFERENTIAL

- **Inadequate intake:** The most common cause (ie, overdiluting formula). Often 2° to psychosocial issues, with no underlying medical condition. Other causes include mechanical problems such as cleft palate/nasal obstruction or sucking/swallowing dysfunction.
- **Inadequate absorption or ↑ losses:** Examples include malabsorption, infectious diarrhea, vomiting, biliary atresia, intestinal obstruction, necrotizing enterocolitis, and short gut.
- **↑ metabolic demand or ineffective utilization:** Examples include inborn errors of metabolism, CF/lung disease, HIV/infection, endocrine disorders, and congenital heart disease.

DIAGNOSIS

- The H&P will dictate the extent of lab workup needed.
- First-line lab evaluation should include a CBC, electrolytes, BUN/creatinine, a lead level if appropriate, and a UA.
- If the child is severely malnourished, also evaluate albumin (to assess protein status), alkaline phosphatase, calcium, and phosphorus (to evaluate for rickets).

TREATMENT

- Treat the underlying cause.
- If the H&P does not suggest an organic cause, start a calorie count and consider nutritional supplementation.
- Hospitalization may be necessary for severe malnourishment or if there is concern for neglect.

Developmental Milestones

You are seeing an infant in clinic for a routine well-child checkup. The mother reports that the infant recently started crawling. In addition, she is reportedly saying "mama" and "dada" to everyone and waving "bye-bye."

If the infant is developmentally on target, how old should she be?

Nine months.

Table 16-1 highlights major developmental milestones. Red flags include the following:

- Persistent primitive reflexes by six months.
- Handedness before one year.
- No pointing by 18 months.

TABLE 16-1. Developmental Milestones

Age	Gross Motor	Fine Motor	Language	Social/Cognitive
2 months	Lifts head/chest when prone.	Tracks past midline.	Alerts to sound; coos.	Recognizes parent; social smile.
4–5 months	**Rolls** front to back and back to front (5 months).	Grasps rattle.	Orients to voice; "ah-goo"; razzes.	Enjoys looking around; laughs.
6 months	**Sits unassisted** (7 months).	**Transfers objects;** raking grasp.	Babbles.	**Stranger anxiety.**
9–10 months	Crawls; pulls to stand.	Uses three-finger pincer grasp.	Says **"mama/dada"** (nonspecific).	Waves "bye-bye"; plays pat-a-cake.
12 months	Cruises (11 months); **walks alone.**	Uses two-finger pincer grasp.	Says **"mama/dada"** (specific).	Imitates actions.
15 months	Walks backward.	Uses cup.	Uses 4–6 words.	Temper tantrums.
18 months	Runs; kicks a ball.	Builds tower of 2–4 cubes.	Names common objects.	Copies parent in tasks (eg, sweeping).
2 years	Walks up/down steps with help; jumps.	Builds tower of six cubes.	Uses **two-word** phrases.	Follows **two-step** commands; removes clothes.
3 years	Rides **tricycle;** climbs stairs with alternating feet (3–4 years).	Copies a circle; uses utensils.	Uses **three-word** sentences.	Brushes teeth with help; washes/dries hands.
4 years	Hops.	Copies a cross.	Counts to 10.	Cooperative play.

(Adapted with permission from Le T et al. *First Aid for the USMLE Step 2 CK,* 7th ed. New York: McGraw-Hill, 2010: 402.)

PREVENTION OF ILLNESS

Immunizations

Figure 16-1 summarizes the recommended timetable for childhood immunizations. Schedules may vary for children who are behind and require catch-up immunizations.

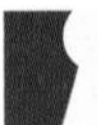

KEY FACT

The HPV vaccine is recommended for girls 11–12 years of age or for girls 13–26 years of age who have not previously been vaccinated as a catch-up.

SAFETY

General Principles

- Car seats should be placed in the rear seat of the car, rear-facing, until the child weighs > 20 lbs **and** is > 1 year of age. Car seats should not be placed in seats with active air bags. Car seats have a finite useful life, and seats that are more than a few years old are not considered safe.
- The **B-HEADSS** interview (see mnemonic) can be used to gauge psychosocial risk.

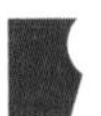

KEY FACT

All infants should go "back" to sleep (ie, sleep on their backs) to ↓ the risk of sudden infant death syndrome (SIDS).

Child Abuse

A three-month-old infant is brought to the pediatric ER with a broken left femur. Her parents explain that they had just left her alone for a minute when she rolled off the couch. In addition to x-rays of her leg, what other evaluation would you want to perform on this child?

Three-month-old infants generally cannot roll on their own, and a fall from a couch should not result in a broken femur. You should thus order a skeletal survey and an ophthalmologic exam as well as a CBC, PT/PTT, AST, ALT, amylase, lipase, calcium, phosphorus, alkaline phosphatase, electrolytes, BUN/creatinine, and UA—in other words, you should perform a full workup for medical causes of unusual fractures in this age group, as well as for additional injuries that might be the result of abuse.

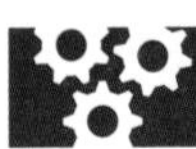

MNEMONIC

Use the B-HEADSS interview for adolescents:

Body image
Home
Education and **E**mployment
Activities
Drugs
Sexuality
Suicidality/depression

Vaccine ▼ Age ▶	Birth	1 month	2 months	4 months	6 months	12 months	15 months	18 months	19–23 months	2–3 years	4–6 years
Hepatitis B	HepB	HepB				HepB					
Rotavirus			RV	RV	RV						
Diphtheria, Tetanus, Pertussis			DTaP	DTaP	DTaP		DTaP				DTaP
Haemophilus influenzae type b			Hib	Hib	Hib	Hib					
Pneumococcal			PCV	PCV	PCV	PCV				PPSV	
Inactivated Poliovirus			IPV	IPV		IPV					IPV
Influenza							Influenza (Yearly)				
Measles, Mumps, Rubella						MMR					MMR
Varicella						Varicella					Varicella
Hepatitis A							HepA (2 doses)			HepA Series	
Meningococcal										MCV	

Range of recommended ages for all children except certain high-risk groups

Range of recommended ages for certain high-risk groups

FIGURE 16-1. Pediatric immunization timetable. (Reproduced from the Centers for Disease Control and Prevention, Atlanta, GA.)

TABLE 16-3. ToRCHeS Infections

Infection	Description	Treatment	Prevention
Toxoplasmosis	Hydrocephalus, seizures, chorioretinitis, intracranial calcifications, and ring-enhancing lesions on head CT.	Pyrimethamine, sulfadiazine, spiramycin.	Avoid exposure to cats and cat feces during pregnancy; avoid raw/undercooked meat; treat women with 1° infection.
Rubella	"Blueberry muffin" rash, cataracts, hearing loss, PDA and other cardiac defects, encephalitis.	None.	Immunize mothers prior to pregnancy.
Cytomegalovirus (CMV)	Petechial rash, periventricular calcifications, microcephaly, chorioretinitis.	Ganciclovir.	Avoid exposure.
Herpes simplex (HSV)	Skin, eye, and mouth vesicles; can progress to severe CNS/systemic infection.	Acyclovir.	Perform a C-section if the mother has active lesions at the time of delivery. The highest risk is from mothers with 1° infection.
Syphilis	Maculopapular skin rash on palms and soles, lymphadenopathy, "snuffles," osteitis.	Penicillin.	Treat seropositive mothers with penicillin.

TABLE 16-4. Common Congenital Anomalies and Malformations

Lesion	Description	Age at Presentation	Symptoms/Signs	Treatment
Cleft lip/palate	Abnormal ridge/division.	Presents at birth.	Poor feeding; aspiration; severe, recurrent otitis media. May be associated with other anomalies.	Surgical repair of the lip/palate.
Tracheoesophageal fistula	Four different types. Blind esophageal pouch with fistula between the distal esophagus and trachea is the most common.	Usually presents in the first few hours of life, but other types can present later in infancy.	Copious secretions, choking/coughing with feeds, cyanosis, respiratory distress/aspiration.	Suctioning of the pouch with an NG tube; reflux precautions; supportive care; surgical repair.
Abdominal wall defects	Gastroschisis (the intestine extrudes through the defect); omphalocele (a membrane-covered herniation of abdominal contents).	Presents antenatally or at birth.	A visible defect. Associated anomalies are common in omphalocele but are rare in gastroschisis.	Coverage of abdominal contents with sterile dressing. NG decompressions, antibiotics, supportive care, and stabilization followed by 1° or staged closure.

TABLE 16-4. Common Congenital Anomalies and Malformations *(continued)*

Lesion	Description	Age at Presentation	Symptoms/Signs	Treatment
Intestinal atresias	Intestinal obstruction.	Present antenatally or at birth.	Abdominal distention, bilious vomiting, obstipation/failure to pass meconium, polyhydramnios. With Down syndrome, look for the characteristic "double bubble" sign of duodenal atresia (see Figure 16-3).	Surgical resection.
Hirschsprung's disease	Absence of ganglion cells in the colon leads to narrowing of the aganglionic segment with dilation of the proximal normal colon. Can be a short (75%) or long segment.	Presents at infancy or usually within the first two years of life.	Failure to pass meconium, vomiting, abdominal distention, chronic constipation.	Diagnose by rectal biopsy at the anal verge to look for ganglion cells. A staged procedure with an initial diverting colostomy followed by resection when the infant is > 6 months of age.
Neural tube defects	Includes anencephaly (incompatible with life) and spina bifida (myelomeningocele, meningocele).	Presents at birth, but may be detected prenatally. Associated with ↑ maternal and **amniotic fluid α-fetoprotein.**	Depends on the defect. Ranges from incompatibility with life to hydrocephalus, paralysis, and neurogenic bowel and bladder. Associated with an ↑ risk of latex allergy.	Risk ↓ with folate ingestion during the first trimester. Surgical repair.

- Physiologic jaundice usually presents within the first 36–48 hours of life and reaches peak total bilirubin levels of 10–15 mg/dL at 5–7 days of life. Visible jaundice starts at the head (or eyes) and travels down the body with increasing bilirubin levels.

Differential

- Initial bilirubin evaluation should include both total and direct bilirubin to establish whether direct or indirect hyperbilirubinemia is the problem.
- Jaundice is less likely to be **physiologic** if it is severe or prolonged, occurs within the first 24 hours of life, or is associated with an elevated direct (conjugated) component.

Treatment

- **↑ feeding:** Most normal babies will be able to excrete bilirubin on their own with time, additional intake, and improved intestinal motility.

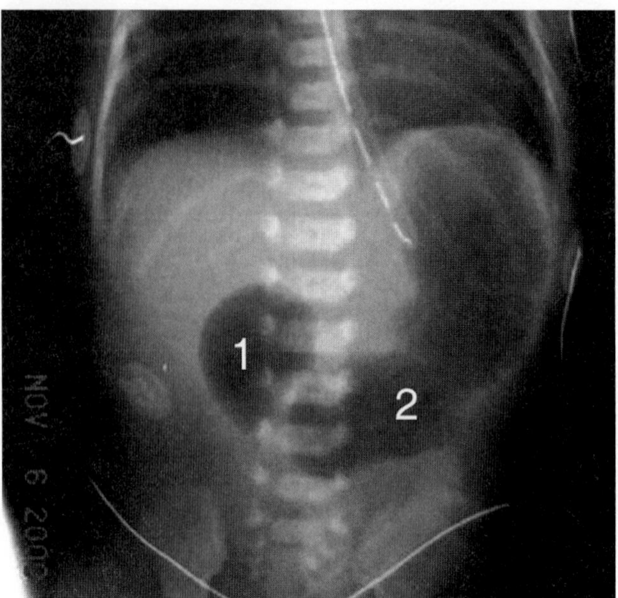

FIGURE 16-3. Duodenal atresia. Note the characteristic "double-bubble" appearance of the duodenal bulb (1) and stomach (2) in a neonate with duodenal atresia presenting with bilious emesis. (Reproduced with permission from Brunicardi FC et al. *Schwartz's Principles of Surgery,* 9th ed. New York: McGraw-Hill, 2010, Fig. 39-13.)

- **UV phototherapy:** Phototherapy is more likely to be necessary if the mother's blood type is O negative or if the infant suffered birth trauma, is of Asian descent, was born preterm, or has a nonphysiologic form of jaundice. Phototherapy modifies the bilirubin molecule into a water-soluble form that can be more easily excreted.
- Exchange transfusion is indicated for severe jaundice.
- Follow total serum bilirubin at least daily while treating for hyperbilirubinemia.

Breast Milk Jaundice

- Breast milk contains an enzyme that further delays hepatic bilirubin conjugation and can prolong jaundice in newborns.
- **Sx/Exam:** Occurs in exclusively breast-fed infants. Jaundice presents after the first 3–5 days of life and peaks at two weeks of age. Total bilirubin levels may reach 19–20 mg/dL and may persist for 1–2 months.
- **Dx:** A diagnosis of exclusion.
- **Tx:** Rarely requires phototherapy. Once the diagnosis is made, breast-feeding should be encouraged, as the problem will go away on its own.

Pathologic Jaundice

Jaundice is considered pathologic if it is severe or prolonged, occurs within the first 24 hours of life, or is associated with an elevated direct (conjugated) bilirubin component. Very high levels of unconjugated bilirubin (> 30 mg/dL) can cross the blood-brain barrier and deposit in the basal ganglia, causing kernicterus, an irreversible, potentially fatal encephalopathy.

- Causes of pathologic **indirect hyperbilirubinemia** include the following:
  - Disorders that ↑ bilirubin production (hemolysis, sepsis, severe bruising/hematoma).

  - Disorders that affect bilirubin conjugation (hepatic enzyme deficiencies, hepatic dysfunction).
  - Disorders that affect bilirubin excretion (intestinal obstruction, poor motility).
- Causes of pathologic **direct** hyperbilirubinemia include the following:
  - **Intrahepatic:** Biliary obstruction/atresia (most common), choledochal cysts, neonatal hepatitis, Dubin-Johnson syndrome, Rotor's syndrome, Alagille syndrome, α_1-antitrypsin deficiency, TPN cholestasis (affects premature infants on TPN).
  - **Extrahepatic:** Sepsis, UTIs, hypothyroidism, CF, inborn errors of metabolism, RBC abnormalities.

Symptoms/Exam

- Look for hepatomegaly, acholic (white) stools, signs of anemia or sepsis, growth abnormalities, and congenital abnormalities.
- **Kernicterus** (usually caused by extremely high levels of indirect hyperbilirubinemia) presents with jaundice, lethargy, poor feeding, a high-pitched cry, hypertonicity, and seizures.

Diagnosis

- Order a CBC (to assess for anemia), a reticulocyte count, and a peripheral blood smear (to rule out hemolysis).
- A Coombs' test can distinguish antibody-mediated disease (eg, ABO incompatibility) from non-immune-related disorders (eg, G6PD deficiency, hereditary spherocytosis).
- Additional testing should be guided by the patient's H&P.

Treatment

- Phototherapy/exchange transfusion.
- Treat associated conditions (eg, hemolysis, sepsis, hypothyroidism, biliary obstruction).

Dermatology

NEONATAL RASHES

The vast majority of skin findings in the neonatal period are benign. Nonetheless, they are often a cause for concern among new parents. Table 16-5 describes common neonatal rashes.

ECZEMA

A chronic inflammatory skin condition that affects nearly 20% of children in the United States. Onset is generally before age five. Also known as atopic dermatitis.

Symptoms/Exam

Presents with dry, itchy, often erythematous skin. May be papular or excoriated in severe cases. In infants, it is usually found on the trunk, cheeks, and scalp. In older children, it is generally found on flexor surfaces and may include lichenified plaques.

TABLE 16-5. Presentation and Treatment of Common Neonatal Rashes

Rash	Presentation	Treatment
Erythema toxicum neonatorum	Erythematous macules and papules that progress to pustules (see Figure 16-4A). Lesions usually appear within 24–48 hours after birth and resolve in 5–7 days.	None.
Transient neonatal pustular melanosis	There are three types of lesions: (1) pustules with a nonerythematous base; (2) erythematous macules with a surrounding scaly area; and (3) hyperpigmented macules. Lesions present at birth and resolve within weeks to months.	None.
Neonatal acne	Papules and pustules appearing on the face and/or scalp (see Figure 16-4B) at three weeks of age. Generally resolves by four months.	Gentle cleansing with soap and water; avoidance of oils and lotions. Ketoconazole or hydrocortisone may help speed resolution of lesions.
Milia	White papules composed of retained keratin and sebaceous material. Present at birth; usually found on the cheeks and nose. Resolves within the first few weeks of life.	None.
Miliaria (crystallina, rubra, pustulosa, profunda)	Vesicles, papules, or pustules caused by the accumulation of sweat beneath sweat ducts blocked by keratin. More common in warm climates and among infants in incubators. Usually appears during the first week of life.	Provision of a cooler environment; loose clothing and cool baths.
Seborrheic dermatitis	Erythema and greasy scales, usually on the face and scalp (see Figure 16-4C). Resolves within weeks to months.	Application of emollient overnight followed by massage and shampooing with baby shampoo to loosen scales; use of a soft brush to remove scales. If gentle cleansing methods do not work, ketoconazole, selenium sulfide, or hydrocortisone may be tried.

Treatment

Treatment consists of the following steps:

- **Avoid triggers** such as heat, perspiration, and dry climates. Triggers may also include specific foods such as eggs, nuts, chocolate, peanut butter, milk, and seafood.
- **Maintain hydration** by daily bathing followed by the application of thick creams (eg, Eucerin, Cetaphil) or ointments (eg, petroleum jelly, Aquaphor) to lock in the skin's moisture.
- **Control itching** by using antihistamines such as diphenhydramine, hydroxyzine, and cyproheptadine. Cool baths may also help alleviate pruritus. Wet cotton dressings applied after bathing and emollients covered with dry, loose cotton dressings can further reduce pruritus.
- **Treat inflammation** with topical corticosteroids (hydrocortisone for mild inflammation; triamcinolone or fluocinolone for more severe cases). Other treatment measures for severe disease include antibiotics, systemic corticosteroids, topical or oral calcineurin inhibitors, and phototherapy.
- **Aggressively treat superinfections** (impetigo or cellulitis), as patients with eczema are more susceptible to bacterial, viral, and fungal skin infections.

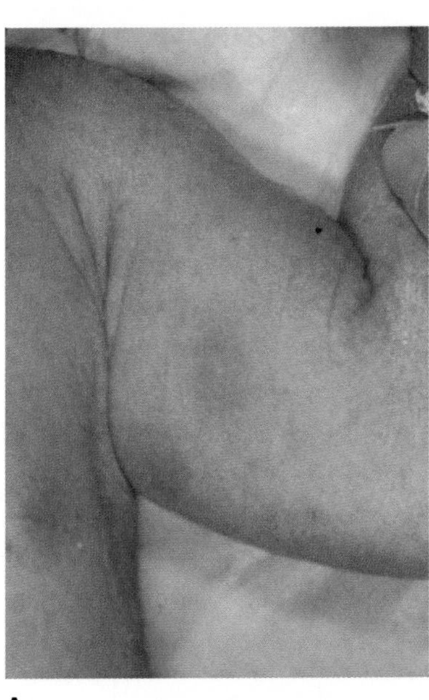
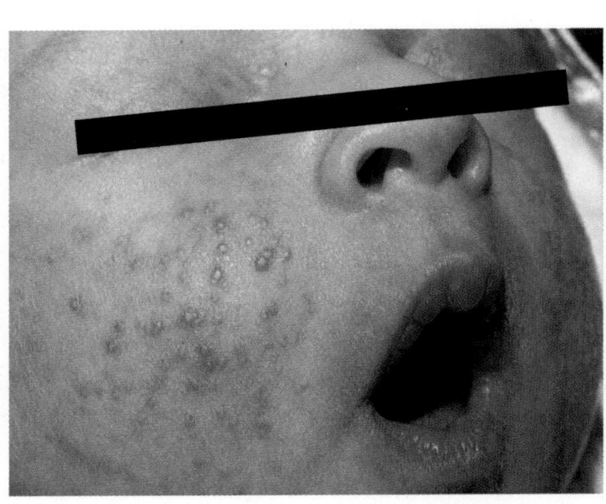
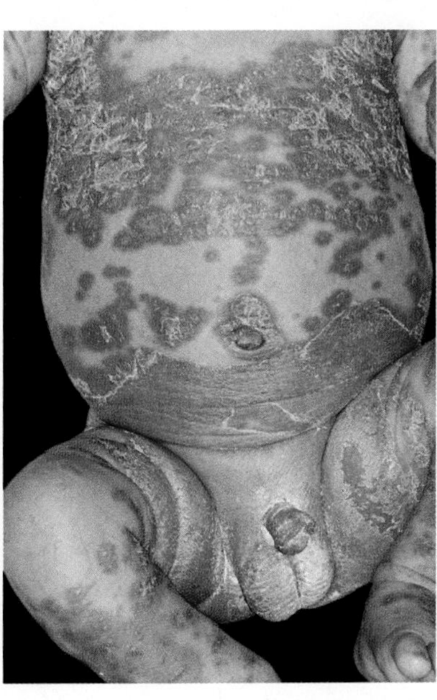

A B C

FIGURE 16-4. Common neonatal rashes. (A) **Erythema toxicum neonatorum.** Erythematous macules are seen on the arm of a one-day-old newborn. (B) **Neonatal acne.** Tiny papulopustules are seen on the face of a three-week-old infant. (C) **Seborrheic dermatitis.** (Reproduced with permission from Wolff K et al. *Fitzpatrick's Dermatology in General Medicine,* 7th ed. New York: McGraw-Hill, 2008, Figs. 106-3, 106-5, and 22-1.)

Endocrinology

CONGENITAL ADRENAL HYPERPLASIA (CAH)

A 10-day-old male infant is brought to the urgent care clinic because his parents feel that he has been "acting funny." On exam, you note that the infant has poor skin turgor and dry lips. He is lethargic and has a sunken fontanelle. You plot his height and weight and discover that he is down 10% from his birth weight despite frequent breast-feeding with a good latch. You order a set of electrolytes that reveal hyponatremia and hyperkalemia. In addition to a sepsis workup, which lab tests should you consider?

You should order a 17-hydroxyprogesterone level and an androstenedione level. In addition, you would want to see newborn screening results looking for congenital adrenal hyperplasia.

A group of disorders caused by a defect in one or more of the enzymes required for cortisol synthesis. These defects lead to overproduction of the precursors in the pathway and to an excess of ACTH as the body attempts to stimulate the adrenal gland. The most common defect, which accounts for 90–95% of all cases, is in the 21-hydroxylase enzyme. Defects in 11β-hydroxylase and 17α-hydroxylase, as well as other enzymes in the pathway for adrenal steroid synthesis, are less common.

SYMPTOMS/EXAM

- **Classic form:** Has two variants, **salt-losing** and **non-salt-losing** CAH.
  - **Girls with either variant:** Present as infants with ambiguous genitalia caused by excess androgen production in utero.
  - **Boys with the salt-losing variant:** Present in the first 1–2 weeks of life with hyponatremia, hyperkalemia, dehydration, and FTT.
  - **Boys with the non-salt-losing variant:** Present with early virilization, including the development of pubic hair, adult body odor, and a growth spurt at 2–4 years of age.
- **Nonclassic form:** Typically presents later with signs of excess androgen production such as hirsutism, acne, early pubarche, irregular menses, and premature closure of the physes.

TREATMENT

KEY FACT

Any illness can lead to an adrenal crisis in children with congenital adrenal hyperplasia. Glucocorticoid doses 2–3 times the maintenance dose should be administered promptly.

- **Glucocorticoid replacement** with hydrocortisone (in infants and younger children) or with dexamethasone or prednisone (in older adolescents) to replace cortisol and suppress androgen production.
- **Mineralocorticoid replacement** with fludrocortisone to normalize sodium and potassium concentrations. Infants should be given supplemental sodium chloride, which can be tapered as they begin to eat table food.
- **Monitoring:** Serum levels of 17-hydroxyprogesterone (17-OHP) and androstenedione, as well as plasma renin activity, should be measured every three months in infants and every 4–12 months in children. In addition, bone-age films should be taken every six months.

PRECOCIOUS PUBERTY

Defined as the development of 2° sex characteristics prior to age eight in girls and age nine in boys. The lower limit of normal for girls is somewhat controversial; some use seven years for Caucasian girls and six years for African American girls. Classified as follows:

- **Gonadotropin-dependent precocious puberty (GDPP):** A result of early activation of the hypothalamic-pituitary-gonadal (HPG) axis. Development occurs in the proper sequence and over a normal interval but begins early. Roughly 80% of cases are idiopathic. Other possible etiologies include CNS lesions; therefore, GDPP patients require brain imaging (CT or MRI).
- **Gonadotropin-independent precocious puberty (GIPP):** Not due to early activation of the HPG axis but rather to the secretion of sex hormones from the adrenals or the gonads.
  - Possible causes in both boys and girls include exogenous estrogen, CAH, adrenal androgen-secreting tumors, pituitary gonadotropin-secreting tumors, and McCune-Albright syndrome (GIPP, café-au-lait spots, and fibrous dysplasia of bone).
  - For girls, additional causes include ovarian cysts and ovarian tumors such as Leydig cell/granulosa cell tumors and gonadoblastomas.
  - For boys, Leydig cell tumors, hCG-secreting germ cell tumors, and a rare disorder known as familial GIPP, in which a mutation in the LH receptor gene causes early Leydig cell maturation, are other possible causes.

DIAGNOSIS

- **Imaging:** X-rays of the wrist to determine bone age.
- **Labs:** Serum estradiol or testosterone level; 17-OHP; basal and GnRH-stimulated LH; dehydroepiandrosterone (DHEA).

TREATMENT

- **GDPP:** GnRH agonists are the therapy of choice if the projected height or rate of development results in a decision to treat.
- **GIPP:** Does not respond to GnRH agonists; treatment depends on the etiology.

Infectious Disease

FEVER WITHOUT A SOURCE (FWS)

An 18-month-old girl who is up to date on all her immunizations is brought to urgent care with a temperature of 39.2°C (102.6°F). She is somewhat more irritable than usual but is consolable and otherwise well. Her physical exam is unremarkable. What workup, if any, should you perform in this child?

Obtain a UA and urine culture. You should consider adding a CBC if the child has not received at least two doses of pneumococcal vaccine and if her temperature is > 39.5°C (103.1°F). If the child were really irritable or lethargic, an LP would be indicated.

Roughly 20% of children with a fever do not have signs or symptoms of a bacterial or viral infection on history or exam. FWS is a concern because it may represent an occult serious bacterial infection (SBI). The concern for SBI, and therefore the recommended workup for FWS, is age dependent:

- **0–28 days:** See the discussion of neonatal sepsis.
- **1–3 months:** Obtain a CBC, a blood culture, and a UA and urine culture. Consider an LP if the infant is irritable or lethargic. Treat with empiric antibiotics (usually ceftriaxone) if the WBC is > 15 or < 5.
- **3–36 months:** If the infant has been vaccinated and appears well, the risk of bacteremia and/or meningitis is low. Obtain a UA and urine culture if the infant is an uncircumcised boy < 1 year of age or a girl < 2 years of age, especially if the fever is > 39°C (102.2°F) or the child has presented with fever for > 48 hours. If the infant is unvaccinated, obtain a CBC and a blood culture. Obtain a blood culture and treat with ceftriaxone if the WBC count is > 15.

UTI is the most common bacterial cause of FWS. In infants < 3 months of age, uncircumcised boys are at highest risk. Among infants > 3 months of age, girls are at highest risk. Some guidelines recommend evaluation of the first febrile UTI in a child < 2 years of age with a renal ultrasound +/– VCUG to rule out structural renal disease or vesicoureteral reflux (see Figure 16-5). These disorders are most likely to occur in very young infants (< 3 months) and those with recurrent UTIs.

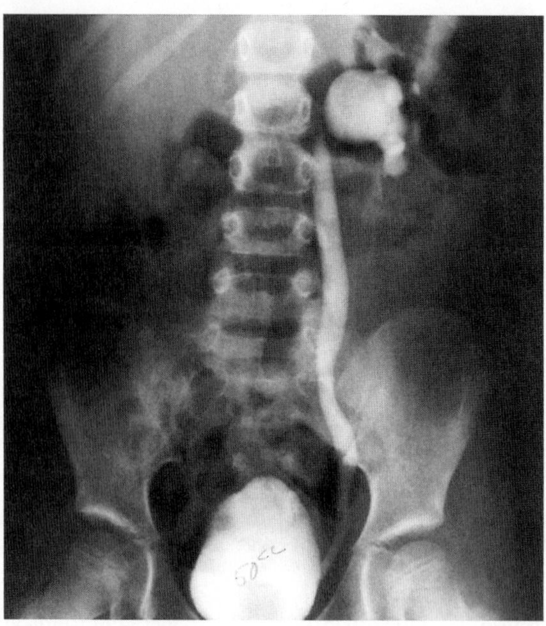

FIGURE 16-5. Vesicoureteral reflux. Frontal radiograph from a voiding cystourethrogram shows reflux to the left ureter and intrarenal collecting system with hydronephrosis. Note the absence of reflux on the normal right side. (Reproduced with permission from Doherty GM. *Current Diagnosis & Treatment: Surgery,* 13th ed. New York: McGraw-Hill, 2010, Fig. 38-7.)

Immunology

IMMUNODEFICIENCY SYNDROMES

A two-year-old girl is brought in by her parents with a high fever and a cough of two days' duration. She is hypoxic and in respiratory distress, and your exam is suggestive of a right lower lobe pneumonia, which is confirmed on CXR. You review her chart and note that the girl was hospitalized at 6 months for mastoiditis and was then hospitalized again at 15 months with a left-sided pneumonia that was complicated by an empyema and a ⊕ blood culture. You also note that her weight is less than the third percentile for age. Aside from the workup needed for her acute infection, what additional tests would you consider in this patient?

It is unusual for a healthy child to have recurrent severe bacterial infections. The fact that each infection has been in a different location argues against an anatomic cause; therefore, a 1° immunodeficiency should be considered. A basic starting evaluation might include a CBC to screen for cellular immunodeficiencies or malignancy; immunoglobulin levels; antibody titers to organisms against which the patient has been vaccinated (including both protein antigens and polysaccharide antigens); and a CH_{50} to evaluate for complement deficiencies. Additional, more specific tests (eg, for HIV or CF) should be guided by the results of this initial evaluation.

Present as recurrent or severe infections. In general, the frequency is roughly 1 in 10,000. Table 16-6 outlines the clinical presentation, diagnosis, and treatment of common pediatric immunodeficiency disorders.

TABLE 16-6. Pediatric Immunodeficiency Disorders

DISORDER	DESCRIPTION	SYMPTOMS	DIAGNOSIS	TREATMENT
		B-CELL DISORDERS		
	Most common.	Present with recurrent **URIs** and **bacteremia with encapsulated organisms** (pneumococcus, *Staphylococcus, H influenzae*) after age six (when maternal antibodies taper).	**Quantitative Ig levels** (subclasses) and specific antibody responses.	Prophylactic antibiotics and IVIG.
X-linked (**B**ruton's agammaglobulinemia)	A profound **B**-cell deficiency found only in **B**oys.	May present before age six. Patients are at risk for pseudomonal infection.		
Common variable immunodeficiency (CVID)	Ig levels drop in the second and third decades of life.	Associated with an ↑ risk of lymphoma and autoimmune disease.		
IgA deficiency (most common)	Low IgA.	Usually asymptomatic. Recurrent infection may be seen.		
		T-CELL DISORDERS		
		Viral infection, fungal infection, intracellular bacteria (broader range of infections). Present at 1–3 months of age.	**Absolute lymphocyte count,** mitogen stimulation response, and delayed hypersensitivity skin testing.	
Thymic aplasia (DiGeorge syndrome)	Patients are unable to generate T cells owing to lack of a thymus.	**Tetany** (due to hypocalcemia) in the first few days of life.		Consider thymus transplant instead of bone marrow transplant (BMT).
Ataxia-telangiectasia	A DNA repair defect.	Oculocutaneous telangiectasias and progressive cerebellar ataxia.		**BMT** for severe disease; **IVIG** for antibody deficiency.

(continues)

TABLE 16-6. Pediatric Immunodeficiency Disorders *(continued)*

DISORDER	DESCRIPTION	SYMPTOMS	DIAGNOSIS	TREATMENT
		COMBINED DISORDERS		
			Absolute lymphocyte count and quantitative Ig levels.	
Severe combined immunodeficiency (SCID)	Severe lack of B and T cells.	Frequent and severe bacterial infections, chronic candidiasis, and opportunistic infections.		**BMT or stem-cell transplant;** IVIG for antibody deficiency; **PCP prophylaxis.**
Wiskott-Aldrich syndrome	An X-linked disorder with less severe B- and T-cell dysfunction.	**Eczema,** ↑ IgE, ↑ IgA, ↓ IgM, and **thrombocytopenia.**		**Supportive treatment:** IVIG and aggressive antibiotics. Patients rarely survive to adulthood.
		PHAGOCYTIC DISORDERS		
		Commonly caused by catalase-⊕ (*S aureus*) and enteric gram-⊖ organisms.	Absolute neutrophil count; adhesion, chemotactic, phagocytic, and bactericidal assays.	
Chronic granulomatous disease (CGD)	An X-linked or autosomal recessive disorder with deficient superoxide reduction by PMNs and macrophages.	Chronic GI and GU infections; osteomyelitis, hepatitis. Anemia, lymphadenopathy, and hypergamma-globulinemia.	A **nitroblue tetrazolium** test is diagnostic.	**Daily TMP-SMX,** judicious use of antibiotics, γ-interferon.
Chédiak-Higashi syndrome	An autosomal recessive defect in neutrophil chemotaxis.	**Recurrent pyogenic skin** and **respiratory infections.** Oculocutaneous albinism, neuropathy, neutropenia.	Blood smear shows PMNs with **giant cytoplasmic granules.**	Aggressive treatment of bacterial infections; corticosteroids, splenectomy.
		COMPLEMENT DISORDERS		
		Recurrent **sinopulmonary infections,** bacteremia, and/or **meningitis** due to **encapsulated organisms** (*S pneumoniae, H influenzae* type b, *Neisseria meningitidis*).		

TABLE 16-6. Pediatric Immunodeficiency Disorders *(continued)*

Disorder	Description	Symptoms	Diagnosis	Treatment
C1 esterase deficiency (hereditary angioneurotic edema)	An autosomal dominant disorder with recurrent angioedema lasting 21–72 hours.	Presents in late childhood or early **adolescence.** Provoked by stress, trauma, or puberty/menses. Can lead to **life-threatening airway edema.**	Measurement of complement components.	Daily prophylactic antifibrinolytic agents or **danazol.** Purified C1 esterase and FFP prior to surgery.
Terminal complement deficiency (C5–C9)	A deficiency of components of the membrane attack complex (C5–C9). Associated with meningococcal and gonococcal infection.	**Mild, recurrent** infection by *Neisseria* spp. **(meningococcal or gonococcal).** Rarely, SLE or glomerulonephritis.	**Total hemolytic complement (CH_{50}):** assess the quantity and function of complement pathway components.	Meningococcal vaccine and appropriate antibiotics.

(Adapted with permission from Le T et al. *First Aid for the USMLE Step 2 CK,* 7th ed. New York: McGraw-Hill, 2010: 411–413.)

KAWASAKI DISEASE (MUCOCUTANEOUS LYMPH NODE SYNDROME)

A relatively common medium-vessel vasculitis of childhood that predisposes to coronary artery aneurysms and to the subsequent development of myocardial ischemia. More common in children < 5 years of age and among those of **Asian,** particularly Japanese, ethnicity.

Symptoms/Exam

Presents as an acute illness characterized by the symptoms outlined in the **CRASH and BURN** mnemonic.

Diagnosis

- A clinical diagnosis.
- Patients must have **fever** for > **5 days** and meet 4–5 of the other criteria.
- Occasional findings include arthritis, excessive irritability, scrotal swelling, pericarditis, and gallbladder inflammation.
- Labs may reveal sterile pyuria, ↑ **ESR/CRP,** and thrombocytosis during the second week of illness.

Treatment

- Give anti-inflammatory, **high-dose ASA** during the acute phase to ↓ the incidence of cardiac abnormalities.
- Administer **IVIG** to prevent coronary artery aneurysms and to preserve myocardial contractility (given as a single infusion within the first 7–10 days of illness; repeat if the patient is still febrile 24 hours later).
- During the convalescent phase, switch to low-dose ASA for its antiplatelet effect.
- Follow patients with regular echocardiography.

Complications

Myocarditis; pericarditis; coronary artery aneurysm predisposing to myocardial ischemia.

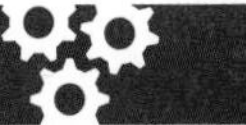

MNEMONIC

Kawasaki symptoms—

CRASH and BURN

Conjunctivitis (bilateral, nonpurulent)
Rash (truncal)
Adenopathy (at least one cervical node > 1 cm)
Strawberry tongue (or any change in oropharyngeal mucosa, including an injected pharynx or lip fissuring)
Hand/foot swelling/desquamation
BURN (fever for > 5 days)

Rheumatology

JUVENILE IDIOPATHIC ARTHRITIS (JIA)

Can be classified into three categories: systemic, pauciarticular, and polyarticular.

Systemic JIA

- **Sx/Exam:** Patients present with intermittent fever, rash (classically described as macular and salmon-pink), lymphadenopathy, and arthritis (usually of the knees, wrists, and ankles, but can affect other joints as well). Affects boys and girls equally.
- **Dx:**
  - Patients are generally worked up for infectious processes and leukemia before a diagnosis is made.
  - WBC count, ESR, CRP, and platelets are elevated.
  - In order for the diagnosis of JIA to be made, the patient must have a daily fever for two weeks, typically above 38.5°C (101.3°F), and arthritis. Arthritis may develop after the initial fever and rash.
- **Tx:**
  - **First line:** NSAIDs.
  - **Second line:** Corticosteroids or methotrexate.
  - **Other:** Agents such as monoclonal antibodies to IL-1 or IL-6, thalidomide, IVIG, hydroxychloroquine, sulfasalazine, cyclosporine, and TNF inhibitors have been used with varying degrees of success.
- **Cx:** A typical course for a first episode of JIA may last 4–6 months. Some children will continue to have fever and rash for years. The long-term sequelae vary from none at all to severe destruction requiring joint replacement.

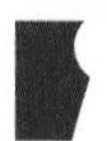

KEY FACT

Children with JIA are at risk for developing macrophage activation syndrome.

Pauciarticular JIA

- The most common form of JIA; affects girls more often than boys.
- **Sx/Exam:** Involves < 5 joints (generally large joints); usually presents at 2–3 years of age.
- **Dx:**
  - See above.
  - Patients are ANA ⊕.
- **Tx:**
  - **First line:** NSAIDs and/or glucocorticoids injected into affected joints.
  - **Second line:** Methotrexate, TNF inhibitors (rarely used).
- **Cx:**
  - Usually resolves within six months.
  - More than 50% of patients will not have relapses; however, severe destructive arthritis may occur.
  - Children with pauciarticular JIA are at risk for uveitis, so routine screening by an ophthalmologist should be done every 3–12 months depending on the age of onset and ANA status.

Polyarticular JIA

- Involves > 4 joints; affects girls more often than boys. Age of onset is 2–5 years and 10–14 years.

- Dx:
  - See above.
  - Patients may be ANA and/or RF ⊕.
  - Lab findings may include anemia, elevated ESR, and hypergammaglobulinemia.
- Tx:
  - NSAIDs are first line but are unlikely to yield long-term control when used as a single agent.
  - **Disease-modifying antirheumatic drugs (DMARDs)** such as methotrexate, leflunomide, sulfasalazine, TNF inhibitors, cyclosporine, azathioprine, rituximab, corticosteroids (systemic and injected), and gold compounds should be added early in the course of treatment.
- Cx:
  - The prognosis is generally better for RF-seronegative patients than for those who are seropositive.
  - RF-seronegative patients often respond to NSAID therapy, while seropositive patients require treatment with DMARDs.
  - Patients are at risk for uveitis and require screening by an ophthalmologist.

REACTIVE ARTHRITIS

Formerly known as Reiter's syndrome, reactive arthritis has three components: postinfectious arthritis, urethritis, and conjunctivitis. Typical pathogens include *Campylobacter, Yersinia, Salmonella, Shigella, Chlamydia trachomatis,* and possibly *C difficile* and *C pneumoniae.* Often, no pathogen is recovered.

SYMPTOMS/EXAM

- Usually affects the lower extremities asymmetrically, presenting as a mono- or oligoarthritis.
- Onset occurs days to weeks after initial infection.

TREATMENT

- **NSAIDs** are first line and may also afford relief from intra-articular glucocorticoid injections.
- If the patient is unresponsive to NSAIDs alone, consider adding a DMARD.

HENOCH-SCHÖNLEIN PURPURA (HSP)

An eight-year-old boy presents to the ER with severe abdominal pain that began this morning. He has had four episodes of emesis over the past eight hours and reports that he continues to have nausea. While you are examining him, you note that he has a nonblanching, palpable erythematous rash on his legs and buttocks. His parents report that the rash was much worse last week. Additional history reveals that the boy was recently diagnosed with Henoch-Schönlein purpura. What is your concern, and which studies should you order?

Intussusception should be a concern, for which you should order an abdominal ultrasound.

The most common small-vessel vasculitis of childhood. Usually affects children 3–15 years of age.

KEY FACT

In cases of HSP with severe, intermittent abdominal pain, obtain an ultrasound to evaluate for intussusception (often ileoileal).

Symptoms/Exam

- Presents with palpable purpura (see Figure 16-6), arthritis/arthralgia, abdominal pain, and glomerulonephritis.
- One-half to two-thirds of patients report having had a URI a few weeks before.
- Arthritis is usually oligoarthritis and migratory, affecting the large joints of the lower extremities more often than the upper extremities.
- If renal involvement occurs, it is usually seen within four weeks of presentation and is typically self-limited.
- Abdominal pain is a result of GI tract inflammation and may be treated with systemic corticosteroids if severe.

Diagnosis

Diagnosis is usually clinical. In cases where the clinical presentation is not clear, a biopsy from the skin or kidney with evidence of IgA deposits confirms the diagnosis.

Treatment

Acetaminophen or NSAIDs for pain control +/– glucocorticoids.

Complications

Recurs in roughly one-third of cases, generally within four months of initial presentation. Recurrences are usually milder than the initial episode.

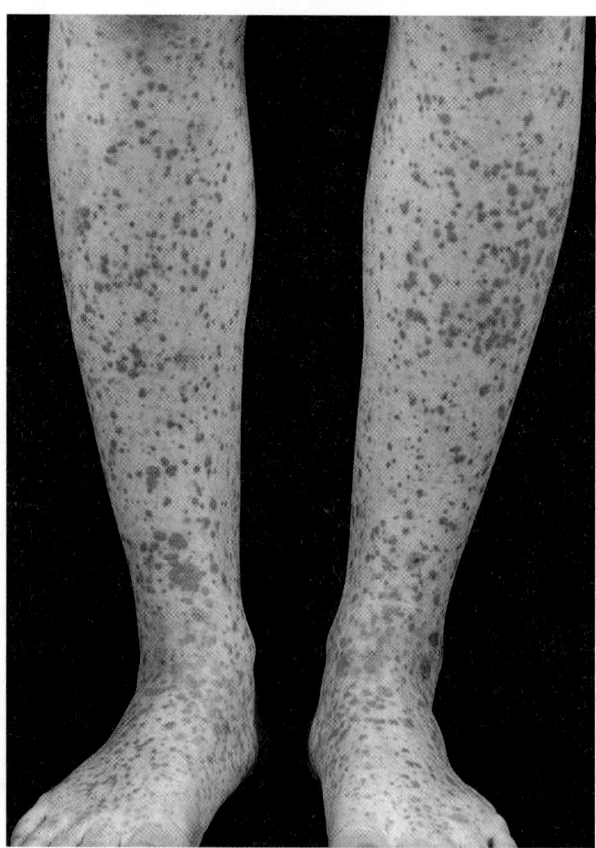

FIGURE 16-6. Classic palpable purpura in Henoch-Schönlein purpura. (Reproduced with permission from Wolff K, Johnson RA. *Fitzpatrick's Color Atlas & Synopsis of Clinical Dermatology,* 6th ed. New York: McGraw-Hill, 2009, Fig. 14-35.)

Cardiology

The incidence of congenital heart disease is approximately 1%. The most common congenital heart lesion is VSD, followed by ASD. The most common cyanotic lesion is transposition of the great arteries (TGA).

VENTRICULAR SEPTAL DEFECT (VSD)

A hole in the ventricular septum. Can be membranous (least likely to close spontaneously), perimembranous, or muscular (most likely to close spontaneously).

SYMPTOMS/EXAM

- May be asymptomatic at birth if the lesion is small.
- Cardiac exam may reveal a **pansystolic, vibratory murmur** at the left lower sternal border **without radiation** to the axillae.
- May become symptomatic between two and six months of age. Symptoms result from flow across the defect, usually from the left to the right ventricle.
- If the lesion is large, it may present with symptoms of **CHF** (shortness of breath, pulmonary edema), frequent **respiratory infection,** FTT, and **exercise/feeding intolerance** (sweating with feeds).
- Look for cardiomegaly and crackles on exam (signs of right heart failure).

DIAGNOSIS

- ECG shows RVH and LVH.
- CXR may show pulmonary edema.
- Echocardiography is definitive.

TREATMENT

- Treat CHF if present.
- Follow small, asymptomatic VSDs annually.
- Surgically repair large or membranous VSDs to prevent later development of heart failure and pulmonary hypertension.

COMPLICATIONS

If left untreated, VSD may lead to irreversible Eisenmenger's syndrome (pulmonary hypertension, RVH, and reversal of left-to-right shunt).

ATRIAL SEPTAL DEFECT (ASD)

A hole in the atrial septum.

SYMPTOMS/EXAM

- Typically asymptomatic until late childhood or early adulthood.
- Cardiac exam may reveal a **systolic murmur** at the **left upper sternal border.**
- A wide and fixed, split S2 and a heaving cardiac impulse at the left lower sternal border are characteristic signs.
- Progression to CHF and cyanosis may occur in the second to third decade of life and depends on the size of the lesion.

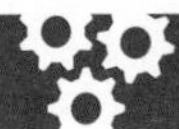

MNEMONIC

Right-to-left shunts (causes of cyanotic congenital heart disease)–

The 5 T's

Truncus arteriosus (1 common artery off of both ventricles)
Transposition of the great arteries (2 vessels switched)
Tricuspid atresia (3 leaflets not well formed)
Tetralogy of Fallot (4 problems present)
Total anomalous pulmonary venous return (5 words)

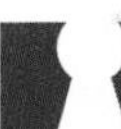

KEY FACT

Patients with VSDs and ASDs no longer require prophylactic antibiotics prior to dental work. Patients who do require antibiotic prophylaxis include those with:

- Unrepaired or incompletely repaired cyanotic CHD.
- Repaired CHD with a residual defect at or adjacent to the site of a prosthetic patch or device.
- Repaired CHD with prosthetic patches or devices within the first six months following the procedure.

Diagnosis

- ECG shows left-axis deviation.
- CXR shows cardiomegaly and ↑ pulmonary vascularity (if defect is large).
- Echocardiography is definitive.

Treatment

Treat CHF if present; follow small ASDs. Surgically repair large ASDs in patients with CHF, and repair before the third decade to prevent symptoms.

Complications

Eisenmenger's syndrome.

PATENT DUCTUS ARTERIOSUS (PDA)

Failure of the ductus arteriosus (the connection between the pulmonary artery and aorta) to close in the first few days of life. Usually results in a **left-to-right shunt** (from aorta to pulmonary artery). Risk factors include **prematurity,** high altitude, and maternal first-trimester **rubella** infection.

Symptoms/Exam

- Presentation ranges from asymptomatic to CHF.
- Cardiac exam may reveal a **wide pulse pressure;** a continuous **"machinery" murmur** at the **left upper sternal border;** and bounding peripheral pulses.
- A loud S2 is characteristic.

Diagnosis

Echocardiography is definitive, showing shunt flow as well as left atrial and left ventricular enlargement.

Treatment

- If diagnosed within days of birth, use **indomethacin** to close the PDA.
- Surgical repair is indicated if the infant is > 6–8 months of age or if indomethacin fails.

Complications

- In the case of pulmonary hypertension of the newborn (such as in meconium aspiration syndrome), flow may be right to left across a PDA, resulting in persistent cyanosis/hypoxia. The reduction of pulmonary hypertension is required to reduce the right-to-left flow.
- Remember that some cyanotic heart lesions (eg, TGA) are dependent on a patent ductus, so do not close the PDA in such cases. To keep the ductus open in such ductal-dependent lesions, medication may be indicated until definitive repair can be performed. Alprostadil (a form of prostaglandin E) is usually used for this purpose.

TETRALOGY OF FALLOT

Consists of four lesions (see the mnemonic **PROVe**).

SYMPTOMS/EXAM

- Presentation ranges from acyanotic ("pink tet") to profound cyanosis. Most patients have some cyanosis, depending on the severity of pulmonary stenosis and the relative right and left ventricular pressures (which determine the direction of flow across the VSD).
- Cyanotic "tet spells" may occur in a child who is crying or overheated. These children need to be calmed and given oxygen, and squatting or other measures can be used to ↑ systemic vascular resistance and restore left-to-right flow across the VSD.
- Cardiac exam may reveal a **systolic ejection murmur** at the left sternal border along with **right ventricular lift.**
- A single S2 is characteristic.

DIAGNOSIS

- **Echocardiography** is definitive.
- CXR shows a **boot-shaped heart.**

TREATMENT

- If a newborn infant with this condition is cyanotic, administer **prostaglandin E** to maintain the PDA.
- Surgical repair is necessary.
- Treat tet spells with **O_2**, a **squatting position, fluids, morphine,** propranolol, and phenylephrine if severe.

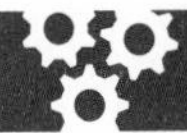

MNEMONIC

Anatomy of tetralogy of Fallot—

PROVe

Pulmonary stenosis (RV outflow obstruction)
RVH
Overriding aorta
VSD

TRANSPOSITION OF THE GREAT ARTERIES (TGA)

The aorta arises from the right ventricle and the pulmonary artery from the left ventricle.

SYMPTOMS/EXAM

- Presents with extreme cyanosis from birth.
- May have no murmur.
- **A single, loud S2** is characteristic.

DIAGNOSIS

- **Echocardiography** is definitive.
- CXR shows an **"egg on a string."**
- An O_2 saturation monitor on the right arm (measuring "preductal" saturation) will show a lower O_2 saturation than one on the lower extremity ("postductal" saturation).

TREATMENT

- Administer **prostaglandin E** to maintain the PDA.
- If necessary, a "balloon septostomy" or Rashkind procedure may be performed to rupture the atrial septum in order to improve mixing of venous and arterial blood as well as to ensure that adequately saturated blood enters the aorta.
- Surgical repair is necessary.

COARCTATION OF THE AORTA

You are on call in the nursery and are asked to evaluate a term male infant who has been doing well over the first 12 hours of life. You examine the infant and find him to be extremely irritable, diaphoretic, and pale with ↑ work of breathing. You listen to his chest and do not appreciate a murmur, and his lungs have a few crackles. You feel his pulses and note that his femoral pulses are difficult to palpate. What simple test can you perform quickly to confirm your suspected diagnosis?

Four-limb blood pressures. His presentation suggests coarctation of the aorta, and higher blood pressure in the upper (vs. lower) extremities is consistent with this diagnosis.

Narrowing of the lumen of the aorta, leading to ↓ blood flow below the obstruction and ↑ flow above it. Risk factors include **Turner's syndrome** and male gender; also associated with **bicuspid aortic valve.**

Symptoms/Exam

- Presents with dyspnea on exertion, syncope, and systemic hypoperfusion/shock.
- Cardiac exam may reveal **hypertension in the upper extremities** and a **lower BP in the lower extremities.**
- **↓ femoral and distal lower extremity pulses** are characteristic.

Diagnosis

- **Echocardiography** or **catheterization** is definitive.
- CXR shows **rib notching** due to collateral circulation through the intercostal arteries.

Treatment

- Surgical repair or balloon angioplasty +/– stent placement.
- Patients require prophylactic antibiotics prior to dental work even after surgical repair.

Complications

Often recurs.

Gastroenterology

PYLORIC STENOSIS

Hypertrophy of the pylorus, leading to gastric outlet obstruction.

Symptoms/Exam

- Occurs at **3–4 weeks of life** (range: two weeks to four months), predominantly in term, **firstborn** male infants.
- Presents with progressively **projectile, nonbilious emesis** that may lead to dehydration.
- Exam may reveal an **olive-shaped mass** in the epigastrium along with visible peristaltic waves.

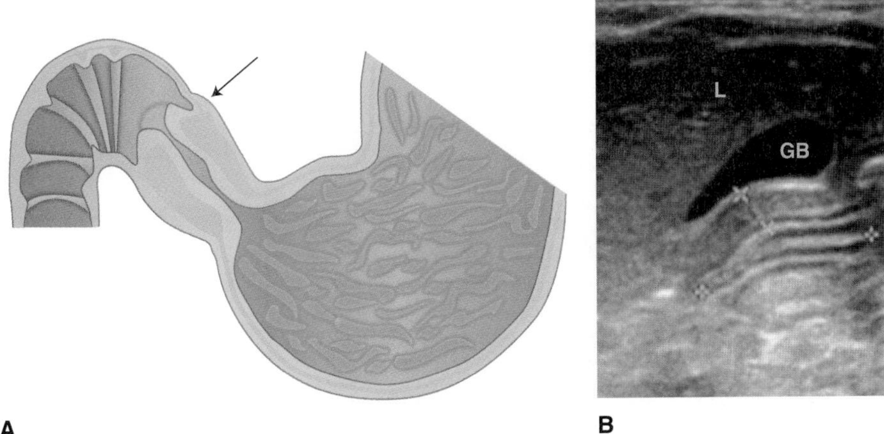

FIGURE 16-7. Hypertrophic pyloric stenosis. (A) Schematic representation of a hypertrophied pylorus. The arrow denotes protrusion of the pylorus into the duodenum. (B) Longitudinal ultrasound of the pylorus showing a thickened pyloric musculature (X's) over a long pyloric channel length (plus signs). L = liver; GB = gallbladder. (Image A adapted with permission from Doherty GM. *Current Diagnosis & Treatment: Surgery,* 13th ed. New York: McGraw-Hill, 2010. Image B reproduced with permission from USMLERx.com.)

Diagnosis

- Electrolytes show **hypochloremic, hypokalemic metabolic alkalosis** 2° to emesis.
- Ultrasound is the gold standard and shows a **hypertrophied pylorus** (see Figure 16-7).
- Barium studies show a **"string sign"** (a narrow pylorus) or a pyloric beak.

Treatment

- First, **correct dehydration and electrolyte abnormalities.**
- Surgical repair consists of pyloromyotomy and is usually well tolerated.

INTUSSUSCEPTION

Telescoping of a bowel segment into itself (see Figure 16-8) may lead to edema, arterial occlusion, gut necrosis, and death. Intussusception is the most common cause of bowel obstruction in the first two years of life. It is usually idiopathic in children < 2 years of age and often has an identifiable "lead point" (eg, a lymph node) in children > 5 years of age. Ileocecal intussusception is the most common type, while ileoileal intussusception is likely due to a pathologic cause.

Symptoms/Exam

- The classic presentation is bouts of **paroxysmal abdominal pain.** The child is often completely comfortable between paroxysms. Vomiting and heme-⊕ stools may be seen. "Currant jelly" stool is a late finding.
- May also present with altered mental status (lethargy or even obtundation), and may be preceded by a viral illness.
- Abdominal exam may reveal a **palpable, sausage-shaped mass.**

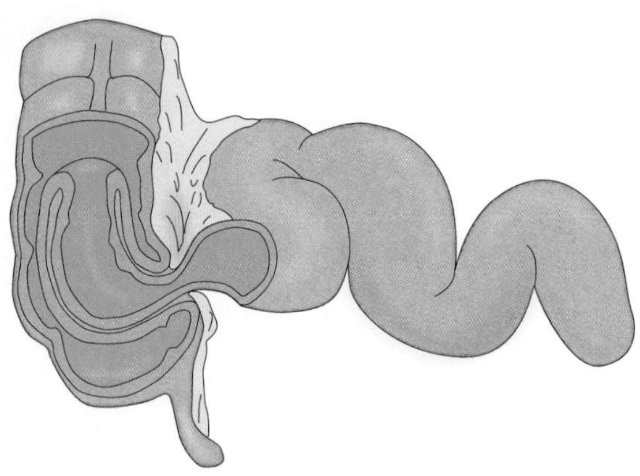

FIGURE 16-8. Intussusception.

Diagnosis

- Abdominal ultrasound is generally part of the initial workup in suspected cases.
- An air-contrast enema or a water-soluble contrast enema is both **diagnostic and therapeutic;** however, abdominal ultrasound is usually performed prior to the enema.

Treatment

- Following reduction via enema, treat with supportive care.
- If reduction fails or if perforation is suspected, surgical intervention may be required.

Complications

Associated with HSP and CF.

MALROTATION/VOLVULUS

Distinguished as follows:

- **Malrotation:** Failure of normal embryologic rotation as the gut returns to the abdominal cavity (during the 10th week of gestation). Results in abnormal location of intestinal contents in the abdomen, as well as incomplete fixation to the posterior abdominal wall. May predispose to intestinal obstruction (by a tissue called "Ladd's bands" that abnormally lies over the proximal duodenum in malrotation) or volvulus.
- **Volvulus:** A complication of malrotation in which the malrotated gut twists on the axis of the superior mesenteric artery, resulting in intestinal obstruction as well as ischemia.

SYMPTOMS/EXAM

- **First three weeks of life:** Volvulus presents as acute onset of **bilious emesis,** small bowel obstruction, or bowel necrosis.
- **Later in infancy/early childhood:** Malrotation may present as acute or intermittent intestinal obstruction, malabsorption, protein-losing enteropathy, or diarrhea.

DIAGNOSIS

- **Malrotation:** An **upper GI series** shows the duodenojejunal junction on the right side of the spine (see Figure 16-9). Barium enema shows a mobile cecum that is not in the RLQ.
- **Volvulus:** Contrast studies show a **"bird's beak"** where the gut is twisted.

TREATMENT

- Volvulus is a **surgical emergency** because the gut may necrose as a result of SMA occlusion.
- Surgical repair is necessary in asymptomatic patients who are diagnosed with malrotation because of the risk of complications such as volvulus.

COMPLICATIONS

- The 1° complication of volvulus is "short bowel syndrome," which occurs when < 30 cm of short bowel is left.
- If a large segment of bowel is lost as a result of bowel ischemia or surgery, the condition may also lead to malnutrition, TPN dependence, and liver failure.

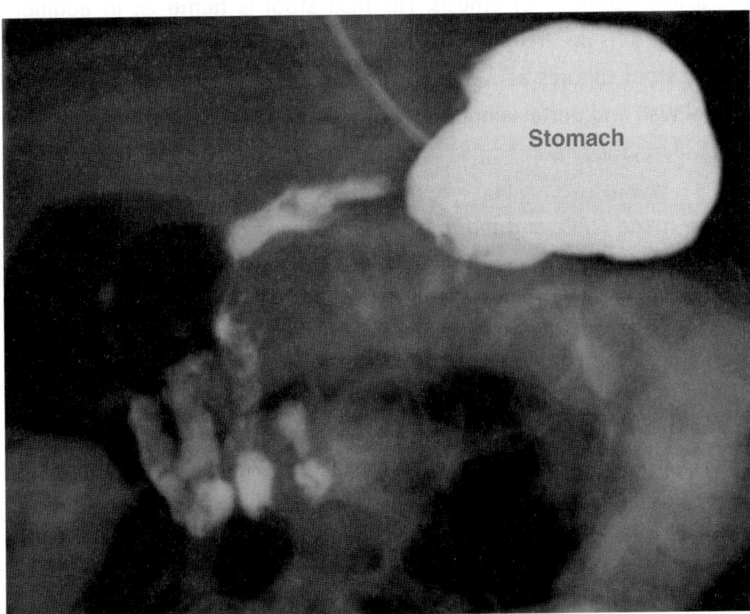

FIGURE 16-9. Midgut malrotation. Frontal radiograph from an upper GI study shows a spiral pattern of duodenal and proximal jejunal loops in the right abdomen, consistent with midgut malrotation. The duodenal-jejunal junction should normally be to the left of the patient's spine. (Reproduced with permission from USMLERx.com.)

TABLE 16-8. Common Pediatric Epilepsy Syndromes

Syndrome	Symptoms/Exam	Diagnosis	Treatment
Absence seizures	Multiple, brief staring episodes.	A generalized, **3-Hz, spike-and-wave** pattern on EEG.	Ethosuximide.
Infantile spasms (West syndrome)	Affects infants < 1 year of age, presenting with **"jackknife"** spasms and psychomotor arrest/ **developmental regression.**	**Hypsarrhythmia** on EEG. Associated with tuberous sclerosis.	ACTH.
Lennox-Gastaut syndrome	The first seizure occurs between one and seven years of age. Presents with multiple, progressive, difficult-to-treat seizure types, including generalized tonic-clonic seizures (GTCS) and drop attacks.	An atypical **spike-and-wave** pattern, primarily in the frontal region, on EEG. Progressive mental retardation. Associated with refractory infantile spasms and tuberous sclerosis.	No effective treatment.
Juvenile myoclonic epilepsy	Affects healthy adolescents, presenting with myoclonic jerks or GTCS in the **early-morning hours/upon awakening.**	May have a genetic basis; patients often have a ⊕ family history.	Easily treated with a variety of antiepileptic medications.
Benign partial epilepsy	Affects healthy children, presenting with partial seizures during wakefulness (oral, vocal, upper extremity symptoms). May spread to GTCS during sleep.	Classic **interictal** spikes from the centrotemporal (rolandic) region.	Seizures usually disappear by adolescence.
Landau-Kleffner syndrome	Those affected are developmentally normal children who **lose language ability** between three and six years of age. Often confused with autism.	A bilateral temporal spike and sharp waves on EEG.	Antiepileptic medications may improve the long-term prognosis but cannot reverse language loss.

(Data from Hay WW et al. *Current Pediatric Diagnosis & Treatment,* 18th ed. New York: McGraw-Hill, 2007: 721–725.)

Oncology

Hematologic malignancies (leukemia and lymphoma) are the most common form of malignancy in children. Solid tumors in pediatrics most commonly occur in the CNS, bone, and kidneys. These topics are covered in Chapter 9.

WILMS' TUMOR

An embryonal tumor of renal origin. Wilms' tumor is the most common renal tumor in children and is usually seen in those 1–4 years of age. Risk factors include a ⊕ family history, neurofibromatosis, aniridia (WAGR syndrome), Beckwith-Wiedemann syndrome, and congenital GU anomalies (eg, Denys-Drash syndrome).

SYMPTOMS/EXAM

- Patients may have abdominal pain or may present with a painless abdominal or flank mass.
- Hematuria and hypertension are commonly seen.
- Systemic symptoms include weight loss, nausea, emesis, bone pain, dysuria, and polyuria.

DIAGNOSIS

- Initially, an abdominal CT or ultrasound should be obtained.
- CXR, chest CT, CBC, LFTs, and BUN/creatinine can be used to assess severity and spread.
- Excisional biopsy to confirm.

TREATMENT

- Transabdominal nephrectomy followed by postoperative chemotherapy (vincristine/dactinomycin).
- Flank irradiation is of benefit in some cases.
- The prognosis is usually good but depends on staging and tumor histology.

NEUROBLASTOMA

A tumor of neural crest cell origin that most commonly affects children < 5 years of age; the most common solid tumor during infancy. Risk factors include neurofibromatosis, tuberous sclerosis, pheochromocytoma, and Hirschsprung's disease.

SYMPTOMS/EXAM

- Lesions can appear anywhere in the body (eg, the skin or skull).
- Presentations include abdominal mass/distention/hepatomegaly, anorexia, weight loss, respiratory distress, fatigue, fever, diarrhea, irritability, or neuromuscular symptoms (if paraspinal).
- Other symptoms include leg edema, hypertension, and periorbital bruising ("raccoon eyes").

DIAGNOSIS

- Definitive diagnosis is based on a tumor tissue sample with or without elevated urine catecholamines (VMA and HVA) **or** on metastases to bone marrow with elevated urine catecholamines.
- The initial workup generally includes a CBC, electrolytes, LDH, ferritin, LFTs, a coagulation screen, urine catecholamines, and BUN/creatinine.
- For staging and assessing severity, obtain bilateral iliac crest bone marrow biopsies, an abdominal CT or MRI, a CXR, bone radiographs, and a technetium radionuclide scan or ^{131}I-metaiodobenzylguanidine (MIBG) scan.

TREATMENT

- Localized tumors are usually cured with excision.
- Chemotherapy includes cyclophosphamide, carboplatin or cisplatin, etoposide or teniposide, vincristine, and doxorubicin.
- Radiation can be used as an adjunct.
- The prognosis is improved if the diagnosis is made before one year of age. Staging is based on the International Neuroblastoma Staging System.

TABLE 16-9. Common Genetic Syndromes *(continued)*

Syndrome	Symptoms	Exam	Diagnosis	Prognosis
Turner's syndrome (45,XO) (incidence 1:10,000)	Short female with shield chest, wide-spaced nipples, webbed neck, and congenital lymphedema.	Mental retardation, gonadal dysgenesis, renal anomalies, cardiac defects (coarctation of the aorta), hearing loss.	Karyotype for diagnosis. Baseline echocardiogram, renal ultrasound, BP, hearing screen.	Infertility; normal life span.
Fragile X syndrome (incidence 1:1500 males)	Boys present with macrocephaly, large ears, macroorchidism, and tall stature. Girls may have only learning disabilities.	Mild to profound mental retardation, autism.	DNA analysis shows expansion of a CGG nucleotide repeat in the FMR1 gene. The size of the repeat correlates with disease severity.	Normal life span.
Marfan's syndrome (incidence 1:10,000)	Tall stature, low upper-to-lower-segment ratio, arachnodactyly, joint laxity, scoliosis, pectus excavatum or carinatum, lens dislocation, retinal detachment, dilation of the aortic root, mitral valve prolapse, lumbosacral dural ectasia, high-arched palate.	Normal intelligence.	Slit-lamp examination, echocardiography, genetic evaluation. Diagnosis is made clinically.	With treatment/corrective surgery of aortic root dilation, patients have a normal life span.

(Data from Hay WW et al. *Current Pediatric Diagnosis & Treatment,* 18th ed. New York: McGraw-Hill, 2007: 721–725.)

CHAPTER 17

PSYCHIATRY

Diagnostic and Statistical Manual of Mental Disorders (DSM)

Psychiatric disorders affect (but do not always limit) a person's ability to handle daily living and/or social or occupational situations. The American Psychiatric Association's ***Diagnostic and Statistical Manual of Mental Disorders*** (DSM) provides diagnostic criteria for mental disorders. The sixth edition, DSM-IV-TR, was released in the year 2000.

The DSM organizes psychiatric diagnoses into five levels, or axes, relating to different aspects of disorder or disability:

- **Axis I:** Clinical disorders.
- **Axis II:** Personality disorders, mental disorders.
- **Axis III:** General medical conditions.
- **Axis IV:** Psychosocial/environmental problems.
- **Axis V:** Global assessment of functioning (GAF).

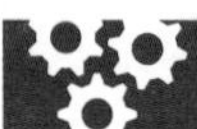

MNEMONIC

Characteristics of personality disorders–

MEDIC

Maladaptive
Enduring
Deviate from cultural norms
Inflexible
Cause impairment in social or occupational functioning

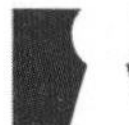

KEY FACT

To differentiate between schizoid and schizotypal, remember that schiz**OID**s feel like "**O**h, **I D**on't care."

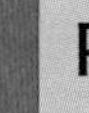

Personality Disorders

Defined as enduring patterns of inner experience and behavior that deviate from cultural standards; are pervasive and inflexible; begin in adolescence or early adulthood; are stable and predictable over time; and lead to distress or impairment (see Table 17-1). In some cases, however (eg, OCPD), personality disorders are more annoying to others than to the person they affect. Treat with psychotherapy; pharmacotherapy is generally used only if psychiatric comorbidities exist.

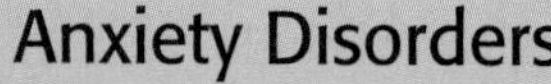

Anxiety Disorders

GENERALIZED ANXIETY DISORDER (GAD)

Lifetime prevalence is 5%; the male-to-female ratio is 1:2. Clinical diagnosis is usually made in the early 20s.

Symptoms

- Characterized by **excessive and pervasive worry** about a number of activities or events that leads to significant impairment or distress.
- Patients may seek medical care for somatic complaints.

Differential

Substance-induced anxiety disorder, anxiety disorder due to a general medical condition (eg, hyperthyroidism), panic disorder, OCD, depression, social phobia, hypochondriasis, somatization disorder.

TABLE 17-1. Signs and Symptoms of Personality Disorders

Cluster	Disorders	Characteristics	Clinical Dilemma/Strategies
Cluster A: **"weird"**	Paranoid	Distrustful and suspicious; interpret others' motives as malevolent. Litigious.	Patients are suspicious and distrustful of doctors and rarely seek medical attention.
	Schizoid	Isolated, detached "loners." Have restricted emotional expression.	Be clear, honest, noncontrolling, and nondefensive. Avoid humor. Maintain emotional distance.
	Schizotypal	Odd behavior/appearance. Exhibit cognitive or perceptual distortions (eg, magical thinking, ideas of reference).	
Cluster B: **"wild"**	Borderline	Unstable mood/relationships and feelings of emptiness. Impulsive. Have a history of suicidal ideation or self-harm.	Patients change the rules, demand attention, and feel they are special. Will manipulate staff and doctor ("splitting").
	Histrionic	Excessively emotional and attention seeking. Sexually provocative.	Be firm: Stick to the treatment plan. Be fair: Do not be punitive or derogatory.
	Narcissistic	Grandiose; need admiration; have sense of entitlement. Lack empathy.	Be consistent: Do not change the rules.
	Antisocial	Violate the rights of others, social norms, and laws. Impulsive; lack remorse. May have a criminal history. **Begins in childhood as conduct disorder.**	
Cluster C: **"worried and wimpy"**	Obsessive-compulsive	Preoccupied with perfectionism, order, and control. Miserly. Have inflexible morals and values.	Patients are controlling and may sabotage their treatment. Words may be inconsistent with actions.
	Avoidant	Socially inhibited; sensitive to rejection. Have fear of being disliked or ridiculed.	Avoid power struggles. Give clear recommendations, but do not push patients into decisions.
	Dependent	Submissive, clingy, need to be taken care of. Have difficulty making decisions. Feel helpless.	

Diagnosis

Diagnostic criteria are as follows:

- **Anxiety/worry on most days for at least six months.**
- **Three or more somatic symptoms,** including restlessness, fatigue, difficulty concentrating, irritability, muscle tension, and sleep disturbance.

Treatment

- Pharmacologic therapy includes venlafaxine, SSRIs, benzodiazepines, and buspirone; second-line treatment with TCAs is appropriate if other antidepressants are ineffective or are not tolerated.
- Benzodiazepines offer acute relief, but tolerance and dependence may result from their use. Use them as a bridge to chronic treatment with SSRIs, as above.
- Psychotherapy and relaxation training are important adjuncts.

OBSESSIVE-COMPULSIVE DISORDER (OCD)

A 30-year-old high school guidance counselor presents to her dermatologist for irritation of her hands. She states that she washes her hands under hot water about 20 times a day and uses a variety of alcohol-based hand sanitizer products to avoid picking up germs. What is the most likely origin of her dermatitis?

Obsessive-compulsive disorder.

Lifetime prevalence is 2–3%. Typically presents in late adolescence or early adulthood, and can lead to severe functional impairment.

Symptoms

- Obsessions are **persistent, intrusive thoughts, impulses, or images** that lead to anxiety/distress and interfere with daily life. Common themes are contamination and fear of harm to oneself or to others.
- Compulsions are **conscious, repetitive behaviors** (eg, hand washing) or mental acts (eg, counting) that patients feel driven to perform to neutralize anxiety from obsessions.

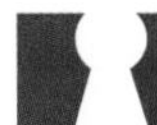

KEY FACT

In general, OCD is ego dystonic, whereas OCPD is ego syntonic.

Differential

OCPD, other anxiety disorders, Tourette's syndrome (multiple motor and vocal tics), depression, schizophrenia, medical conditions (eg, brain tumor, temporal lobe epilepsy, group A β-hemolytic streptococcal infection).

Diagnosis

Patients recognize that their obsessions and/or compulsions are excessive, unreasonable productions of their own minds (rather than thought insertion). Nonetheless, their behaviors cause marked distress and are time-consuming (take > 1 hour/day).

Treatment

Pharmacotherapy (eg, SSRIs, clomipramine, fluvoxamine) and **behavioral therapy** (eg, exposure and response prevention).

PANIC DISORDER

More common in women, with a mean age of onset of 25. Lifetime prevalence is 1.5–3.5%. Often accompanied by **agoraphobia** (30–50% of cases), a fear of being in places or situations from which escape is difficult; of being outside the home alone; or of being in public places (see the discussion of phobias).

Symptoms

Presents as **panic attacks**—discrete periods of intense fear or discomfort in which at least four of the following symptoms develop abruptly and peak within 10 minutes: palpitations, sweating, trembling, shortness of breath, chest pain, nausea, dizziness, numbness, depersonalization, or fear of losing control.

Differential

Medical conditions (eg, angina, hyperthyroidism, hypoglycemia), substance-induced anxiety disorder, other anxiety disorders.

Diagnosis

Recurrent, unexpected panic attacks followed by at least **one month** of worry about and/or behavioral change to avoid subsequent attacks.

Treatment

- Behavioral therapy.
- Pharmacotherapy includes SSRIs, either alone or in combination with benzodiazepines. TCAs or MAOIs should be used only if SSRIs are not tolerated or are ineffective.
- Benzodiazepines (eg, alprazolam, clonazepam) are effective for immediate relief but have abuse potential.

PHOBIAS

The three categories of phobia are agoraphobia, social phobia, and specific phobia. Lifetime prevalence is 10%.

Symptoms

- Phobias are persistent, excessive, or unreasonable fear and/or avoidance of an object or situation that leads to significant distress or impairment.
- Exposure to the object or stimulus may precipitate **panic attacks.**

Differential

Other anxiety disorders, depression, avoidant and schizoid personality disorders, schizophrenia, appropriate fear, normal shyness.

Diagnosis

- **Social phobia** is characterized by unreasonable, marked, and persistent **fear of scrutiny and embarrassment in social or performance situations** (also referred to as social anxiety disorder). It usually begins in adolescence.
- **Specific phobia** is immediately **cued by an object or a situation** (eg, spiders, animals, heights). It usually begins in childhood.
- In adults, the **duration is six or more months.**
- As in OCD, symptoms interrupt the patient's life, and patients recognize that their fears are excessive.

Treatment

- Cognitive-behavioral therapy (CBT) and pharmacotherapy (eg, SSRIs, benzodiazepines, β-blockers) are effective for social phobias.
- **Behavioral therapy** that uses exposure and desensitization is best for specific phobia.

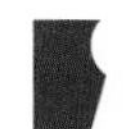

KEY FACT

Cognitive-behavioral therapy is a type of therapy that helps patients learn new ways to cope by:

- Identifying automatic thoughts, or "cognitive distortions."
- Testing the automatic thoughts.
- Identifying and testing the validity of maladaptive assumptions.
- Strategizing on alternative ways to deal with problems.

POSTTRAUMATIC STRESS DISORDER (PTSD)

A 22-year-old war refugee presents to establish care at a local free clinic. She is soft-spoken and gives only brief responses to questions despite being fluent in English. The physician is unable to conduct a pelvic exam because of her obvious physical and emotional discomfort. The patient hesitantly admits to having vivid nightmares and flashbacks of the war. What psychiatric diagnosis should be considered in this patient?

Posttraumatic stress disorder.

Results from exposure to a traumatic event that involved **actual or threatened death or serious injury** and evoked **intense fear, helplessness, or horror.** The lifetime prevalence is 8%.

SYMPTOMS

- Examples of traumatic events include war, torture, natural disasters, assault, rape, and serious accidents.
- Patients with PTSD may have experienced the trauma personally, or they may have witnessed the event in a way that leads them to feel personally threatened, helpless, and horrified (eg, a child witnessing a parent being assaulted).
- Nightmares and flashbacks are common.
- Watch for **survival guilt,** personality change, substance abuse, depression, and suicide.

DIFFERENTIAL

- **Acute stress disorder:** Symptoms are the same as or similar to those of PTSD but last < **1 month,** occur within one month of a trauma, and are primarily dissociative.
- **Adjustment disorder with anxiety:** Emotional or behavioral symptoms occurring within three months of a stressor and lasting < 6 months.
- **Other:** Depression, OCD, acute intoxication or withdrawal, factitious disorders, malingering, borderline personality disorder.

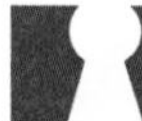

KEY FACT

Victims of human trafficking may present with symptoms similar to those of PTSD.

DIAGNOSIS

Symptoms persist for > **1 month** and include the following:

- **Reexperiencing** of the event (eg, nightmares, flashbacks).
- Avoidance of trauma-related stimuli or **numbing** of general responsiveness.
- **Hyperarousal** (eg, hypervigilance, exaggerated startle, irritability, difficulty falling or staying asleep).

TREATMENT

- Pharmacotherapy includes first-line treatment with SSRIs; if SSRIs are not tolerated or are ineffective, use TCAs or MAOIs.
- Second-generation antipsychotics (eg, risperidone, olanzapine, quetiapine), anticonvulsants (eg, divalproex, topiramate), α_2-adrenergic agonists (clonidine), or β-blockers (propranolol) may be helpful for some patients.
- CBT and group therapy are also effective.

Cognitive Disorders

DELIRIUM

Delirium is common in hospitalized medical or surgical patients (15–70%) and is a medical, not psychiatric, disorder. However, since delirium may mimic psychosis, psychiatrists are often consulted on this problem. Risk factors include advanced age, hospitalization, medications (benzodiazepines, anticholinergics, opioids), starting multiple new medications at once, pre-existing cognitive deficits, electrolyte abnormalities, malnutrition, hypoxia, a windowless ICU environment, infections, vision or hearing deficits, and severe illness.

SYMPTOMS

- Characterized by the following:
  - **Disturbance of consciousness** and/or perception.
  - **Altered cognition** (memory, orientation, language)—eg, **diminished attention span,** impaired short-term memory, or unclear speech.
  - **Acute onset.**
  - A history suggesting a probable medical cause of delirium.
- Symptoms "wax and wane" during the day and feature lucid intervals.

DIFFERENTIAL

In contrast to delirium, dementia usually has an insidious onset; includes chronic memory and executive function deficits; and is characterized by symptoms that tend not to fluctuate during the day (see Table 17-2).

DIAGNOSIS

- The number of potential causes of delirium is extensive. First evaluate for recent medication changes, hypoglycemia, hepatic encephalopathy, or UTI.

TABLE 17-2. Delirium vs. Dementia

	DELIRIUM	DEMENTIA
Course	**Acute** (abrupt onset), lasting hours to days; usually reversible.	**Chronic** (progressive degradation), lasting months to years; usually irreversible.
Functionality	Fluctuating ability to focus and shift attention. **Clouded consciousness.**	Alert. Intact consciousness.
Cognition	Similar to dementia, but more likely to include perceptual disturbances (hallucinations) and paranoia.	Disrupted memory, orientation, and language. Hallucinations are present in about 30% of those with advanced disease.
Causes	Evidence of a general medical condition causing the problem (seizures, postictal state, infections, thyroid disorders, UTI, vitamin deficiencies); substances (eg, cocaine, opioids, PCP); head trauma, kidney disease, sleep deprivation.	Insidious processes such as Alzheimer's disease, Huntington's disease, vascular dementia, AIDS dementia, and major depressive disorder in the elderly.

- Workup may include a CBC, electrolytes, BUN/creatinine, glucose, LFTs, UA, urine toxicology, vitamin B_{12}/folate, TSH, RPR, HIV, blood culture, serum calcium/phosphorus/magnesium, pulse oximetry, ABGs, CSF, or serum drug screening.

Treatment

- Treat the underlying medical condition.
- Minimize or discontinue delirium-inducing drugs (eg, benzodiazepines, anticholinergics), and simplify medication regimens if possible.
- Recommend reorientation techniques (eg, clocks or wall calendars), and provide an environment that will facilitate healthy sleep/wake cycles.
- Pharmacotherapy may be beneficial and includes **low-dose antipsychotics** (haloperidol, risperidone, olanzapine, quetiapine), usually for short-term use. Physical restraints may be necessary to prevent physical harm to self/others.

DEMENTIA

General deterioration of function 2° to **chronic, progressive cognitive decline** with intact attention and consciousness. Most common among the elderly (those > 85 years of age), and most often caused by Alzheimer's disease (50%) or multi-infarct dementia (25%). Refer to the Dementia section of Chapter 13 for further detail.

DEPRESSION AND ANXIETY DUE TO A GENERAL MEDICAL CONDITION

- Depression can be 2° to drug intoxication (alcohol or sedative-hypnotics; antihypertensives such as methyldopa, clonidine, and propranolol) or to stroke, hypothyroidism, MS, or SLE.
- Anxiety may be caused by drugs (caffeine, sympathomimetics, steroids), endocrinopathies (pheochromocytoma, hypercortisolism, hyperthyroidism, hyperparathyroidism), metabolic disorders (hypoxemia, hypercalcemia, hypoglycemia), or SLE.

Mood (Affective) Disorders

MAJOR DEPRESSIVE DISORDER (MDD)

Untreated episodes of MDD can last for four or more months, and the risk of recurrence is 50% after only one episode. The average age of onset is in the mid-20s; lifetime prevalence is 10–25% for females (the highest risk is in the childbearing years) and 5–12% for males. The male-to-female ratio is 1:2. MDD is often associated with a life stressor, and up to 15% of those affected die by suicide.

Symptoms

Diagnosis requires depressed mood or **anhedonia** (loss of interest or pleasure) and at least five of the following symptoms during a two-week period:

- Insomnia or hypersomnia.
- Feelings of worthlessness or excessive guilt.
- Fatigue or loss of energy.

- ↓ ability to concentrate, or indecisiveness.
- Significant weight loss or weight gain, or change in appetite.
- Psychomotor agitation or retardation.
- Recurrent thoughts of death or suicide.

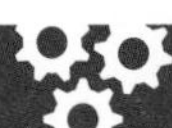

MNEMONIC

Symptoms of depression–

SIG E CAPS

Sleep (↓/↑)
Interest (↓)
Guilt
Energy (↓)
Concentration
Appetite (↓/↑)
Psychomotor agitation or retardation
Suicidal ideation

Differential

- **Dysthymia:** A milder, chronic depressed state of two or more years' duration.
- **Bereavement:** Does not involve severe impairment or suicidality; usually improves within two months, but can last up to a year. Symptoms may vary on the basis of cultural norms. For example, visual and auditory hallucinations (such as thinking the deceased is still alive) are common and can be considered normal. Similarly, feelings of grief around anniversaries and other special events beyond the one-year period are also quite common.
- **Adjustment disorder with depressed mood:** Has fewer symptoms; occurs within three months of a stressor; lasts < 6 months.
- **Other:** Substance-induced mood disorder (eg, illicit drugs, β-blockers, OCPs); mood disorder due to a medical condition (eg, hypothyroidism, ACA stroke); dementia.

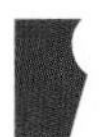

KEY FACT

Cognitive decline is a common sign of major depressive disorder in the elderly ("pseudodementia").

Diagnosis

Symptoms last two or more weeks and must lead to significant dysfunction or impairment.

Treatment

- **Pharmacotherapy:**
  - The effectiveness of antidepressants is similar between and within classes (50–70% of patients), and these drugs take at least 3–4 weeks to have an effect. Thus, the selection of an antidepressant should be based on side effect profiles, the safety and tolerability of side effects, patient preference, cost, and the patient's previous response to specific antidepressants.
  - Continue treatment for six or more months. Avoid abrupt discontinuation of medications even if the patient "feels better"; instead, taper over 6–12 months unless the patient has had adverse side effects (eg, ↑ thoughts of suicide).
- **Electroconvulsive therapy (ECT):**
  - Safe and effective.
  - Best for refractory or catatonic depression, but may also be used for acute mania or acute psychosis and when the patient refuses to eat or drink (eg, severely depressed elderly) or is suicidally depressed.
  - Adverse effects include postictal confusion, arrhythmias, headache, and **retrograde amnesia** (inability to recall memories prior to the event).
  - Relative contraindications include intracranial mass, aneurysm, and recent MI/stroke. **Pregnancy is not a contraindication.**
- **Psychotherapy:** Psychotherapy combined with antidepressants is more effective than either modality alone.

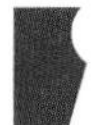

KEY FACT

Severe MDD can present with psychotic symptoms, in which case an antipsychotic in addition to an antidepressant may be temporarily required.

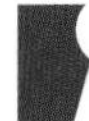

KEY FACT

Seasonal affective disorder (SAD), which is typified by fall/winter depression, is treated with bright-light therapy (phototherapy).

BIPOLAR DISORDER

A family history of bipolar illness significantly ↑ risk. Prevalence is 1%. The male-to-female ratio is 1:1, but women more often seek treatment. Symptoms usually appear around age 20, and the number of cycles actually ↑ with age. About 10–15% of those affected die by suicide.

SYMPTOMS

- A **manic episode** is defined as follows:
  - **One week** of an abnormally and persistently **elevated ("euphoric"), expansive, or irritable mood.**
  - At least three of the following (four if the mood is irritable), as remembered by the mnemonic **DIGS FAR:**
    - **D**istractibility
    - **I**nsomnia (↓ need for sleep)
    - **G**randiosity (inflated self-esteem)
    - Pressured **S**peech
    - **F**light of ideas (racing thoughts)
    - Psychomotor **A**gitation/↑ goal-directed **A**ctivity
    - **R**ecklessness/pursuit of pleasurable but **R**isky behaviors (eg, gambling, sexual indiscretions)
- A **mixed episode** must meet the criteria for both manic and depressive episodes for one week or more.
- Mania and mixed episodes are considered **psychiatric emergencies** 2° to impaired judgment and the risk of hurting oneself or others.

> **KEY FACT**
>
> Catatonia may be observed in both schizophrenia and mood disorders. Of the latter, it is more often associated with mania than depression.

DIFFERENTIAL

- **Hypomania:** Features no marked functional impairment or psychosis. Symptoms last for four days or less. Does not require hospitalization.
- **Cyclothymic disorder:** Chronic cycles of mild depression (dysthymia) and hypomania for two or more years. Effectively a milder form of bipolar II disorder.
- **Other:** Substance-induced mood disorder, schizophrenia, schizoaffective disorder, personality disorders, medical conditions (eg, temporal lobe epilepsy, hyperthyroidism), ADHD.

DIAGNOSIS

- **Bipolar I disorder:** Diagnosis is made after just **one mixed or manic episode.** Depressive episodes are common but are not required for diagnosis.
- **Bipolar II disorder:** Characterized by at least **one hypomanic** (rather than manic) **episode** alternating with at least **one major depressive episode.**

TREATMENT

- **Acute mania:** Lithium, anticonvulsants, antipsychotics, benzodiazepines, ECT.
- **Bipolar depression:** Mood stabilizers (lithium or lamotrigine are first line) +/– antidepressants. **Monotherapy with an antidepressant is not recommended.** If the patient does not respond to first-line treatment, the next step may include adding lamotrigine (if started with lithium), bupropion, or SSRIs. In severe cases, consider ECT.

> **KEY FACT**
>
> Screen for bipolar disorder before starting antidepressants, as they can induce acute mania or psychosis in bipolar patients.

Psychotic Disorders

SCHIZOPHRENIA

Thought to be related to dysregulation of dopamine (↑ in the limbic system and ↓ in the frontal cortex). Lifetime prevalence is 1%. Family history ↑ risk, and an ↑ incidence is seen in those born during winter/early spring. Peak onset is 18–25 years for men and 25–35 years (and perimenopausally) for women. Few patients have a complete recovery. As with other psychiatric disorders, social/occupational dysfunction can be significant. There is a high incidence of substance abuse, and > 75% of patients smoke cigarettes. The suicide rate is 10%.

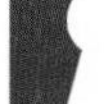

KEY FACT

A **bizarre delusion** is defined as an absurd, totally implausible, fixed false belief that is not shared by other members of that society/culture—eg, the conviction that aliens from another planet have implanted electrodes into one's brain.

SYMPTOMS

At least two of the following are required for one or more months, with continuous signs for six or more months:

- **Positive symptoms:** Bizarre delusions, hallucinations, disorganized thoughts/speech/behavior. Hallucinations are usually auditory (eg, running commentary/monologues or conversations between two voices) but may also be visual, tactile, or, rarely, olfactory.
- **Negative symptoms:** Affective flattening, avolition, apathy, alogia.

DIFFERENTIAL

- **Brief psychotic disorder:** Symptoms are of < **1 month's duration;** onset often follows a psychosocial stressor. Associated with a better prognosis. (Postpartum psychosis can last up to three months.)
- **Schizophreniform disorder:** Diagnostic criteria are the same as those for schizophrenia, but symptoms have a duration of **1–6 months.**
- **Schizoaffective disorder:** Mood symptoms are present for a significant portion of the illness, but psychotic symptoms have been present without a mood episode.
- **Delusional disorder: Nonbizarre delusions for one or more months** in the absence of other psychotic symptoms; often chronic.
- **Other:** Mood disorder with psychotic features (contrast with schizoaffective disorder); substance-induced psychosis (eg, amphetamines) or drug withdrawal (eg, alcoholic hallucinosis); psychosis due to a general medical condition (eg, brain tumor); delirium or dementia; shared psychotic disorder.

DIAGNOSIS

There are several subtypes of schizophrenia, classified by their predominant symptoms:

- **Paranoid:** Marked by delusions and hallucinations. Carries the best prognosis.
- **Disorganized (hebephrenic):** Characterized by disinhibition and poor contact with reality. Carries the worst prognosis.
- **Catatonic:** Involves a marked ↑ or ↓ in speech and motor function. Rare (10–15% of cases).
- **Residual:** Entails eventual loss of positive symptoms but persistence of negative ones in long-term, untreated schizophrenics.
- **Undifferentiated:** A constellation of symptoms that is too inconsistent to be classified according to the above subtypes.

TREATMENT

Antipsychotic medications (neuroleptics). Hospitalize when the patient is a danger to himself/herself or to others. Psychosocial treatments, individual supportive psychotherapy, and family therapy help prevent relapse.

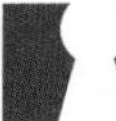

KEY FACT

Negative symptoms are harder to treat.

DISSOCIATIVE IDENTITY DISORDER

A condition in which a person presents with **two or more distinct personalities** (aka "alters"). Each of these identities interprets and interacts with the world differently—eg, they may be of different ages, levels of intelligence, or even genders. The individual usually claims no memory when the other identities take over but sometimes reports internal quarreling between the "alters." Often associated with severe and prolonged abuse and/or neglect in childhood. Comorbid PTSD is common. Formerly known as multiple personality disorder.

DISSOCIATIVE FUGUE

Temporary amnesia for one's own identity, typically lasting hours to days, and **usually precipitated by acute stressors.** Classically, the affected individual is found after having traveled to a different city or state and having established a new identity. Upon recovery, he or she is amnestic for the fugue episode as well as for the original stressor that caused it. Like other dissociative disorders, fugue cannot be attributed to ingestion of illicit substances or other psychiatric conditions such as delirium.

Somatoform Disorders

SOMATIZATION DISORDER

Chronic pain symptoms in four or more sites/organ systems that are **not intentionally produced** and cannot be explained by a general medical condition. Onset is before age 30, and the condition is much more prevalent in women.

CONVERSION DISORDER

- Presents with **sensory symptoms, motor deficits, or "psychogenic seizures"** that are not intentionally produced and cannot be explained by an organic etiology.
- **Relation to a stressful event** suggests association with psychological factors (eg, complete right arm paralysis after a fight).
- Symptoms usually subside spontaneously.

HYPOCHONDRIASIS

An 18-year-old student presents to the ER with a chief complaint of dyspareunia. Although she reports having experienced a bicycle accident approximately one year ago, she has had multiple diagnostic workups that have always been negative. She is now particularly concerned that she has contracted an STD and does not appear relieved when the physician states that her exam and blood work are normal. What diagnosis should be considered in this patient?

Hypochondriasis.

Preoccupation over > 6 months with **fear of having a serious disease** based on **misinterpretation of symptoms** (rather than delusions). Patients usually recognize that their concerns are excessive, but they are not reassured by negative medical evaluations. Men and women are affected equally.

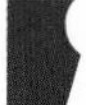

KEY FACT

Medical students are prone to thinking that they have the symptoms of whatever disease they are studying. It has been suggested that this is nosophobia, or fear of contracting disease, rather than true hypochondriasis.

PAIN DISORDER

- Pain intensity or a pain profile that is inconsistent with physiologic processes. More common in women than in men, with a peak onset at 40–50 years of age.
- **Sx/Exam:** Symptoms are exacerbated by or related to psychological factors, especially depression.
- **Tx:** Treat with physical therapy, psychotherapy, and antidepressants. Analgesics rarely provide relief.

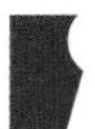

KEY FACT

Fibromyalgia, a pain disorder that features chronic pain and allodynia, is often accompanied by other psychiatric comorbidities. It is treated with antidepressants, muscle relaxants, anticonvulsants (eg, pregabalin), and dopamine agonists (eg, ropinirole).

BODY DYSMORPHIC DISORDER

Preoccupation with an imagined defect in appearance. Multiple visits to surgeons and dermatologists are common. Slightly more common in women than in men. Associated with depression. Treat with SSRIs.

Volitional/Intentional Disorders

Unlike somatoform disorders, which have no conscious mechanism or motivation for symptoms, volitional disorders feature a **conscious mechanism** for illness (eg, self-harm, intentional ingestion of toxins) and a 1° or 2° gain.

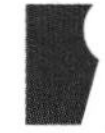

KEY FACT

Munchausen's syndrome refers to repeated episodes of factitious disorders (either the same or new complaints). The sufferer feels a deep psychological need to play the role of patient and feels comforted by assuming such a role.

FACTITIOUS DISORDER

- Symptoms are intentionally caused or exaggerated for 1° gain (eg, assuming a sick role), although patients do not understand why they do this (ie, **unconscious motivation**).
- The disorder is more common in men and among health care workers.

MALINGERING

Feigning of symptoms for anticipated external (2°) gain (eg, money, food, shelter).

Sleep Disorders

1° INSOMNIA

Significant **difficulty falling or staying asleep.** Affects up to one-third of the general population. The disorder cannot be attributed to physical or mental conditions but is often precipitated by anxiety. Symptoms occur three or more times a week for at least one month.

NARCOLEPSY

Has a prevalence of approximately 0.16%, and usually presents before age 30.

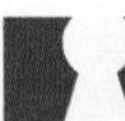

KEY FACT

HypnaGOgic hallucinations occur when you **GO** to sleep. HypnoPOMPic hallucinations occur when you awaken and **"PUMP"** yourself up for the day.

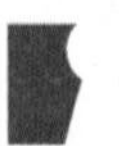

KEY FACT

Cataplexy is sudden loss of muscle tone leading to collapse, usually in the setting of strong emotions or excitement. It is treated with SSRIs.

May be familial. Often associated with mood disorders, substance abuse, and GAD.

Symptoms

- Presents with excessive daytime sleepiness and daytime **sleep attacks** characterized by ↓ REM sleep latency. Symptoms occur daily for three or more months.
- May involve hypnagogic (just before sleep) or hypnopompic (just before awakening) hallucinations.

Treatment

Amphetamines **(methylphenidate)** or nonamphetamine stimulants (modafinil).

SLEEP APNEA

Disturbances to the normal sleep cycle 2° to **airflow obstruction** +/– **pauses in respiratory effort,** leading to **excessive daytime somnolence.** Both central (CSA) and obstructive sleep apnea (OSA) can be diagnosed via polysomnography (a sleep study), but OSA is strongly associated with snoring and is usually observed in obese men. Therapy usually includes continuous positive airway pressure (CPAP) while sleeping and treatment of underlying/associated medical problems (eg, heart failure, obesity).

CIRCADIAN RHYTHM SLEEP DISORDER

Discrepancy between when the patient would like to sleep and when he or she actually does so. Often 2° to jet lag or shift work.

Substance-Related Disorders

KEY FACT

Exercise caution when diagnosing mood disorders in patients who are acutely intoxicated/impaired.

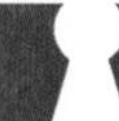

KEY FACT

Dependence ≈ abuse + tolerance and/or withdrawal.

SUBSTANCE ABUSE/DEPENDENCE

The lifetime prevalence of substance abuse is approximately 20%. The lifetime prevalence of using one or more illicit substances in the United States is roughly 40%. Comorbid psychiatric disorders are common.

Symptoms

The signs, symptoms, and physical findings of acute intoxication and withdrawal are outlined in Table 17-3.

Diagnosis

- Check urine and serum toxicology. Offer HIV testing; check LFTs and consider hepatitis testing.
- **Diagnostic criteria:**
  - Individuals display maladaptive patterns of behavior (ie, reliance on substances) to cope with stressors, leading to clinically significant impairment and, in general, to an overall worsening of the situation.
  - **Substance abuse** (one or more criteria in one year): Failure to meet obligations, substance use during hazardous activities, substance-related legal problems, or continued use despite social problems.

- **Substance dependence** (three or more criteria in one year): Tolerance, ↑ use, desire to ↓ use, withdrawal, spending a significant amount of time obtaining the substance, disinterest in other activities.

TABLE 17-3. Signs and Symptoms of Intoxication and Withdrawal

Drug	Intoxication	Withdrawal
Alcohol	Disinhibition/impaired judgment, emotional lability, slurred speech, ataxia, aggression, hallucinations, hypoglycemia, blackouts (retrograde amnesia), coma.	Tremor, tachycardia, hypertension, malaise, nausea, seizures, DTs, agitation, hallucinations. **May be life-threatening and require hospitalization.**
Opioids	Euphoria leading to apathy, CNS depression, nausea, vomiting, constipation, pupillary constriction, seizures, respiratory depression (life-threatening in overdose). Naloxone/naltrexone will block opioid receptors and reverse effects (beware of the antagonist clearing before the opioid, particularly with long-acting opioids such as methadone).	Anxiety, insomnia, anorexia, diaphoresis, dilated pupils, fever, rhinorrhea, piloerection, nausea, stomach cramps, diarrhea, yawning, myalgias. Extremely uncomfortable, but rarely life-threatening.
Amphetamines, cocaine	Psychomotor agitation, impaired judgment, tachycardia, pupillary dilation, fever, diaphoresis, hypertension, paranoia, angina, arrhythmias, seizures, hallucinations, sudden death. Treat with haloperidol for severe agitation and symptom-targeted medications.	Post-use "crash" with hypersomnolence, dysphoria/nightmares, depression, malaise, severe craving, suicidality.
Phencyclidine hydrochloride (PCP)	Belligerence, psychosis, **violence,** impulsiveness, psychomotor agitation, fever, tachycardia, vertical/horizontal nystagmus, ataxia, seizures, delirium. Give benzodiazepines or haloperidol for severe symptoms; otherwise reassure.	Recurrence of intoxication symptoms due to reabsorption in the GI tract; sudden onset of severe, random violence.
LSD	Marked anxiety or depression, delusions, visual hallucinations, flashbacks, pupillary dilation. Give benzodiazepines or traditional antipsychotics for severe symptoms.	–
Marijuana (THC)	Euphoria, slowed sense of time, impaired judgment, "heightened senses," social withdrawal, ↑ appetite, dry mouth, diaphoresis, conjunctival injection, hallucinations, anxiety, paranoia, tachycardia, hypertension, amotivational syndrome.	–
Barbiturates	Low safety margin; respiratory depression.	Anxiety, seizures, delirium, life-threatening cardiovascular collapse.
Benzodiazepines	Interactions with alcohol, amnesia, ataxia, somnolence, mild respiratory depression.	Rebound anxiety, seizures, tremor, insomnia, hypertension, tachycardia.
Caffeine	Restlessness, insomnia, diuresis, muscle twitching, arrhythmias, psychomotor agitation.	Headache, lethargy, depression, weight gain, irritability, craving.
Nicotine	Restlessness, insomnia, anxiety, arrhythmias.	Irritability, headache, anxiety, weight gain, craving.

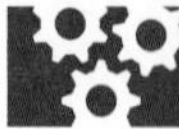

MNEMONIC

CAGE questions:

1. Have you ever felt the need to **C**ut down on your drinking?
2. Have you ever felt **A**nnoyed by criticism of your drinking?
3. Have you ever felt **G**uilty about your drinking?
4. Have you ever had a morning **E**ye opener?

More than one "yes" on the CAGE questionnaire makes alcohol abuse likely.

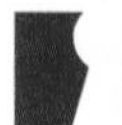

KEY FACT

Alcoholism can to**AST** your liver.

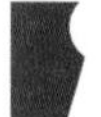

KEY FACT

DTs are a medical emergency with an untreated mortality rate of 20%. Give IV lorazepam.

KEY FACT

Alcohol use is related to 50% of all homicides and automobile fatalities.

Treatment

Group therapy, Narcotics Anonymous, recovery housing. Hospitalization may be necessary for acute withdrawal. Consider methadone maintenance for opiate dependence.

ALCOHOLISM

The lifetime prevalence of alcohol abuse is roughly 10% in women and approximately 20% in men. The lifetime prevalence of alcohol dependence is 3–5% in women and 10% in men. Evidence of a problem usually begins to surface between 21 and 34 years of age. Family history ↑ risk. Common causes of death include suicide, cancer, heart disease, and hepatic disease.

Diagnosis

- Screen with the CAGE questionnaire.
- Monitor vital signs for tachycardia and elevated BP associated with withdrawal; look for stigmata of liver disease such as palmar erythema or spider angiomata.
- Labs may reveal macrocytosis and an **elevated AST** and GGT.

Treatment

- Rule out medical complications; correct electrolyte abnormalities and hydrate.
- Start a **benzodiazepine taper** (eg, chlordiazepoxide, lorazepam) for withdrawal symptoms—ie, the CIWA protocol.
- Give multivitamins and folic acid; **administer thiamine before glucose** to prevent Wernicke's encephalopathy.
- Individual or group counseling, Alcoholics Anonymous, disulfiram, naltrexone, or acamprosate may be of benefit.

Complications

- **GI bleeding** (eg, gastritis, varices, Mallory-Weiss tears), **pancreatitis, liver disease,** delirium tremens (DTs), alcohol-induced psychosis, peripheral neuropathy, cerebellar degeneration.
- **Wernicke's encephalopathy:** Acute and usually reversible ataxia accompanied by confusion and ophthalmoplegia.
- **Korsakoff's syndrome:** A chronic and often irreversible condition marked by anterograde amnesia +/– confabulation.

Eating Disorders

ANOREXIA NERVOSA

A 15-year-old boy presents to his family doctor for a routine well-child exam. The father is concerned that his son has been eating poorly ever since he and his wife filed for divorce. The son, for his part, states that he has been trying to exercise more and eat less so that he can make the basketball team at school. The boy's growth curve reveals a drop from the 50th to the 15th percentile for weight. What psychiatric diagnoses should be considered?

Depression and anorexia nervosa. (Although eating disorders are much less common in males, the diagnosis should still be considered in male patients.)

Females account for 90% of cases. Peak incidences are at age 14 and age 18. Risk factors include family history, higher socioeconomic status (SES), poor self-esteem, psychiatric comorbidities (eg, major depression, OCD, anxiety), and body-conscious careers/activities such as modeling, ballet, and wrestling. Mortality from suicide or medical complications is 10%.

SYMPTOMS

Classified as **restricting type** (excessive dieting or exercising) or **binge-eating/purging type** (vomiting, laxatives, diuretics). Presents with the following:

- **Refusal to maintain normal body weight** (ie, the patient is < 85% of ideal body weight).
- Intense fear of weight gain.
- Distorted body image.
- Amenorrhea (three missed cycles).

DIAGNOSIS

- Measure height and weight. Check CBC, electrolytes, TSH/free T_4, and an ECG.
- Look for **lanugo** (fine body hair), dry skin, lethargy, bradycardia, hypotension, and peripheral edema.

TREATMENT

Patients often deny the health risks of their behavior. Monitor caloric intake and **focus on slow weight gain.** Individual, family, and group psychotherapy are crucial. SSRIs (fluoxetine) have been used successfully, but avoid bupropion in light of the risk of seizure.

BULIMIA NERVOSA

Affects 1–3% of young adult females. The prognosis is more favorable than that of anorexia nervosa. Associated with an ↑ frequency of affective disorders, substance abuse, and borderline personality disorder.

Symptoms

Patients have normal weight or are overweight but engage in the following behaviors twice a week for three or more months:

- **Binge eating** with a sense of lack of self-control.
- **Compensatory behavior** to prevent weight gain (eg, self-induced vomiting, laxatives, diuretics, overexercise).

Diagnosis

- The same as that for anorexia nervosa. Look for poor dentition, **enlarged parotid glands,** scars on the dorsal hand surfaces (from finger-induced vomiting), **electrolyte imbalances**, and **metabolic alkalosis.**
- In contrast to anorexia nervosa, **patients are typically distressed about their symptoms and behaviors** and are consequently easier to treat.

Treatment

Restore the patient's nutritional status and electrolytes and then rebuild his/her weight. **CBT** is the most effective treatment. Antidepressants are useful even in nondepressed patients, but **avoid bupropion** in light of its seizure risk.

Childhood Disorders

AUTISM SPECTRUM DISORDERS

More common in males, and symptoms usually appear before age three. Subtypes include the following:

- **Autism:** Characterized by **delayed and aberrant communication** (language); cognitive dysfunction; **abnormal social interaction;** and restricted, repetitive, and **stereotyped patterns of behavior,** interests, and activities.
- **Asperger's disorder:** Similar to autistic disorder, but involves **normal language and cognition.**
- **Rett's disorder:** A neurodegenerative disorder that **affects girls only.** It is marked by **normal development until five months of age** followed by deceleration of head circumference, stereotyped hand movements (wringing, hand washing), loss of social engagement, poor gait and truncal movements, severely impaired language development, severe psychomotor retardation, and an ↑ risk of seizure.
- **Childhood disintegrative disorder:** Severe **developmental regression** after > 2 years of normal social/motor/language development.

DISRUPTIVE BEHAVIORAL DISORDERS

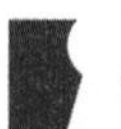

KEY FACT

Conduct disorder is diagnosed in **C**hildren and can eventually lead to in**C**arceration. **A**dults suffer from **A**ntisocial personality disorder.

- **Oppositional defiant disorder:** A **negative, hostile, and defiant attitude toward authority figures** of six or more months' duration. May lead to conduct disorder.
- **Conduct disorder:** A disorder in which a patient repeatedly and significantly **violates societal norms and the rights of others** (eg, bullies, tortures animals, steals/destroys property) for one or more years. Considered a precursor to antisocial personality disorder.

ATTENTION-DEFICIT HYPERACTIVITY DISORDER (ADHD)

- The most common childhood psychiatric disorder.
- **Sx/Exam:** Involves six or more symptoms of either **inattention** (eg, easy distractibility, difficulty following instructions/finishing tasks, tendency to make careless mistakes) or **hyperactivity/impulsivity** (eg, interrupts others/has difficulty waiting) **in two or more settings** (school, work, home). Causes impairment before seven years of age.
- **Dx:** Although parents often immediately think of this diagnosis, first consider physical and social factors that may contribute to the problem (eg, the child has poor vision and can't see the chalkboard).
- **Tx:** Initial treatment generally includes behavior modification. Pharmacologic approaches include psychostimulant (eg, amphetamines, **methylphenidate**) or nonstimulant medications (eg, **bupropion, atomoxetine,** SSRIs, α_2-agonists).

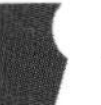

KEY FACT

Approximately 50% of patients diagnosed in childhood continue to have ADHD into adulthood.

OTHER CAUSES OF LEARNING IMPAIRMENT

- **Learning disabilities:** Weaker academic performance than expected for age, intelligence, and education. May involve specific deficits such as dyslexia or more general problems with understanding and processing new information. Tend to occur more frequently in males and in those of lower SES, and may have a familial pattern. As with ADHD, consider physical and social factors prior to making a diagnosis.
- **Mental retardation:** Global deficits in intellectual and adaptive/social function. **Eighty-five percent of cases are mild,** with an IQ between 50 and 70. Associated with chromosomal abnormalities, congenital infections, teratogens, and inborn errors of metabolism.
- **Tourette's syndrome:** Multiple **motor and vocal tics** such as blinking, grimacing, or grunting that occur many times a day for > 1 year and cause functional impairment. Associated with ADHD, learning disorders, and OCD. Treated with **dopamine receptor antagonists** (eg, haloperidol, pimozide), clonidine, behavioral therapy, and counseling. Stimulants can worsen or precipitate tics.

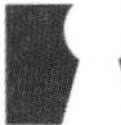

KEY FACT

Fetal alcohol syndrome is the number-one preventable cause of mental retardation; Down syndrome is the number-one cause overall.

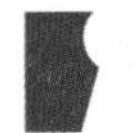

KEY FACT

Tourette's syndrome is often depicted in popular media as including coprolalia (the repetition of obscene words), but this tic is found in only 10–30% of cases.

ENURESIS

Enuresis (bed-wetting) is not a clinical disorder until a child is > 5 years of age (the child may not feel/understand neurologic impulses until then). It should initially be treated with behavioral therapy (eg, bed alarms); imipramine should be reserved for refractory cases.

Psychiatric Emergencies

SUICIDE RISK ASSESSMENT

- The eighth leading overall cause of death in the United States. Risk factors include the following:
  - **Gender:** Men **complete** suicide three times more often than do women, whereas women **attempt** suicide three times more frequently. Men also prefer more violent methods (eg, hanging, firearms, jumping from high places) as opposed to overdose.

- **Age:** Those > 75 years of age account for 25% of completed suicides. Suicide is also the third leading cause of death in 15- to 24-year-olds, after homicides and accidents.
- **Ethnicity:** Two-thirds of completed suicides are Caucasian males.
- **Psychiatric illness:** MDD, bipolar disorder, psychotic disorder, substance abuse or dependence.
- **Other risk factors:** Include unemployment or job dissatisfaction; chronic, debilitating illness; a history of prior suicide attempts; and a family history of suicide.

- Protective factors include religious affiliation or civic groups, married status, and parenthood.

NEUROLEPTIC MALIGNANT SYNDROME

A life-threatening complication of antipsychotic treatment. May also be precipitated in patients with Parkinson's disease following the abrupt withdrawal of the dopamine precursor levodopa. Mortality is 10–20%.

Symptoms

- **Can occur at any time** during the course of treatment.
- Presents with **muscular rigidity** and dystonia, akinesia, mutism, obtundation, and agitation.
- Autonomic symptoms include **high fever,** diaphoresis, hypertensive episodes, and tachycardia.
- Look for extremely **elevated CK** and **elevated liver enzymes.** May progress to **rhabdomyolysis** and/or renal dysfunction.

Treatment

Stop the offending medication; give **dantrolene,** bromocriptine, or amantadine.

SEROTONIN SYNDROME

Caused by the use of MAOIs with SSRIs or MAOIs with venlafaxine. Less commonly, it may involve SSRIs with lithium, SSRIs with levodopa, or SSRIs with an atypical antipsychotic.

Symptoms

- Presents with delirium, agitation, tachycardia, diaphoresis, and diarrhea.
- Exam reveals myoclonus and hyperreflexia. In severe cases, patients may present with hyperthermia, seizures, rhabdomyolysis, renal failure, cardiac arrhythmias, and DIC.

Treatment

Stop the offending medications; give supportive care. Administer a serotonin antagonist or cyproheptadine.

Pharmacotherapy

ANXIOLYTICS AND SEDATIVE-HYPNOTICS

Benzodiazepines

- **Applications:** Used for anxiety, alcohol withdrawal, insomnia, anesthesia, seizures, and muscle spasms. Have **rapid onset of action; augment sedation and respiratory depression** from other CNS depressants (eg, alcohol). Where possible, use on a short-term basis only (eg, no more than 2–3 months) or occasionally PRN.
- **Interactions:** P-450 inhibitors (eg, cimetidine, fluoxetine) ↑ levels; carbamazepine and rifampin ↓ levels.
- **Relative contraindications:** Disadvantages include a risk of abuse, tolerance, dependence, and withdrawal. May also induce delirium in elderly and/or critically ill patients. Avoid in patients who are at high risk for falling.

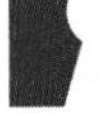

KEY FACT

Diazepam is longer-acting than lorazepam.

Buspirone

- **Mechanism of action:** A 5-HT_{1A} partial agonist.
- **Applications:** Used for GAD and chronic anxiety; for the augmentation of depression or OCD therapy; and for patients with a history of substance abuse. May also be used when sedation poses a potential risk. Unlike benzodiazepines, it has **no anticonvulsant or muscle-relaxant properties.** Also characterized by few side effects and no tolerance, dependence, or withdrawal.
- **Relative contraindications:** Has slow onset of action and lower efficacy than benzodiazepines. Should not be used with MAOIs. **Not effective as a PRN anxiolytic** (chronic ↑ in 5-HT are anxiolytic, but acute ↑ cause anxiety).

Antihistamines

Used for the short-term management of insomnia and for preoperative sedation.

Zolpidem

A nonbenzodiazepine used for insomnia. ↓ sleep latency and ↑ total sleep time. Has rapid onset; withdrawal is rare.

ANTIDEPRESSANTS

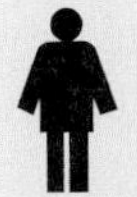

A 29-year-old attorney is being treated for depression. He blushingly admits that since starting SSRIs, he has noticed diminished interest in sex and difficulty maintaining an erection. What other antidepressant medications should be considered to prevent these sexual side effects?

Bupropion or mirtazapine.

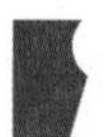

KEY FACT

Use of antidepressant medications during pregnancy carries the risk of abstinence syndrome and pulmonary hypertension in the neonate. However, untreated depression carries the risk of low birth weight.

Selective Serotonin Reuptake Inhibitors (SSRIs)

- Include **fluoxetine, sertraline, paroxetine, citalopram, escitalopram,** and **fluvoxamine.**
- **Applications:** First-line therapy for **depression** and **many anxiety disorders.** Well tolerated, effective, and relatively safe in overdose.
- **Interactions:** Can ↑ warfarin levels because of P-450 interactions.
- **Side effects: Sexual dysfunction,** nausea, diarrhea, anorexia, headache, anxiety, tremor, sleep disturbance.

Atypical Antidepressants

- **Bupropion:**
  - **Mechanism of action:** Dopamine reuptake inhibition. Metabolite weakly blocks norepinephrine (NE) reuptake.
  - **Applications:** Constitutes first-line therapy for depression and smoking cessation. Effective for patients who have had sexual side effects from other antidepressants.
  - **Side effects:** Common side effects include anxiety, agitation, and insomnia. Can worsen tics. Also **lowers seizure threshold,** especially in the setting of rapid or large dose increases or immediate-release preparations. Not associated with weight gain.
  - **Relative contraindications:** A history of seizure disorder, eating disorders, or head trauma.
- **Venlafaxine:**
  - **Mechanism of action:** The main action is 5-HT and NE reuptake inhibition.
  - **Applications:** Used for major depression and GAD. Has a more rapid response than SSRIs.
  - **Side effects:** Adverse effects include **diastolic hypertension (monitor BP),** insomnia, nervousness, sedation, **sexual dysfunction,** anticholinergic effects, and nausea.
- **Mirtazapine:**
  - **Mechanism of action:** An α_2-antagonist that enhances NE and 5-HT. Does not affect the P-450 system. More effective as part of dual therapy.
  - **Side effects:** Sedation (worse in **lower** doses) and **weight gain.** Has little effect on sexual function.
- **Trazodone:**
  - **Mechanism of action:** Primarily inhibits 5-HT reuptake. At lower doses, may be helpful in insomnia.
  - **Side effects:** Sedation, **priapism.**

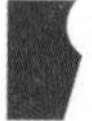

KEY FACT

Duloxetine has a profile similar to that of venlafaxine but has a smaller effect on blood pressure.

KEY FACT

Antidepressants are the preferred long-term treatment for anxiety, but they can be anxiogenic initially. Bupropion, in particular, should not be used with anxiety disorders.

Tricyclic Antidepressants (TCAs)

- Include **nortriptyline, desipramine, imipramine, amitriptyline, clomipramine,** and **doxepin.** TCAs are considered to be **second-line agents** owing to their relatively poor side effect profile compared with the newer antidepressants, along with the risk of dysrhythmias, and even death, from an overdose.
- **Mechanism of action:** Block the reuptake of NE and serotonin.
- **Applications:** Useful for chronic pain and migraines. OCD responds to clomipramine.
- **Interactions:** Levels ↑ when used with SSRIs because of P-450 competition. Also interact with ranitidine and warfarin.

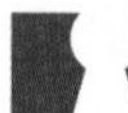

KEY FACT

TCAs may be lethal in an overdose.

KEY FACT

TCA toxicity:

- Trembling (convulsions)
- Coma
- Arrhythmias

- **Side effects:**
  - **Anticholinergic:** Dry mouth, blurry vision, constipation, urinary retention.
  - **Cardiac: Orthostatic hypotension; cardiac conduction delays with prolonged PR and QRS intervals.** TCAs are contraindicated in patients with a history of heart block and in those at high risk of suicide. Obtain a baseline ECG prior to initiating therapy, and use with caution in the elderly.
  - **Other:** Sedation, weight gain.

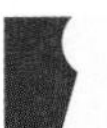

KEY FACT

Ingestion of fermented foods (eg, aged cheeses, red wine, beer) can precipitate a hypertensive crisis in patients taking MAOIs.

Monoamine Oxidase Inhibitors (MAOIs)

- Include **phenelzine, selegiline,** and **tranylcypromine.** MAOIs are also considered to be **second-line agents** owing to their relatively poor side effect profile compared to the newer antidepressants.
- **Side effects:**
  - Common side effects include orthostatic hypotension, insomnia, weight gain, edema, and sexual dysfunction.
  - May lead to **tyramine-induced hypertensive crisis.** Dietary restrictions include aged cheeses, sour cream, yogurt, pickled herring, cured meats, and certain alcoholic beverages such as chianti.
  - Potentially fatal **serotonin syndrome** can occur if MAOIs are combined with SSRIs, TCAs, meperidine, fentanyl, or indirect sympathomimetics (eg, those found in **OTC cold remedies**).

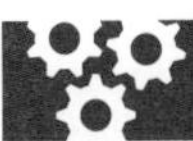

MNEMONIC

Side effects of MAOIs–

The 6 H's

Hepatocellular jaundice/necrosis
Hypotension (postural)
Headache
Hyperreflexia
Hallucinations
Hypomania

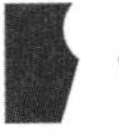

KEY FACT

"Activating" antidepressants: bupropion, venlafaxine, and SSRIs and MAOIs in general.

ANTIPSYCHOTICS

First-Generation ("Typical") Antipsychotics

- **Mechanism of action:** Act through dopamine receptor blockade.
- **Applications:** Used for psychotic disorders and acute agitation. Cheap and effective. Include the following:
  - **High-potency agents** (haloperidol, fluphenazine): ↓ only positive symptoms of psychosis. Associated with more extrapyramidal symptoms (EPS).
  - **Low-potency agents** (thioridazine, chlorpromazine): Associated with more sedation, anticholinergic effects, and hypotension.
- **Side effects:** Key side effects include the following:
  - **EPS:** Result from excessive cholinergic effect (see Table 17-4).
  - **Hyperprolactinemia** (amenorrhea, gynecomastia, galactorrhea).
  - **Anticholinergic effects** (dry mouth, blurry vision, urinary retention, constipation).
  - **Neuroleptic malignant syndrome.**
  - **Other:** Cardiac arrhythmias, weight gain, sedation.

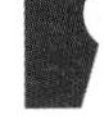

KEY FACT

"Sedating" antidepressants: trazodone, mirtazapine, and amitriptyline.

Second-Generation ("Atypical") Antipsychotics

- **Mechanism of action:** Act through 5-HT_2 and dopamine antagonism.
- **Applications:** Currently first-line therapy for schizophrenia. Benefits are **fewer EPS and anticholinergic effects than first-generation agents.**
  - **Risperidone, olanzapine, quetiapine, ziprasidone,** and **aripiprazole** are commonly used.
  - **Clozapine** is second-line therapy and is used for treatment-refractory patients.

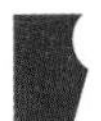

KEY FACT

"Augmentation" strategies for antidepressants:

1. Lithium (with TCA)
2. Triiodothyronine (with TCA or SSRI)
3. Mirtazapine
4. Aripiprazole (with SSRI)
5. Buspirone
6. Bupropion

KEY FACT

Evolution of EPS—

- 4 hours: Acute dystonia
- 4 days: Akinesia
- 4 weeks: Akathisia
- 4 months: Tardive dyskinesia

KEY FACT

Metoclopramide is actually a more common cause of tardive dyskinesia than antipsychotics.

TABLE 17-4. Extrapyramidal Symptoms and Treatment

Symptom	Description	Treatment
Acute dystonia	Involuntary muscle contraction or spasm (eg, torticollis, oculogyric crisis). More common in young men.	Give an anticholinergic (benztropine) or diphenhydramine. To prevent, give prophylactic benztropine with an antipsychotic.
Dyskinesia	Pseudoparkinsonism (eg, shuffling gait, cogwheel rigidity).	Give an anticholinergic (benztropine) or a dopamine agonist (amantadine). ↓ the dose of neuroleptic or discontinue (if tolerated).
Akathisia	Subjective/objective restlessness.	↓ neuroleptic and try β-blockers (propranolol). Benzodiazepines or anticholinergics may help.
Tardive dyskinesia	Stereotypic oral-facial movements. Likely from dopamine receptor sensitization. Often irreversible (50%). More common in older women.	Discontinue or ↓ dose of neuroleptic, attempt treatment with more appropriate drugs, and consider changing neuroleptic (eg, changing to clozapine or risperidone). Treat symptoms with β-blockers or benzodiazepines. Giving anticholinergics or decreasing neuroleptics may initially worsen tardive dyskinesia.

- **Side effects:**
  - May cause **sedation, weight gain, anticholinergic effects,** and **QT prolongation.** Obtain baseline values, and monitor the patient's weight, lipid profile, and glucose levels.
  - Olanzapine carries the risk of **diabetogenesis.**
  - Common side effects of clozapine include sedation, constipation, weight gain, and sialorrhea (drooling). **Clozapine may also cause agranulocytosis and seizures** (requires weekly CBCs during the first six months followed by biweekly monitoring).

MOOD STABILIZERS

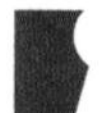

KEY FACT

When using lithium, monitor renal and thyroid function. Chronic use can lead to hypothyroidism and nephrotoxicity.

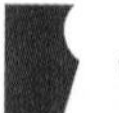

KEY FACT

Lithium toxicity treatment may include hemodialysis.

Lithium

- **Applications:** Used for long-term maintenance or prophylaxis of bipolar disorder. Effective in mania and in augmenting antidepressants in depression and OCD. ↓ suicidal behavior/risk in bipolar disorder. Has a **narrow therapeutic index** and requires monitoring of serum levels.
- **Side effects:**
  - Include thirst, polyuria, fine tremor, weight gain, diarrhea, nausea, acne, and hypothyroidism.
  - Lithium toxicity presents with a **coarse tremor, ataxia,** vomiting, confusion, seizures, and arrhythmias.
  - Teratogenic.

Valproic Acid

- **Applications:** First-line agent for **acute mania** and bipolar disorder; effective in **rapid cyclers** (those with four or more episodes per year).
- **Side effects:**
  - Sedation, weight gain, hair loss, tremor, ataxia, GI distress.
  - Pancreatitis, thrombocytopenia, and fatal hepatotoxicity are uncommon. Do not use in patients with hepatitis or cirrhosis.
  - Monitor platelets, LFTs, and serum drug levels.
  - Teratogenic.

Carbamazepine

- **Applications:** Second-line agent for acute mania and bipolar disorder.
- **Side effects:**
  - Common side effects include nausea, sedation, rash, and ataxia.
  - Rare side effects include hepatic toxicity, SIADH (leading to hyponatremia), **bone marrow suppression** (leading to life-threatening dyscrasias such as aplastic anemia), and **Stevens-Johnson syndrome.**
  - Monitor blood counts, transaminases, and electrolytes. Drug interactions complicate its use (eg, cannot be used with MAOIs).
  - Teratogenic.

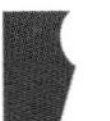

KEY FACT

Lamotrigine or lithium may be used as first-line agents for bipolar depression.

Other Anticonvulsants

- Include **oxcarbazepine, lamotrigine, gabapentin,** and **topiramate.**
- Efficacy is not well documented.
- Do not require blood level monitoring and do not cause weight gain.
- **Lamotrigine is associated with Stevens-Johnson syndrome and toxic epidermal necrolysis.**

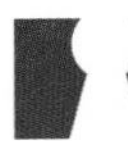

KEY FACT

The bioavailability of gabapentin actually ↓ with larger doses.

NOTES

CHAPTER 18

PULMONARY

Pulmonary Function Tests (PFTs)

The two measurements most often used in pulmonary function testing are FEV_1 (forced expiratory volume in one second) and FVC (forced vital capacity). Findings are categorized as follows:

- **Obstructive pattern** (eg, COPD, chronic bronchitis, bronchiectasis, asthma):
  - An FEV_1/FVC ratio of < 70% (the normal ratio in adults is generally > 75%).
  - Total lung capacity (TLC) will be ↑ in some obstructive processes, such as COPD, whereas it may be normal or ↑ in asthma.
  - The severity of FEV_1 is used to grade obstructive airway diseases.
- **Restrictive pattern** (eg, obesity, kyphosis, inflammatory/fibrosing lung disease, interstitial lung disease):
  - While FEV_1 and FVC will each be low, the FEV_1/FVC ratio will be normal or ↑.
  - TLC will be ↓ in restrictive processes.
  - An FVC of < 80% is suggestive of restriction when the FEV_1/FVC ratio is normal.

KEY FACT

Asthma, while obstructive in nature, is a reversible condition. It usually has a normal DL_{CO} because the alveoli are unaffected. By contrast, COPD is characterized by a ↓ DL_{CO} because some alveoli are destroyed and unavailable for gas diffusion.

Table 18-1 outlines PFT findings in the setting of common lung conditions.

TABLE 18-1. PFTs in Common Settings

	FEV_1/FVC	TLC	DL_{CO}[a]
Asthma	Normal/↓	Normal/↑	Normal/↑
COPD	↓	↑	↓
Fibrotic disease	Normal/↑	↓	↓
Extrathoracic restriction	Normal	↓	Normal

[a] DL_{CO}, defined as the diffusing capacity of carbon monoxide, measures the gas exchange capacity of the capillary-alveolar interface.

Hypoxia and Hypoxemia

Defined as a room-air O_2 saturation of < 88% or a PaO_2 of < **55 mm Hg** on ABG measurement or evidence of cor pulmonale. Think about the **cause of hypoxia** in order to determine the next step:

- **Ventilation-perfusion (V/Q) mismatch:**
  - Examples include asthma, COPD, nonmassive pulmonary embolus (PE), and pneumonia.
  - **Responds to O_2.**
  - Associated with an ↑ **alveolar-arterial oxygen (A-a) gradient.**
- **Hypoventilation:**
  - Commonly due to **oversedation** from medications.
  - **Responds to O_2.**
  - Characterized by a **normal A-a gradient.**
- **Decreased diffusion:**
  - Think about interstitial or parenchymal lung diseases.
  - **Responds to O_2.**
  - Characterized by an ↑ **A-a gradient.**
  - Associated with a **very low DL_{CO}.**
- **High altitude:**
  - **Responds to O_2.**
  - Characterized by a **normal A-a gradient.**
- **Shunt physiology:**
  - Think about **acute respiratory distress syndrome, significant lobar pneumonia,** patent foramen ovale, or **patent ductus arteriosus.**
  - Typically **does not respond to O_2.**
  - Characterized by an ↑ **A-a gradient.**

KEY FACT

Hypoxia due to shunt physiology will **not** correct with supplemental O_2.

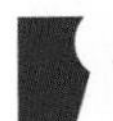

KEY FACT

Hypoxia can lead to apnea in infants, so be sure to use supplemental O_2 to maintain O_2 saturations.

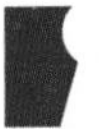

KEY FACT

Think of methemoglobinemia in a patient with a low O_2 saturation on pulse oximetry but a normal PaO_2 on ABG. Treatment is with methylene blue.

TREATMENT

Always treat hypoxic patients with adequate amounts of O_2 to maintain saturations of > 90% or a PaO_2 of > 60 mm Hg. Definitive treatment entails reversing the underlying cause of the hypoxia.

Asthma

A patient with a history of asthma that was previously controlled with once-monthly albuterol states that he has been using his albuterol inhaler 4–5 times a week but denies any nighttime symptoms. How would you adjust his treatment regimen?

Add a low-dose inhaled corticosteroid, as the patient now has mild persistent asthma.

Asthma is defined as chronic inflammation of the airways. Patients may be atopic (the classic triad is eczema, wheezing, and seasonal rhinitis).

Symptoms

- Look for **intermittent wheezing,** coughing, chest tightness, or shortness of breath.
- Symptoms may be seasonal or may occur following exposure to **triggers** (eg, URIs, dust, pet dander, cold air) or with exercise.

Exam

- Determine the severity of the attack by assessing **mental status, the ability to speak in full sentences,** the presence of cyanosis, use of accessory muscles, and, of course, vital signs. O_2 saturation monitoring is not adequate, as ventilation is more important than oxygenation.
- Look for wheezing or rhonchi along with a prolonged expiratory phase. Patients with severe exacerbations may have ↓ **wheezing.** These patients will need prompt assessment of their gas exchange (with ABG analysis) along with aggressive treatment.

KEY FACT

Think of GERD in a patient with chronic cough that worsens when the patient lies supine.

Differential

- **Not all that wheezes is asthma!** Rule out foreign body aspiration, laryngeal spasm or irritation, GERD, and CHF. In patients with chronic cough, think about asthma as well as allergic rhinitis, postnasal drip, or GERD.
- PFTs can help differentiate asthma from COPD and chronic bronchitis (see below), although there are overlapping findings.

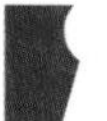

KEY FACT

A ⊖ methacholine challenge generally excludes asthma.

Diagnosis

- CXR may show **hyperinflation** (suggesting air trapping) but can also be normal.
- Definitive diagnosis is made by demonstration of **obstruction** on PFTs:
  - **Reversibility** with bronchodilators as defined by an ↑ **in FEV_1 or FVC by 12% and at least 200 mL.**
  - **Methacholine challenge** testing in a monitored setting can be used to confirm the diagnosis.

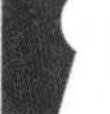

KEY FACT

Inhaled corticosteroids are safe for use in pregnancy.

Treatment

- **Chronic asthma:** See Table 18-2.
- **Acute asthma exacerbations:** Recognizing the severity of the attack and instituting the correct therapy are the keys to treatment.
  - Initiate **short-acting β-agonist** (albuterol) therapy (nebulizer or MDI).
  - Administer a **systemic corticosteroid** such as methylprednisolone or prednisone.
  - Begin **inhaled corticosteroids** as well.
  - Follow patients closely with **peak flows,** and tailor therapy to the response.
  - Chronic antibiotics (without evidence of infection), anticholinergics, cromolyn, and leukotriene antagonists are generally **not useful** in this setting.

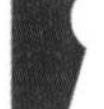

KEY FACT

Be sure to check an ABG in any patient with an asthma exacerbation. A normal Pco_2 suggests that the patient is tiring out and is about to crash.

TABLE 18-2. Medications for the Treatment of Chronic Asthma

Type	Symptoms (Day/Night)	FEV_1	Medications
Severe persistent	Continual Frequent	≤ 60%	High-dose inhaled corticosteroids + long-acting inhaled β-agonists. Possible PO steroids. PRN short-acting bronchodilator.
Moderate persistent	Daily > 1 night/week	60–80%	Low- to medium-dose inhaled corticosteroids + long-acting inhaled β-agonists. PRN short-acting bronchodilator.
Mild persistent	> 2/week but < 1/day > 2 nights/month	≥ 80%	Low-dose inhaled corticosteroids. PRN short-acting bronchodilator.
Mild intermittent	≤ 2 days/week ≤ 2 nights/month	≥ 80%	No daily medications. PRN short-acting bronchodilator.

(Reproduced with permission from Le T et al. *First Aid for the USMLE Step 2 CK,* 7th ed. New York: McGraw-Hill, 2010: 458.)

Chronic Obstructive Pulmonary Disease (COPD)

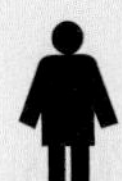

You order PFTs for a patient with worsening shortness of breath. Which of the following values would be consistent with a diagnosis of COPD?

(A) Low FEV_1, low FVC, low FEV_1/FVC, high TLC, low DL_{CO}.
(B) Low FEV_1, low FVC, high FEV_1/FVC, low TLC, low DL_{CO}.

The answer is A. Choice B describes a restrictive pattern.

A combination of emphysema and chronic bronchitis, COPD generally involves the destruction of lung parenchyma. This results in ↓ elastic recoil, which in turn leads to air trapping. **TLC ↑** as a result of a **rise** in the **residual volume.** Chronic bronchitis is defined as chronic productive cough for three or more months in each of two successive years.

Symptoms

Look for cough, dyspnea, wheezing, and a **history of smoking.** Dyspnea is usually progressive. In advanced disease, weight loss may be seen.

Exam

- **Emphysema ("pink puffer"):** ↓ breath sounds, minimal cough, dyspnea, pursed-lip breathing, hypercarbia/hypoxia late, barrel chest.
- **Chronic bronchitis ("blue bloater"):** Rhonchi; productive cough; cyanosis, but with mild dyspnea; hypercarbia/hypoxia early. Patients are frequently overweight with peripheral edema.

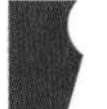

KEY FACT

Think α_1-antitrypsin deficiency in young patients with COPD and bullae.

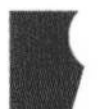

KEY FACT

Only O_2 therapy and smoking cessation have been unequivocally shown to improve survival in patients with COPD.

KEY FACT

Don't forget—empiric antibiotics are indicated for acute COPD exacerbations!

- **Clubbing is generally not present in COPD.**
- Patients may also have evidence of **cor pulmonale** (right heart failure from pulmonary hypertension).
- PFTs may suggest the diagnosis in patients who smoke.
- **FEV_1/FVC** is < **70%** and FEV_1 < 80% of predicted.
- The condition is **not reversible** with bronchodilators.
- **DL_{CO}** tends to be low in emphysema and mildly reduced in chronic bronchitis.
- **TLC** is ↑.
- CXR shows hyperlucent, **hyperinflated** lungs with **flat diaphragms** and a narrow cardiac silhouette (see Figure 18-1).

Treatment

- Chronic COPD:
  - The mainstays of treatment are inhaled **β-agonists** (albuterol) and **anticholinergics** (ipratropium).
  - **O_2 therapy** is indicated for patients with an O_2 saturation of < **88% or a PaO_2 of < 55 mm Hg** or a PaO_2 of 55–60 mm Hg and evidence of cor pulmonale. It is also indicated with desaturations of < 88% during exercise or at night.
  - **Smoking cessation and O_2 therapy have been proven to ↓ mortality in COPD.**
  - Inhaled corticosteroids **do not** play a major role unless PFTs reveal significant reversible airway disease.
  - Remember to **vaccinate** COPD patients against influenza (yearly) and pneumococcal pneumonia (at least once).
- **Acute COPD exacerbations:**
  - Defined as ↑ **dyspnea** or a **change in cough or sputum production.**
  - Check a **CXR** to look for causes of the exacerbation (pneumonia, CHF).
  - Administer O_2 to maintain a saturation of 90–95% (no need to go higher!).

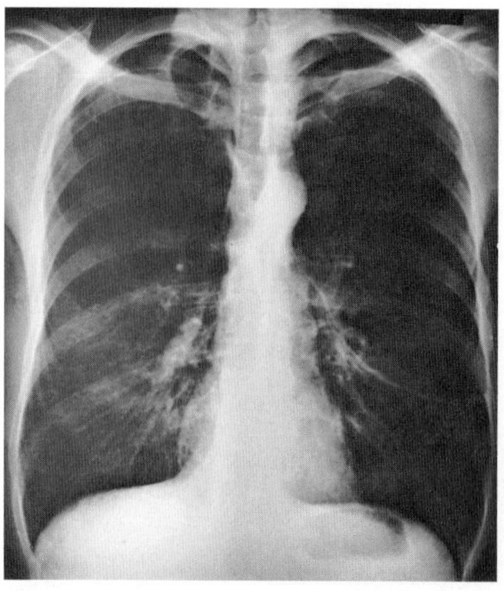

A

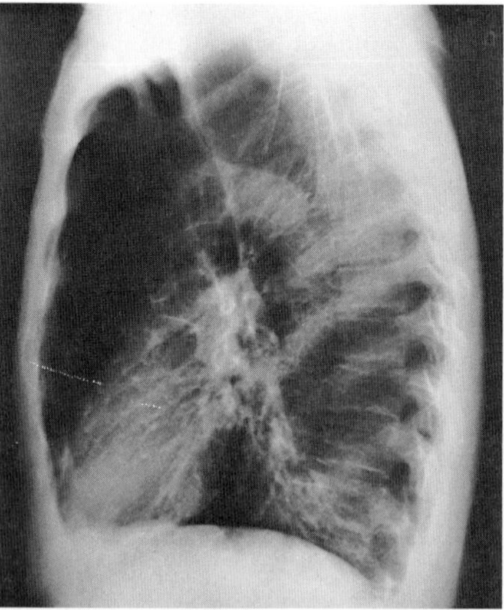

B

FIGURE 18-1. Chronic obstructive pulmonary disease. Note the hyperinflated and hyperlucent lungs, flat diaphragms, increased AP diameter, narrow mediastinum, and large upper lobe bullae on AP (**A**) and lateral (**B**) CXR. (Reproduced with permission from Stobo JD et al. *The Principles and Practice of Medicine*, 23rd ed. Stamford, CT: Appleton & Lange, 1996: 135.)

- Start patients on an inhaled **β-agonist** (albuterol) and **anticholinergics** (ipratropium).
- **Systemic corticosteroids** (prednisone) may ↓ the length of hospital stay but should be tapered over 3–14 days.
- **Empiric antibiotics** with coverage of *Streptococcus*, *H influenzae*, and *Moraxella* (eg, amoxicillin, TMP-SMX, doxycycline, azithromycin, clarithromycin) **are indicated** in an acute setting.
- Spirometry in an acute setting is **not helpful** in guiding therapy.

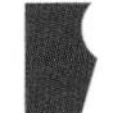

KEY FACT

Always treat hypoxic patients with O_2. CO_2 retention won't kill the patient, but hypoxia will.

Pleural Effusion

A 33-year-old man presents with cough, night sweats, and pleuritic chest pain. A CXR shows a left pleural effusion. A PPD test results in 16 mm of induration. Thoracentesis yields the following lab results: glucose 50, LDH 340, pleural fluid protein 4.6, and serum protein 3.0 mg/dL. A sputum culture for acid-fast bacilli (AFB) is ⊖. What is your next step?

This patient has an exudative pleural effusion with suspected TB. A pleural biopsy is needed to confirm the diagnosis despite the fact that the patient's sputum culture was ⊖ for AFB.

Effusions are characterized as either transudative or exudative on the basis of their composition.

Symptoms/Exam

- Patients are usually short of breath and may complain of pleuritic chest pain. Some may be asymptomatic or have symptoms of an underlying process (eg, CHF, pneumonia, cancer).
- Exam reveals ↓ **breath sounds, dullness** to percussion, and ↓ tactile fremitus on the side with the effusion (see Figure 18-2).

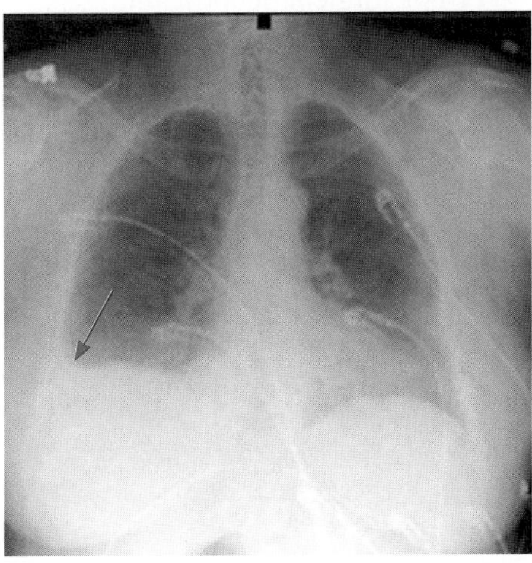

A

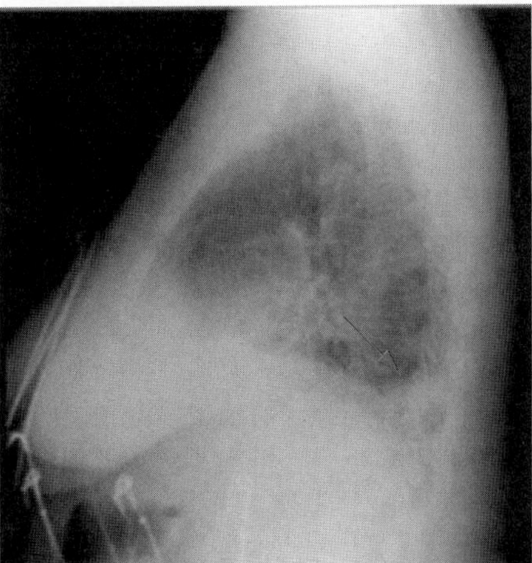

B

FIGURE 18-2. Pleural effusion. PA (A) and lateral (B) CXRs show blunting of the right costophrenic sulcus (arrows). (Reproduced with permission from USMLERx.com.)

TABLE 18-3. Thoracentesis Findings in Transudative vs. Exudative Pleural Effusions

	Pleural/Serum Protein (Ratio)	Pleural/Serum LDH (Ratio)	Pleural LDH
Transudative	< 0.5 ***and***	< 0.6 ***and***	< 200
Exudative	> 0.5 ***or***	> 0.6 ***or***	> 200

Diagnosis

- **Thoracentesis.**
- Obtain the following assays on the pleural fluid to aid in management: Gram stain and culture, AFB, glucose, triglycerides, cell count with differential, and pH. Serum total protein and LDH values will also be needed (see Table 18-3).
  - If the fluid is **transudative,** no further workup is needed; focus on treating the underlying cause (eg, diuresing the patient).
  - If the fluid is **exudative,** refer to Table 18-4 to help determine the cause.

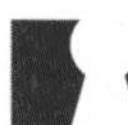

KEY FACT

Thoracentesis is indicated for any effusion > 10 mm thick (or about 100 mL) on decubitus CXR.

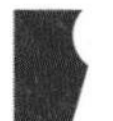

KEY FACT

Consider a pleural biopsy if you suspect TB. Send the fluid for cytology if you suspect malignancy.

Treatment

- If the decubitus CXR shows an effusion > 10 mm thick (or about 100 mL), always do a **thoracentesis.** This may be both therapeutic (to relieve dyspnea) and diagnostic.
- **Indications for a chest tube (any one of these)** are as follows:
  - A pleural WBC count > 100,000 or frank pus, or gram-⊕ fluid.
  - Glucose < 40 mg/dL.
  - pH < 7.0.

Complications

- An untreated pleural effusion in the setting of pneumonia may become infected and turn into an empyema.
- Over time, exudative effusions may become loculated and require drainage by video-assisted thoracoscopy (VATS) or surgical decortication.

TABLE 18-4. Assays for Exudative Fluid and Their Differential Diagnosis

Pleural Assay	Value	Differential
Glucose	< 60	Empyema or parapneumonia, TB, RA, malignancy.
WBCs	> 10,000	Empyema or parapneumonia, RA, malignancy.
RBCs	> 100,000	Gross blood—think of trauma, PE.
Cellular differential	Lymphocytes PMNs Eosinophils	TB, sarcoid, malignancy, chylothorax. Empyema, PE. Bleeding, pneumothorax.
pH	< 7.20	Complicated effusion or empyema.
Triglycerides	> 150	Diagnostic of chylothorax.

- The principal complications of thoracentesis include pneumothorax and bleeding (remember, the neurovascular bundle runs along the inferior side of the rib).

Pneumothorax

Defined as air that becomes trapped in the pleural space. This can be traumatic, spontaneous, or iatrogenic. Spontaneous pneumothorax can be due to underlying lung pathology such as COPD or CF.

KEY FACT

Suspect pneumothorax with shortness of breath and chest pain plus underlying COPD, CF, chest procedures (eg, central lines), or trauma. A 1° pneumothorax may be encountered in young adults with a tall, thin body habitus.

SYMPTOMS/EXAM

- Look for patients who develop acute shortness of breath and pleuritic chest pain.
- Look for **tachypnea,** ↓ tactile fremitus, ↓ breath sounds, **tympany** on percussion on the side involved, and tracheal deviation toward the affected side.

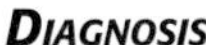

DIAGNOSIS

CXR will reveal the diagnosis. Look for a distinct lack of lung markings within the pneumothorax along with collapse of the lung on that side (see Figure 18-3). Tracheal deviation away from the side of the pneumothorax suggests tension pneumothorax.

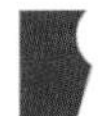

KEY FACT

The differential for shortness of breath/chest pain includes pneumothorax, MI, PE, pleuritis, and aortic dissection.

TREATMENT

- Insertion of a chest tube is required in patients with a pneumothorax of > 30%.
- Smaller pneumothoraces may be managed simply with supplemental O_2 and observation.
- Treat pain with morphine and NSAIDs.
- For patients with recurrent pneumothorax, consider pleurodesis.

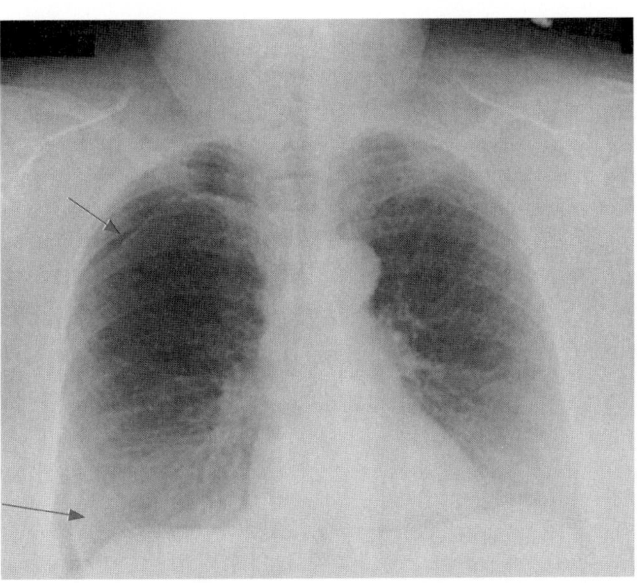

A

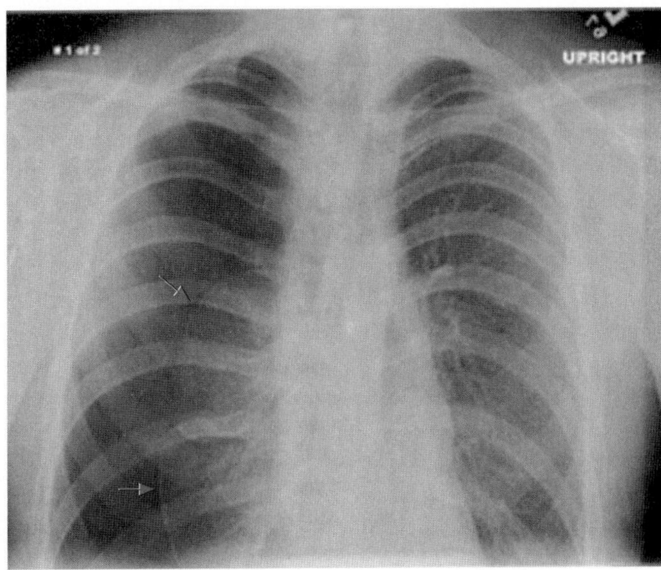

B

FIGURE 18-3. Pneumothorax. (A) Small right pneumothorax. (B) Right tension pneumothorax with collapse of the right lung and shifting of mediastinal structures to the left. Arrows denote pleural reflections. (Reproduced with permission from USMLERx.com.)

TENSION PNEUMOTHORAX

A 34-year-old man with COPD comes to the ER with sudden-onset shortness of breath that requires high levels of supplemental O_2. Physical exam reveals ↓ breath sounds on the left side and a trachea deviated to the right. What is your next step?

Needle decompression for presumed left-sided tension pneumothorax.

- In this emergent complication of pneumothorax, defects in the chest wall act as a one-way valve. This allows air to be drawn into the pleural space and become trapped. The result is **rapid decompensation,** hypotension, and circulatory collapse leading to **shock.**
- Common scenarios in which to think of tension pneumothorax include **penetrating trauma,** positive-pressure ventilation, and COPD.
- **Dx:** Diagnostic clues include those of a **pneumothorax** along with **tachycardia, hypotension,** ↑ O_2 requirements, and ↑ JVP. The trachea deviates **away** from the side with tension.
- **Tx:** If you suspect that the patient has a tension pneumothorax, **don't wait for imaging!** Insert a needle to decompress the chest and then insert a chest tube.

KEY FACT

A tension pneumothorax is an emergency! If you suspect this, don't wait for imaging; insert a needle to decompress the chest.

Pulmonary Embolism (PE)

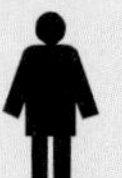

A 72-year-old patient who was admitted to the hospital for a hemorrhagic stroke develops shortness of breath, and imaging reveals a pulmonary embolus as well as a left lower extremity DVT. How do you proceed?

Place an IVC filter.

Remember **Virchow's triad** when thinking of risk factors for venous thromboembolism (VTE):

- **Stasis:** Immobility, CHF, obesity, ↑ JVP.
- **Endothelial injury:** Trauma, surgery, recent fracture, prior DVT.
- **Hypercoagulable state:** Pregnancy, OCP use, coagulation disorders, malignancy, burns.

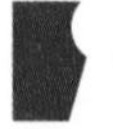

KEY FACT

Consider PE in any hospitalized patient who has dyspnea.

Symptoms

Think about PE or DVT in **any patient with risk factors** and complaints of leg pain or swelling, acute-onset chest pain (especially pleuritic), shortness of breath, or syncope.

Exam

Findings on exam include tachypnea, tachycardia, cyanosis, a loud P2 or S2, ↑ JVP, and signs of right heart failure. Patients may occasionally have hemoptysis or a low-grade fever.

Differential

Most signs and symptoms of PE are nonspecific, so be sure to think about other entities that can present this way, including **acute MI, pneumonia, CHF,** and **aortic dissection.**

DIAGNOSIS

See Figure 18-4 for a diagnostic algorithm. Initial assessment should include the following:

- **ABGs** may show a 1° respiratory alkalosis and an ↑ A-a gradient.
- **CXR** findings may include the following:
  - **Normal** (most common!).
  - A wedge-shaped infarct (Hampton's hump).
  - Oligemia in the affected lobe (Westermark's sign).
  - Pleural effusion.
- **ECG** may reveal an S wave in lead I, a Q wave in lead III, and T-wave inversion in lead III (not very sensitive or specific).
- The **pretest probability** of PE will help determine the diagnostic utility of the V/Q scan.
  - If either the pretest probability or the V/Q scan results are intermediate, some type of confirmatory testing will be needed.
  - V/Q scans are also preferred in patients for whom CT angiography has relative contraindications (eg, renal insufficiency, pregnancy).
- In a nonhospitalized patient, a ⊖ D-dimer assay, when combined with some form of imaging, may help rule out DVT with good negative predictive value.

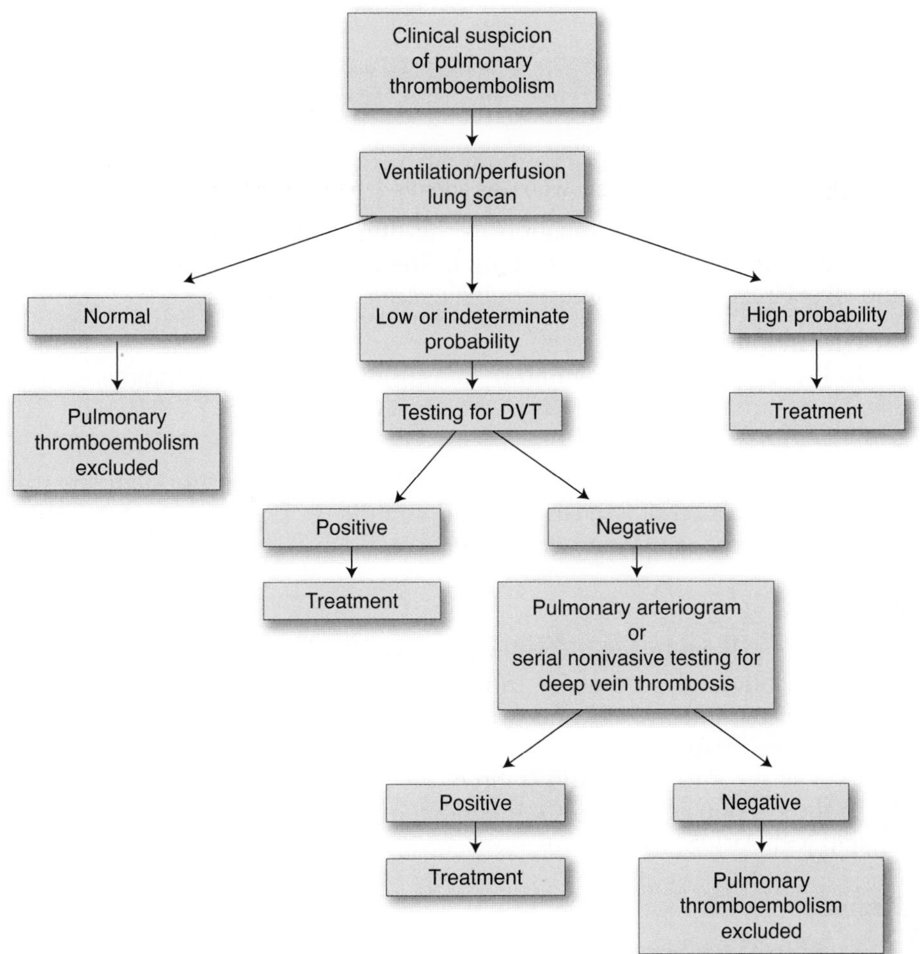

FIGURE 18-4. Diagnostic approach to pulmonary embolism. (Modified with permission from Tierney LM et al. *Current Medical Diagnosis & Treatment: 2005.* New York: McGraw-Hill, 2005: 281.)

KEY FACT

The most common ECG finding in pulmonary embolism is sinus tachycardia.

- **CT angiography** has largely replaced V/Q scanning except in patients with renal insufficiency or dye allergy. It may also be useful as a confirmatory test when the V/Q scan is indeterminate.
- **Pulmonary angiography** can be considered for the diagnosis of PE and may be needed if other testing is intermediate. (It is now rarely necessary.)

Treatment

- Treat VTE patients with anticoagulation.
  - Initially use **IV heparin or low-molecular-weight heparin.**
  - Patients who are not anticoagulated adequately within 24 hours have a high rate of recurrence.
  - Patients should then be transitioned to warfarin therapy with a goal INR of 2.0–3.0.
- In patients with documented large **central PEs** (saddle PEs) and hypotension or shock, consider administering **tPA** along with heparin. The duration of anticoagulation therapy will vary with risk factors:
  - For patients with a **first event** and **reversible** or time-limited risk factors (eg, surgery, pregnancy), treat for at least **3–6 months.**
  - Consider **lifelong anticoagulation** in patients with **chronic risk factors** (malignancy, paraplegia, recurrent DVTs, or PEs).
- In patients who cannot safely be anticoagulated, an IVC filter may be useful. Although these filters can ↓ the risk of PE, they are associated with a **higher risk** of recurrent DVT.

KEY FACT

Don' t forget to order DVT prophylaxis for all of your hospitalized patients!

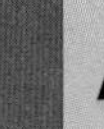

Acute Respiratory Distress Syndrome (ARDS)

ARDS is a common problem in the ICU and is a significant cause of mortality. It can be 2° to a range of underlying conditions, all with a similar end result of widespread inflammation in the lung parenchyma with leaking of fluid into the alveolar spaces, leading to (noncardiogenic) pulmonary edema and alveolar damage. Common etiologies are as follows:

- **Direct:** Pneumonia, aspiration.
- **Indirect:** Sepsis (most common), transfusions, pancreatitis, trauma.

Symptoms/Exam

Look for a patient with risk factors, usually in an **ICU setting.** Patients will have an **acute** onset of hypoxia and will be difficult to oxygenate. Intubation is required to maintain an acceptable Pao_2.

Diagnosis

- Patients will be hypoxic despite maximal O_2 therapy and typically have **diffuse bilateral pulmonary infiltrates with pulmonary edema** on CXR without evidence of volume overload (eg, **normal capillary wedge pressure**) (see Figure 18-5).
- Look at the **Pao_2/Fio_2 ratio** (ratio of the arterial O_2 level on ABG divided by the fraction of inhaled O_2 the patient is on). A ratio of < **200** is consistent with ARDS.

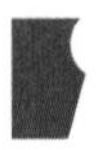

KEY FACT

Think of ARDS in a patient with a Pao_2/Fio_2 ratio < 200, diffuse infiltrates, and normal cardiac function.

Treatment

- Patients typically require intubation and mechanical ventilation for the management of hypoxia.
- **Low tidal volumes** (6 mL/kg) and associated permissive hypercapnia (ie, letting the Pco_2 rise) lead to a ↓↓ risk of barotrauma.

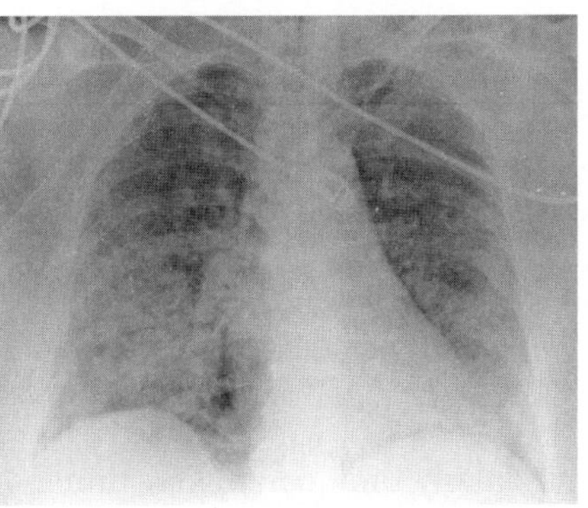

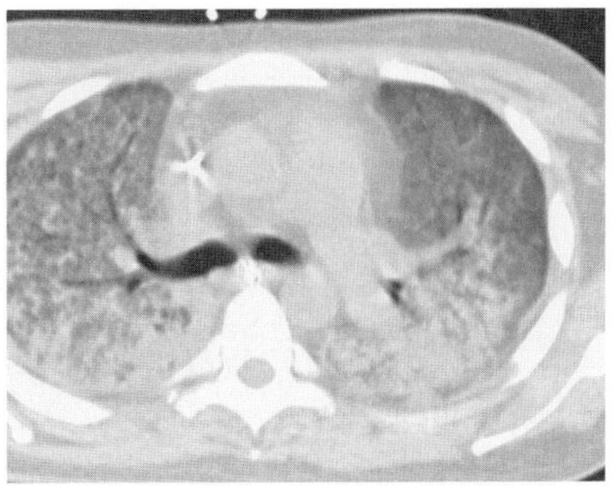

FIGURE 18-5. Acute respiratory distress syndrome. (**A**) Frontal CXR showing patchy areas of airspace consolidation in a patient with ARDS. (**B**) Transaxial CT showing ground-glass opacity anteriorly and consolidations dependently in a patient with exudative-phase ARDS. (Reproduced with permission from Fauci AS et al. *Harrison's Principles of Internal Medicine,* 17th ed. New York: McGraw-Hill, 2008, Figs. 262-2 and 262-4.)

- **Positive end-expiratory pressure (PEEP)** is used to improve oxygenation and thus ↓ the FiO_2 requirement and associated O_2 toxicity.
- Look for the **underlying cause** and focus treatment on that as you are stabilizing the patient and treating hypoxia.

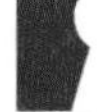

KEY FACT

Remember—use low tidal volumes and PEEP for the treatment of ARDS.

Solitary Pulmonary Nodule (SPN)

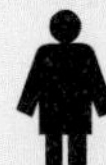

A chest CT of a 61-year-old patient with no smoking history reveals a noncalcified 1.7-cm nodule. What is your next step?

Compare the CT scan with an old CXR.

KEY FACT

The appearance of "popcorn" calcification within an SPN likely represents a benign hamartoma.

Defined as a radiodense lesion seen on chest imaging that is < **3 cm in diameter** and is not associated with infiltrates, adenopathy, or atelectasis. Most SPNs are detected on routine CXR in patients who are otherwise **asymptomatic.**

Symptoms/Exam

- **Benign** processes include histoplasmosis, coccidioidomycosis, TB, and hamartoma. Characteristics and risk factors include the following:
  - **Very fast** or **no growth** on serial imaging two years apart.
  - A **diffuse, dense and central, popcorn-like, or concentric "target" calcification pattern.**
  - Occurrence in patients who are **lifelong nonsmokers,** are < **30 years of age,** and have **no history of malignancy.**
- **Malignant** lesions include lung cancer or metastases. Risk factors include the following:
  - Size > **2 cm.**
  - **Spiculation** (ie, ragged edges).
  - Upper lobe location.
  - Occurence in patients who are **smokers,** are > **40 years of age,** or have a **prior diagnosis of cancer.**

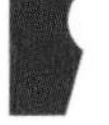

KEY FACT

Benign characteristics of SPN:

- "Bull's-eye" calcification
- "Popcorn" calcification
- "Satellite nodule"

Malignant characteristics of SPN:

- "Sunburst" pattern
- Spiculation

DIAGNOSIS/TREATMENT

- Start by examining old radiographs to determine age and change in size. Lesions with > 1 malignant feature should be further evaluated with CT imaging.
- If imaging points to a malignancy, biopsy tissue via bronchoscopy, needle aspiration, or VATS. If there is a low probability of malignancy, evaluate with serial CXRs or CTs every three months for one year and then every six months for one year.
- **Surgery** is the procedure of choice, particularly **thoracoscopy** or **thoracotomy** if the patient is a surgical candidate.

Sarcoidosis

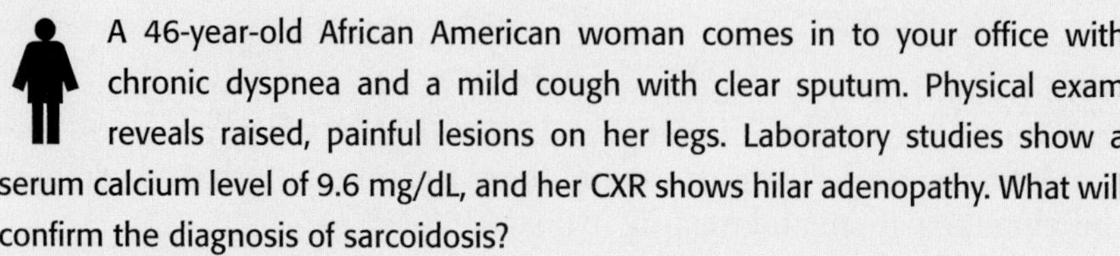

A 46-year-old African American woman comes in to your office with chronic dyspnea and a mild cough with clear sputum. Physical exam reveals raised, painful lesions on her legs. Laboratory studies show a serum calcium level of 9.6 mg/dL, and her CXR shows hilar adenopathy. What will confirm the diagnosis of sarcoidosis?

An endobronchial biopsy revealing a noncaseating granuloma is confirmatory. A biopsy specimen of erythema nodosum will not show granulomatous involvement and is not diagnostically helpful.

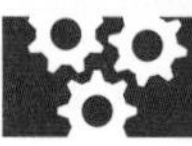

MNEMONIC

Features of sarcoidosis–

GRUELING

Granulomas
Rheumatoid arthritis
Uveitis
Erythema nodosum
Lymphadenitis
Interstitial fibrosis
Negative PPD
Gammaglobulinemia

An idiopathic illness characterized by the formation of **noncaseating granulomas** in various organs. Most patients have pulmonary involvement.

SYMPTOMS/EXAM

Typical features include **fever, cough, malaise, weight loss, dyspnea,** and **arthritis,** particularly of the knees and ankles.

DIFFERENTIAL

Sarcoidosis is a **diagnosis of exclusion,** so be sure to rule out other diseases that present similarly, such as **TB, lymphoma,** fungal infection, idiopathic pulmonary fibrosis, HIV, and berylliosis.

DIAGNOSIS

- Look for **bilateral hilar lymphadenopathy** on CXR and/or infiltrates.
- PFTs will show a **restrictive** or **mixed restrictive-obstructive** pattern. Patients may also have **hypercalcemia.**
- Tissue biopsy will show **noncaseating granulomas without organisms.**

TREATMENT

Therapy includes systemic **corticosteroids** such as prednisone. Gear other medications toward the control of symptoms such as coughing or wheezing.

Obstructive Sleep Apnea (OSA)

Characterized by recurrent episodes of upper airway collapse during sleep that lead to **intermittent hypoxia and recurrent arousals.**

Symptoms

Patients and their bed partners may complain about **snoring.** Patients may also have **excessive daytime sleepiness,** neurocognitive impairment, morning headache, unrefreshing sleep, or impotence. They may report choking or gasping during sleep and may have witnessed apnea episodes at home.

Exam

Patients are typically **obese** and **hypertensive.** They may also have a **large neck circumference.** Look for **micrognathia/retrognathia, a large tongue,** or large tonsils. Patients with severe OSA may have peripheral edema.

Differential

Rule out other causes of excessive daytime sleepiness, including **obesity hypoventilation syndrome,** narcolepsy, and restless leg syndrome.

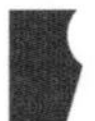

KEY FACT

Overnight polysomnography (sleep study) is the gold standard for the diagnosis of obstructive sleep apnea. An AHI of > 5 is diagnostic.

Diagnosis

Overnight polysomnography (sleep study) is the gold standard for diagnosis. Severity is measured by the apnea-hypopnea index (AHI), defined as the number of apneas and/or hypopneas per hour of sleep. An **AHI of > 5** is diagnostic of OSA.

Treatment

Encourage weight loss. The most effective treatment is with **continuous positive airway pressure (CPAP)** to keep the airways open during sleep. Surgery such as uvulopalatopharyngoplasty (UPPP) is effective in 40–50% of cases.

Complications

Patients with OSA are at ↑ risk of **motor vehicle accidents** as well as for the development of **hypertension, left ventricular dysfunction, pulmonary hypertension,** and insulin resistance.

Bronchiolitis

Involves inflammation in smaller airways; occurs most often in infants from two months to one year of age. **RSV** accounts for the vast majority of cases. Other viral causes include adenovirus, influenza, and parainfluenza.

Symptoms

Patients are typically **infants.** Symptoms begin as those of a **URI** (sore throat, runny nose) and **progress** over the next 3–7 days to lower respiratory symptoms (cough, wheezing).

Exam

Patients may have cough, fever, **tachypnea,** and **intercostal retractions.** Look for cyanosis, expiratory wheezing, and crackles.

DIAGNOSIS

- Look for **hyperinflation** of the lungs on CXR with flattening of the diaphragms and mild interstitial infiltrates.
- RSV may be diagnosed with **ELISA** or a fluorescent antibody test.

KEY FACT

Intubate infants with ↑ P_{CO_2} levels or ↑ O_2 requirements.

TREATMENT

- **Supplemental O_2** (oxygen tent).
- Aerosolized **albuterol.**
- In cases of RSV, use **ribavirin** for patients with severe disease or underlying cardiac or pulmonary problems.

Cystic Fibrosis (CF)

An autosomal recessive disorder with mutations located in the CFTR gene, leading to abnormal transfer of sodium and chloride. Multiple exocrine glands and cilia in various organs become dysfunctional. The **most common** genetic disease in the United States and among **Caucasians, affecting 1 in 3200.**

SYMPTOMS

- Patients typically present in childhood or adolescence. Look for patients with **recurrent pulmonary infections,** sinusitis, **bronchiectasis, infertility,** or **pancreatic insufficiency** (diabetes, malabsorption, steatorrhea).
- Infants may present with **meconium ileus** or **intussusception.**

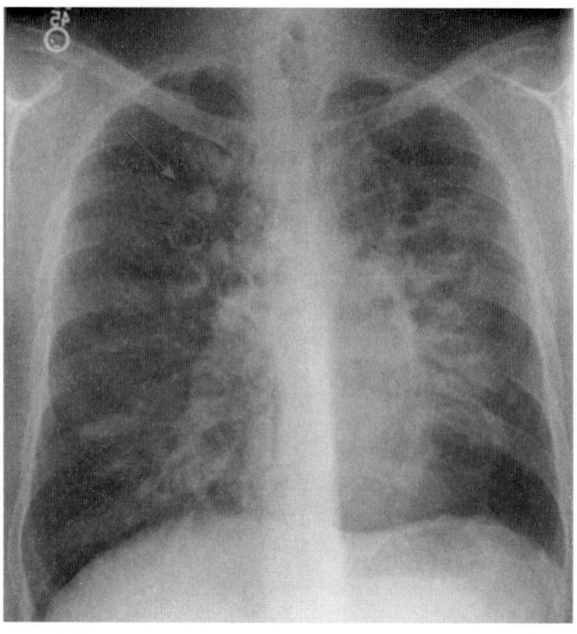

A

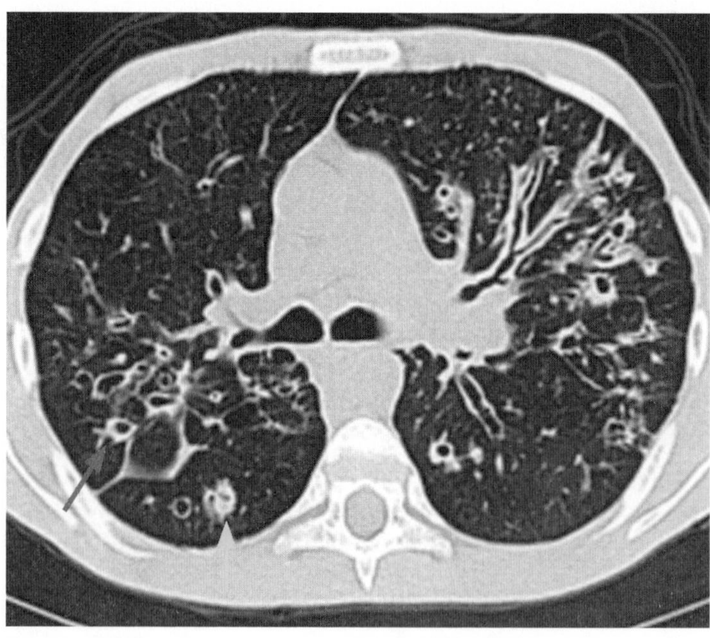

B

FIGURE 18-6. Cystic fibrosis. (**A**) Frontal CXR showing central cystic bronchiectasis (arrow) in a patient with CF. (**B**) Transaxial CT image showing cystic bronchiectasis (red arrow), with some bronchi containing impacted mucus (yellow arrow). (Reproduced with permission from USMLERx.com.)

Exam

- Patients may have short stature and nasal polyps.
- Lung exam often reveals **wheezing, crackles,** or **squeaks. Clubbing** may be present.
- Hyperinflation is seen early, followed by peribronchial cuffing, mucous plugging, and bronchiectasis (see Figure 18-6).

Diagnosis

- Diagnosis is made with a sweat chloride test of > **60 mEq/L** (must be confirmed on two different days).
- Genetic testing can confirm the presence of many of the genetic mutations.

Treatment

- Manage the disease with attention to nutrition, **chest physiotherapy, bronchodilators, pancreatic enzymes, mucolytics** (DNase), and stool softeners (fiber).
- Patients need supplemental **fat-soluble vitamins (A, D, E, K)** to address fat malabsorption.
- **Chronic** and **chronic intermittent oral antibiotics (azithromycin)** or **inhaled antibiotics (tobramycin)** may also be beneficial. ***Pseudomonas aeruginosa*** is common; therapies are tailored to treat the infecting organism.
- In severe end-stage pulmonary disease, bilateral **lung transplantation** should be considered, as it is the **only definitive treatment.**

Complications

Associated with both **pseudomonal** and **staphylococcal** infections.

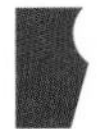

KEY FACT

In patients with cystic fibrosis with signs of pulmonary infection, think *Pseudomonas* and/or *Staphylococcus.*

NOTES

CHAPTER 19

HIGH-YIELD CCS CASES

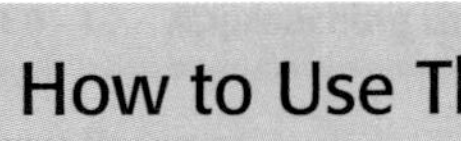

How to Use This Section

In this section are 100 **minicases** reflecting the types of clinical situations encountered on the actual CCS. Each case consists of **columns** that start on the left-hand page and end on the right-hand page with the **Final Diagnosis.** As you read each column, ask yourself what you should do and/or think next (see Table 19-1). If no results are given for a test, assume that is **normal.** To get the most out of these minicases, we **strongly** recommend that you do at least a few of the CCS cases on the USMLE CD-ROM (or from the USMLE Web site) to get a feel for the case flow and key decision points. This will allow you to place the minicases in context. Happy studying!

HEADACHE

CASE 1

HX	PE	DDX
21 yo F presents with a severe headache. She has a history of throbbing left temporal pain that lasts for 2–3 hours. Before these episodes start, she sees flashes of light in her right visual field and feels weakness and numbness on the right side of her body for a few minutes. The headaches are often associated with nausea and vomiting. She has a family history of migraine.	VS: T 37°C (99.2°F), P 70, BP 120/80, RR 15, O_2 sat 100% room air Gen: NAD Lungs: WNL CV: WNL Abd: WNL Ext: WNL Neuro: WNL	▪ Cluster headache ▪ Intracranial neoplasm ▪ Migraine (complicated) ▪ Partial seizure ▪ Pseudotumor cerebri ▪ Tension headache ▪ Trigeminal neuralgia

CASE 2

HX	PE	DDX
29 yo F presents with daily episodes of bilateral bandlike throbbing pain in her frontal-occipital region that last between 30 minutes and a few hours. She usually experiences these episodes when she is either tired or under stress. She denies any associated nausea, vomiting, phonophobia, photophobia, or aura. She also feels pain and stiffness in her neck and shoulder.	VS: Afebrile, P 70, BP 120/80, RR 15 Gen: NAD Lungs: WNL CV: WNL Abd: WNL Ext: WNL Neuro: WNL	▪ Cluster headache ▪ Intracranial neoplasm ▪ Meningitis ▪ Migraine headache ▪ Pseudotumor cerebri ▪ Sinusitis ▪ Tension headache

CASE 3

HX	PE	DDX
65 yo F presents with a severe intermittent headache in the right temporal lobe together with blurred vision in her right eye and pain in her jaw during mastication.	VS: T 37°C (99°F), P 85, BP 140/85, RR 18, O_2 sat 100% room air Gen: NAD HEENT: Tenderness on temporal artery palpation Neck: No rigidity Lungs: WNL CV: WNL Abd: WNL Ext: WNL Neuro: WNL	▪ Cluster headache ▪ Glaucoma ▪ Intracranial neoplasm ▪ Meningitis ▪ Migraine ▪ Temporal arteritis (giant cell arteritis) ▪ Tension headache ▪ Trigeminal neuralgia

INITIAL MGMT	CONTINUING MGMT	F/U
Emergency room W/U ▪ CT–head ▪ CBC ▪ Chem 8 ▪ ESR **Rx** ▪ IV normal saline ▪ IV promethazine, prochlorperazine, or metoclopramide ▪ ASA, NSAIDs, or acetaminophen ▪ Caffeine ▪ IM sumatriptan (if the patient does not improve)		▪ Follow up in one month ▪ Prophylactic therapy if the migraine recurs—eg, β-blockers, antidepressants (SSRIs, TCAs), anticonvulsants (valproic acid, gabapentin), calcium channel blockers

Final Dx: Migraine (complicated)

INITIAL MGMT	CONTINUING MGMT	F/U
Office W/U ▪ CBC with differential ▪ Chem 8 ▪ ESR **Rx** ▪ Cold compresses ▪ Acetaminophen ▪ NSAIDs		▪ Follow up in one month ▪ Relaxation exercises

Final Dx: Tension headache

INITIAL MGMT	CONTINUING MGMT	F/U
Emergency room STAT ▪ IV normal saline ▪ Prednisone **Emergency room W/U** ▪ CBC ▪ Chem 8 ▪ CT–head: ⊖ ▪ CXR: ⊖ ▪ ESR: ↑↑ ▪ CRP: ↑↑	**Ward W/U** ▪ Ophthalmology consult ▪ Temporal artery biopsy: ⊕ for temporal arteritis ▪ ESR every morning ▪ Screen for polymyalgia rheumatica **Rx** ▪ Continue prednisone until ESR normalizes; then taper	▪ Discharge home ▪ Continue low-dose maintenance prednisone ▪ ESR in two weeks ▪ Adequate dietary calcium and vitamin D if steroids are to be used chronically

Final Dx: Temporal arteritis (giant cell arteritis)

CASE 4

HX	PE	DDX
25 yo M presents with a high fever, severe headache, and photophobia.	VS: T 39°C (103°F), P 95, BP 150/85, RR 18, O_2 sat 100% room air Gen: Moderate distress Neck: Nuchal rigidity Lungs: WNL CV: WNL Abd: WNL Ext: WNL Neuro: ⊕ Kernig's and Brudzinski's signs	▪ Encephalitis ▪ Intracranial or epidural abscess ▪ Meningitis ▪ Migraine ▪ Sinusitis ▪ Subarachnoid hemorrhage

CASE 5

HX	PE	DDX
60 yo M with a past medical history of hypertension presents with severe headache, nausea, and vomiting. The patient states that he stopped taking his metoprolol because he thought that he did not need it anymore.	VS: T 37°C (99.3°F), P 100, BP 220/120, RR 20, O_2 sat 95% room air Gen: Severe distress HEENT: Funduscopy reveals papilledema Lungs: WNL CV: WNL Abd: WNL Ext: WNL Neuro: WNL	▪ Cluster headache ▪ Intracranial hemorrhage ▪ Intracranial neoplasm ▪ Malignant hypertension ▪ Migraine ▪ Partial seizure

INITIAL MGMT	CONTINUING MGMT	F/U
Emergency room STAT ▪ IV normal saline ▪ Blood culture ▪ CT—head ▪ Ceftriaxone and vancomycin ▪ LP-CSF: ↑ WBCs, ↑ protein, ↓ CSF/blood glucose ratio, gram-⊕ cocci, ↑ opening pressure ▪ IV dexamethasone **Emergency room W/U** ▪ CBC: ↑ WBC count ▪ Chem 8 ▪ CT—head: ⊖ ▪ CXR: ⊖ **Rx** ▪ Acetaminophen	**Ward W/U** ▪ CSF culture: ⊕ for *S pneumoniae* ▪ Blood culture: ⊖ **Rx** ▪ Continue ceftriaxone + vancomycin + steroids	▪ Improved within 48 hours ▪ Discharge home ▪ Follow up in one month

Final Dx: Bacterial meningitis

INITIAL MGMT	CONTINUING MGMT	F/U
Emergency room STAT ▪ O_2 ▪ IV labetalol ▪ BP in both arms ▪ CT—head: White matter changes consistent with hypertension ▪ ECG: LVH ▪ CXR **Emergency room W/U** ▪ Cardiac/BP monitoring ▪ CPK-MB, troponin × 3: ⊖ ▪ CBC ▪ Chem 8 ▪ UA	**ICU W/U** ▪ Continuous cardiac monitoring ▪ Lipid profile ▪ Echocardiography: EF $< 45\%$ **Rx** ▪ Labetalol or metoprolol if good control previously ▪ ACEIs (low EF) ▪ HCTZ	▪ Transfer to the floor ▪ Counsel patient re medication compliance ▪ Discharge home ▪ Follow up in one week

Final Dx: Hypertensive emergency

ALTERED MENTAL STATUS/LOSS OF CONSCIOUSNESS

CASE 6

HX	PE	DDX
84 yo F brought in by her son complains of forgetfulness (eg, forgets phone numbers, loses her way home) along with difficulty performing some of her daily activities (eg, bathing, dressing, managing money, answering the phone). The problem has gradually progressed over the past few years.	VS: P 90, BP 120/60, RR 12 Gen: NAD Lungs: WNL CV: WNL Abd: WNL Ext: WNL Neuro: On mini-mental status exam, patient cannot recall objects, follow three-step commands, or spell "world" backward; cranial nerves intact; strength and sensation intact	▪ Alzheimer's disease ▪ B_{12} deficiency ▪ Chronic subdural hematoma ▪ Depression ▪ Hypothyroidism ▪ Intracranial tumor ▪ Neurosyphilis ▪ Pressure hydrocephalus ▪ Vascular dementia

CASE 7

HX	PE	DDX
79 yo M is brought in by his family complaining of a seven-week history of difficulty walking accompanied by memory loss and urinary incontinence. Since then he has had ↑ difficulty with memory and more frequent episodes of incontinence.	VS: P 92, BP 144/86, RR 14 Gen: NAD Lungs: WNL CV: WNL Abd: WNL Ext: WNL Neuro: Difficulty with both recent and immediate recall on mini-mental status exam; spasticity and hyperreflexia in upper and lower extremities; problem initiating gait (gait is shuffling, broad-based, and slow)	▪ Alzheimer's disease ▪ B_{12} deficiency ▪ Chronic subdural hematoma ▪ Frontal lobe syndromes ▪ Huntington's disease ▪ Intracranial tumor ▪ Meningitis ▪ Normal pressure hydrocephalus ▪ Parkinson's disease ▪ Vascular dementia

INITIAL MGMT	CONTINUING MGMT	F/U
Office W/U ▪ CBC ▪ Chem 14 ▪ TSH ▪ Serum B_{12} ▪ Serum folic acid ▪ VDRL/RPR ▪ CT—head **Rx** ▪ Donepezil		▪ Patient counseling ▪ Support group ▪ Advance directives ▪ Family counseling

Final Dx: Alzheimer's disease

INITIAL MGMT	CONTINUING MGMT	F/U
Emergency room W/U ▪ CBC ▪ Chem 8 ▪ LFTs ▪ TSH ▪ CT—head: Enlarged lateral ventricles with no prominence of cortical sulci ▪ LP ▪ Serum B_{12} ▪ Serum folic acid	**Ward W/U** ▪ Neurosurgery consult ▪ Neurology consult ▪ Ventriculoperitoneal shunt	▪ Advance directives ▪ Family counseling ▪ Supportive care

Final Dx: Normal pressure hydrocephalus

CASE 8

HX	PE	DDX
The on-call physician is called to see a 46 yo M patient because of seizures. The patient was admitted to the surgical ward two days ago, after emergency trauma surgery. The nurse reports that the patient was anxious, agitated, irritable, and tachycardic last night. Later on, the nurse noted nausea, diarrhea, sweating, and insomnia. The patient had tremors, startle response, and hallucinations earlier tonight.	VS: T 37°C (99°F), P 133, BP 146/89, RR 22, O_2 sat 92% room air Gen: Sweating; cigarette burns on hands; multiple tattoos and rings Chest: WNL Abd: Hepatomegaly Ext: Evidence of recent surgery Neuro: Tremor, confusion, delirium, clouded sensorium, and evidence of peripheral neuropathy	▪ Alcohol withdrawal ▪ Amphetamine psychosis ▪ Delirium ▪ Sedative withdrawal ▪ SLE

CASE 9

HX	PE	DDX
24 yo M is brought to the ER in a drowsy state. His wife reports that he was working at home when he suddenly stiffened, fell backward, and lost consciousness. While he was lying on the ground, he was noted to have no respiration for about one minute, followed by jerking of all four limbs for about five minutes. He was unconscious for another five minutes.	VS: T 37°C (98.2°F), P 90, BP 120/80, RR 12 Gen: NAD Lungs: WNL CV: WNL Abd: WNL Ext: WNL Neuro: In a state of confusion and lethargy but oriented; no focal neurologic deficits	▪ Alcohol withdrawal ▪ Cardioembolic stroke ▪ Frontal lobe epilepsy ▪ Migraine headache ▪ Psychiatric conditions ▪ Seizures ▪ Syncope ▪ Vascular conditions

INITIAL MGMT	CONTINUING MGMT	F/U
Ward W/U ▪ CBC: MCV 110 fL ▪ Chem 8: Hypokalemia, hypomagnesemia ▪ Urine toxicology: WNL ▪ LFTs: GGT 40 U/L ▪ CT–head: Cerebral atrophy, no subdural hematoma **Rx** ▪ Thiamine before IV D_5W NS ▪ Pyridoxine ▪ Folic acid ▪ IV diazepam ▪ Atenolol ▪ Replete K and Mg	**Ward W/U** ▪ Chem 8: Corrected hypokalemia, hypomagnesemia **Rx** ▪ IV normal saline ▪ IV diazepam ▪ Atenolol ▪ Naltrexone (for maintenance therapy if indicated)	▪ Follow up in four weeks ▪ Patient counseling ▪ Smoking cessation ▪ Dietary supplements ▪ Addiction unit consult ▪ Social work consult

Final Dx: Alcohol withdrawal

INITIAL MGMT	CONTINUING MGMT	F/U
Emergency room W/U ▪ CBC ▪ Chem 8 ▪ LFTs ▪ ABG ▪ Serum calcium, magnesium, phosphate ▪ ECG ▪ EEG ▪ CT–head ▪ MRI–brain ▪ UA ▪ Urine toxicology	**Ward W/U** ▪ Continue IV ▪ O_2 **Rx** ▪ Neurology consult	▪ Follow up in 3–4 weeks ▪ Patient counseling ▪ Family counseling ▪ Advise patient to use seat belts ▪ Advise patient not to drive

Final Dx: Grand mal seizure (complex tonic-clonic seizure)

CASE 10

HX	PE	DDX
72 yo M is brought to the ER complaining of syncope. He underwent a coronary artery bypass graft (CABG) three years ago. He reports fatigue and dizziness over the past five days. The patient's fall was broken by his wife, and as a result he has no head trauma. His wife reports loss of consciousness of about three minutes' duration. Prior to the syncopal episode, the patient recalls a prodrome of lightheadedness. His medications include propranolol, digoxin, and diltiazem.	VS: T 37°C (98.1°F), P 35, BP 114/54, RR 15 Gen: NAD Lungs: WNL CV: Irregular S1 and S2, bradycardia Abd: WNL Ext: WNL Neuro: Alert and oriented; CN II–XII intact; 5/5 motor strength in all extremities	▪ Aortic stenosis ▪ Asystole ▪ Dilated cardiomyopathy ▪ Heart block ▪ MI ▪ Myocarditis ▪ Myopathies ▪ Restrictive cardiomyopathy ▪ Vasodepressor/vasovagal response

CASE 11

HX	PE	DDX
25 yo F with no significant past medical history is brought to the ER after having been found unresponsive with an empty bottle lying next to her.	VS: T 38°C (99.8°F), P 50, BP 110/50, RR 9, O_2 sat 92% room air Gen: Drowsy HEENT: Pinpoint pupils Lungs: WNL CV: Bradycardia Abd: WNL Ext: WNL Neuro: Opens eyes to painful stimuli Limited PE with ABCs	▪ Acetaminophen overdose ▪ Narcotic overdose ▪ TCA overdose

INITIAL MGMT	CONTINUING MGMT	F/U
Emergency room W/U ▪ IV normal saline ▪ CBC ▪ Chem 8 ▪ LFTs ▪ ECG: Third-degree AV block ▪ Cardiac enzymes ▪ Serum troponin I ▪ Serum calcium, magnesium, phosphate ▪ CXR ▪ UA ▪ O_2 ▪ Continuous cardiac monitoring **Rx** ▪ Temporary transvenous cardiac pacemaker ▪ Withhold AV nodal agents	**ICU W/U** ▪ Continuous cardiac monitoring ▪ ECG ▪ Lipid profile ▪ Echocardiography **Rx** ▪ Lipid-lowering agents ▪ Cardiology consult ▪ Cardiac catheterization, angiocardiography ▪ Permanent cardiac pacemaker	▪ Cardiac rehabilitation program ▪ Smoking cessation ▪ Counsel patient to limit alcohol intake ▪ Counsel patient not to drive ▪ Low-fat, low-sodium diet

Final Dx: Complete heart block

INITIAL MGMT	CONTINUING MGMT	F/U
Emergency room STAT ▪ Suction airway ▪ Fingerstick blood sugar ▪ IV normal saline ▪ IV naloxone: Patient responded ▪ Dextrose 50% ▪ IV thiamine ▪ ABG **Emergency room W/U** ▪ CBC ▪ ECG ▪ Urine pregnancy ▪ Urine toxicology ▪ UA ▪ Serum acetaminophen, salicylate ▪ INR ▪ Serum lactate ▪ CXR, PA	**ICU W/U** ▪ Gastric lavage: Pill fragments ▪ Continuous monitoring: Patient started to become drowsy again (monitor events) **Rx** ▪ IV naloxone: Patient responded ▪ Psychiatry consult ▪ Suicide precautions	▪ Monitor for at least 24 hours

Final Dx: Narcotic overdose

CASE 12

HX	PE	DDX
60 yo M was found unconscious by his wife, who called the paramedics. She left him in bed at 7 A.M. to go to her volunteer job. When she returned for lunch at 1 P.M., she found an empty bottle of amitriptyline next to him. When paramedics arrived, he was noted to be in respiratory distress and was transferred to the ER.	VS: T 38°C (101°F), P 110, BP 95/45, RR 35, O_2 sat 89% on 100% face mask Gen: Acute distress; shallow, rapid breathing HEENT: Dilated pupils Lungs: WNL CV: Tachycardia Abd: WNL Neuro: Opens eyes to painful stimuli **Limited PE**	▪ Anticholinergic toxicity ▪ TCA intoxication

FATIGUE/WEAKNESS

CASE 13

HX	PE	DDX
68 yo M presents following a 20-minute episode of slurred speech, right facial drooping and numbness, and weakness of the right hand. His symptoms had totally resolved by the time he got to the ER. He has a history of hypertension, diabetes mellitus, and heavy smoking.	VS: T 37°C (98°F), P 75, BP 150/90, RR 16, O_2 sat 100% room air Gen: NAD Neck: Right carotid bruit Lungs: WNL CV: WNL Abd: WNL Ext: WNL Neuro: WNL	▪ Intracranial tumor ▪ Seizure ▪ Stroke ▪ Subdural or epidural hematoma ▪ TIA

INITIAL MGMT	CONTINUING MGMT	F/U
Emergency room STAT ▪ Intubate **Emergency room W/U** ▪ Cardiac/BP monitoring ▪ Chem 14 ▪ CBC ▪ ABG ▪ Serum lactate ▪ Serum osmolality ▪ Blood ketones ▪ Urine toxicology: ⊕ for TCAs ▪ ECG: Widened QRS ▪ Serum magnesium ▪ CXR, PA ▪ Cardiac enzymes ▪ CT—head **Rx** ▪ IV D_5W 0.9 NS ▪ Thiamine ▪ Central line placement ▪ NG tube gastric lavage ▪ Activated charcoal ▪ IV bicarbonate	**ICU W/U** ▪ Continuous monitoring of urine output q 1 h ▪ Continuous BP monitoring ▪ Continuous cardiac monitoring ▪ Neuro check **Rx** ▪ Cardiology consult ▪ Lidocaine for TCA-induced ventricular arrhythmias ▪ IV magnesium sulfate, one time	▪ Psychiatry consult

Final Dx: Tricyclic antidepressant (TCA) intoxication

INITIAL MGMT	CONTINUING MGMT	F/U
Emergency room STAT ▪ Assess ABCs ▪ O_2 ▪ Blood glucose ▪ IV normal saline ▪ CT—head **Emergency room W/U** ▪ Continuous cardiac monitoring ▪ BP monitoring ▪ ECG ▪ CBC ▪ Chem 8 ▪ CXR ▪ PT/PTT, INR ▪ Neurology consult **Rx** ▪ ASA	**Ward W/U** ▪ Repeat neurologic exam ▪ Continuous cardiac monitoring ▪ BP monitoring ▪ Telemetry ▪ Lipid profile, HbA_{1c} ▪ Echocardiography: EF 60% ▪ Carotid duplex: > 75% stenosis in right carotid artery **Rx** ▪ Vascular surgery consult ▪ Patient is scheduled for elective carotid endarterectomy ▪ ASA	▪ Counsel patient re smoking cessation, exercise ▪ Treat hypertension ▪ Treat diabetes ▪ Diabetic diet ▪ Diabetic teaching ▪ Treat cholesterol ▪ Low-fat, low-sodium diet

Final Dx: Transient ischemic attack (TIA)

CASE 14

HX	PE	DDX
40 yo F presents with numbness, lower extremity weakness, and difficulty walking. She reports having had a URI approximately two weeks ago. She says that her weakness started from her lower limbs to her hip and then progressed to her upper limbs. She also complains of lightheadedness on standing and shortness of breath.	VS: Afebrile, P 115, BP 130/80 with orthostatic changes, RR 16 Gen: NAD Lungs: WNL CV: WNL Ext: WNL Neuro: Loss of motor strength in lower limbs; absent DTRs in patella and Achilles tendon; sensation intact	▪ Conversion disorder ▪ Guillain-Barré syndrome ▪ Myasthenia gravis ▪ Paraneoplastic neuropathy ▪ Poliomyelitis ▪ Polymyositis

CASE 15

HX	PE	DDX
40 yo F presents with fatigue, weight gain, sleepiness, cold intolerance, constipation, and dry skin.	VS: T 36°C (97°F), BP 100/60, HR 60 Gen: Obese Skin: Dry HEENT: Scar on neck from previous thyroidectomy Lungs: WNL CV: WNL Neuro: Delayed relaxation of DTRs	▪ Anemia ▪ Depression ▪ Diabetes ▪ Hypothyroidism

CASE 16

HX	PE	DDX
16 yo M complains of myalgia, fatigue, and sore throat. He also reports loss of appetite and nausea but no vomiting. He reports that his girlfriend recently had similar symptoms that lasted a few weeks.	VS: T 38°C (101°F), P 85, BP 125/80, RR 18 Gen: Maculopapular rash HEENT: Posterior and auricular lymphadenopathy and pharyngitis with diffuse exudates and petechiae at junction of hard and soft palates Lungs: WNL CV: WNL Abd: Soft, nontender; mild hepatosplenomegaly Ext: WNL Neuro: WNL	▪ CMV ▪ Hepatitis ▪ Infectious mononucleosis ▪ 1° HIV infection ▪ Streptococcal pharyngitis ▪ Toxoplasmosis

INITIAL MGMT	CONTINUING MGMT	F/U
Emergency room W/U ▪ CBC ▪ Chem 8 ▪ TSH ▪ ESR ▪ CRP ▪ RF ▪ VDRL ▪ Serum B_{12} ▪ Serum folic acid ▪ ECG ▪ Serum CPK ▪ CXR ▪ LP: ↑ CSF protein ▪ HIV testing, ELISA	**Ward Rx** ▪ Immunoglobulins ▪ Plasmapheresis ▪ Rehabilitative medicine consult ▪ Neurology consult ▪ Immunology consult ▪ Spirometry	▪ Follow up in 3–4 weeks ▪ Patient counseling ▪ Family counseling ▪ Advise patient to use seat belts

Final Dx: Guillain-Barré syndrome

INITIAL MGMT	CONTINUING MGMT	F/U
Office W/U ▪ CBC ▪ Chem 14 ▪ TSH: ↑ ▪ FT_4: ↓ ▪ ECG ▪ Lipid profile ▪ Depression index **Rx** ▪ Thyroxine		▪ Check TSH after one month

Final Dx: Hypothyroidism

INITIAL MGMT	CONTINUING MGMT	F/U
Office W/U ▪ CBC: ↑ WBC count ▪ Peripheral smear: Atypical lymphocytes ▪ Chem 14: ↑ SGOT and SGPT ▪ ESR ▪ CRP ▪ Mono test: ⊕ ▪ Serum EBV titer: ↑, rapid strep **Rx** ▪ Acetaminophen or NSAIDs ▪ Hydrate; patient counseling		▪ Follow up in two weeks with CBC ▪ Advise patient to rest at home ▪ Advise patient to avoid sports

Final Dx: Infectious mononucleosis

CASE 17

HX	PE	DDX
40 yo F complains of feeling tired, hopeless, and worthless. She also reports depressed mood, inability to sleep, and impaired concentration. She has been missing work. She denies any suicidal thoughts or attempts and denies having hallucinations. She has no history of alcohol or drug abuse and has not lost a loved one within the last 12 months. She is married and has one child and a supportive husband.	VS: P 70, BP 120/60, RR 12 Gen: NAD Lungs: WNL CV: WNL Abd: WNL Ext: WNL Neuro: WNL	▪ Adjustment disorder ▪ Anemia ▪ Anxiety ▪ Cancer ▪ Chronic fatigue syndrome ▪ Dementia ▪ Depression ▪ Fibromyalgia ▪ Hypothyroidism

COUGH/SHORTNESS OF BREATH

CASE 18

HX	PE	DDX
2 yo M is brought in by his mother because of sudden-onset shortness of breath and cough. He had a URI four days ago. Earlier in the day he was playing with peanuts with his brother. His immunizations are up to date.	VS: T 37°C (98°F), P 110, BP 80/50, RR 38, O_2 sat 99% room air Gen: Respiratory distress; using accessory muscles HEENT: WNL Neck: WNL Lungs: Inspiratory stridor; ↓ breath sounds in right lower base CV: Tachycardia Abd: WNL	▪ Angioedema ▪ Asthma ▪ Croup ▪ Epiglottitis ▪ Foreign-body aspiration ▪ Laryngitis ▪ Peritonsillar abscess ▪ Pneumonia ▪ Retropharyngeal abscess

CASE 19

HX	PE	DDX
75 yo F presents with chest pain and shortness of breath. She reports having fallen five days ago and has a long cast for her femoral fracture.	VS: Afebrile, BP 120/75, HR 100, RR 24 Gen: Respiratory distress HEENT: WNL Lungs: Rales, wheezing, ↓ breath sounds in left lower lung CV: Loud P2 and splitting of S2 Abd: WNL	▪ CHF ▪ Lung cancer ▪ MI ▪ Pericarditis ▪ Pneumothorax ▪ Pulmonary embolism ▪ Syncope

INITIAL MGMT	CONTINUING MGMT	F/U
Office W/U ▪ CBC ▪ Chem 14 ▪ TSH ▪ Urine/serum toxicology **Rx** ▪ Suicide contract ▪ SSRI (eg, sertraline) or ▪ SNRI (eg, mirtazapine) ▪ Psychiatry consult		▪ Follow up in one week ▪ Supportive psychotherapy ▪ Exercise program ▪ Patient counseling

Final Dx: Major depression

INITIAL MGMT	CONTINUING MGMT	F/U
Emergency room STAT ▪ CXR, PA and lateral ▪ XR—neck ▪ Bronchoscopy: Foreign body is removed and patient improves **Rx** ▪ Consider IV methylprednisolone before removal of the foreign body		▪ Follow up in two weeks

Final Dx: Foreign-body aspiration

INITIAL MGMT	CONTINUING MGMT	F/U
Emergency room W/U ▪ IV normal saline ▪ NPO ▪ CBC ▪ Chem 14 ▪ ABG: Hypoxia and hypocapnia ▪ CXR: Left lower lobe atelectasis, Hampton's humps ▪ CT—chest: Pulmonary embolism ▪ ECG ▪ DVT U/S: Venous DVT ▪ Heparin IV and warfarin	**Ward W/U** ▪ Continuous cardiac and BP monitoring ▪ Pulmonary medicine consult ▪ PT/PTT, INR **Rx** ▪ Discontinue heparin two days after INR is therapeutic ▪ Warfarin	▪ Follow up in two weeks with PT/INR ▪ Chest physical therapy ▪ Warfarin ▪ Rehabilitative medicine consult

Final Dx: Pulmonary embolism

CASE 20

HX	PE	DDX
5 yo M is brought to the ER with a harsh barking cough. He has a history of URIs with coryza, nasal congestion, and sore throat. His symptoms have been present for about a week.	VS: T 38°C (101°F), BP 110/65, HR 100, RR 22 Gen: Pallor and mild respiratory distress with intercostal retraction and nasal flaring HEENT: WNL Lungs: Stridor, hoarseness, barking cough CV: WNL Abd: WNL	▪ Bacterial tracheitis ▪ Croup ▪ Diphtheria ▪ Epiglottitis ▪ Measles ▪ Peritonsillar abscess ▪ Retropharyngeal abscess

CASE 21

HX	PE	DDX
75 yo M presents with shortness of breath on exertion along with cough and blood-streaked sputum. He reports progressive malaise and weight loss together with loss of appetite over the past six months. He smokes 40 packs of cigarettes per year.	VS: Afebrile, BP 130/85, HR 90, RR 15 Gen: WNL Chest: Barrel-shaped chest, gynecomastia Lungs: Rales, wheezing, ↓ breath sounds, dullness on percussion in left upper lung CV: WNL Abd: Mild tenderness in RUQ with mild hepatomegaly Ext: Finger clubbing; dark-colored, pruritic rash on both forearms	▪ Lung cancer ▪ Lymphoma ▪ Sarcoidosis ▪ Tuberculosis

INITIAL MGMT	CONTINUING MGMT	F/U
Emergency room W/U ▪ O_2 ▪ CBC ▪ Chem 8 ▪ Throat culture ▪ XR—neck: Subglottic narrowing	**Ward Rx** ▪ Humidified air ▪ Epinephrine ▪ Dexamethasone	▪ Follow up in one month ▪ Family counseling

Final Dx: Croup

INITIAL MGMT	CONTINUING MGMT	F/U
Office W/U ▪ CBC: ↓ hemoglobin ▪ Chem 8 ▪ LFTs: ↑ transaminase ▪ ABG ▪ ESR: ↑ ▪ CXR: Infiltrate and nodules in upper left lobe ▪ Sputum cytology: Adenocarcinoma ▪ Sputum culture ▪ PPD: ⊖ ▪ CT—chest: Left upper lobe mass	**Office W/U** ▪ PFTs ▪ Oncology consult ▪ Surgery consult ▪ Dietary consult ▪ Bronchoscopy with biopsy ▪ CT—abdomen and pelvis ▪ CT—head ▪ Antiemetic medication	▪ Smoking cessation ▪ Patient counseling ▪ Family counseling ▪ Follow up in 3–4 weeks with CXR and CBC ▪ Counsel patient to limit alcohol intake

Final Dx: Lung cancer

CASE 22

HX	PE	DDX
60 yo M presents with ↑ dyspnea, sputum production, and a change in the color of his sputum to yellow over the past three days. He is a smoker with a history of COPD.	VS: T 38°C (100.6°F), P 90, BP 130/70, RR 28, O_2 sat 92% on 2-L NC Gen: Moderate respiratory distress Lungs: Rhonchi at left lower base; diffuse wheezing CV: WNL Abd: WNL Ext: WNL	▪ Bronchitis ▪ CHF ▪ COPD exacerbation ▪ Lung cancer ▪ Pneumonia ▪ URI

CASE 23

HX	PE	DDX
50 yo Mexican immigrant M presents with cough productive of bloody sputum accompanied by night sweats, weight loss, and fatigue of three months' duration.	VS: T 38°C (100°F), BP 130/85, HR 90, RR 22 Gen: Pallor Lungs: ↓ breath sounds in upper lobes of both lungs CV: WNL Abd: WNL	▪ Bronchiectasis ▪ Fungal lung infection ▪ Lung cancer ▪ Lymphoma ▪ Sarcoidosis ▪ TB ▪ Vasculitis

INITIAL MGMT	CONTINUING MGMT	F/U
Emergency room STAT ▪ O_2 ▪ IV normal saline ▪ IV steroids ▪ Albuterol by nebulizer ▪ Ipratropium by nebulizer ▪ Sputum culture ▪ Blood culture **Emergency room W/U** ▪ CBC: ↑ WBC count ▪ CXR: Left lower lobe infiltrate ▪ ECG ▪ ABG ▪ Peak flow: < 200 L/min ▪ Sputum Gram stain: Gram-⊕ cocci ▪ Chem 8 **Rx** ▪ Third-generation cephalosporin + azithromycin vs. levofloxacin or gatifloxacin IV	**Ward W/U** ▪ Peak flow: 300 L/min ▪ FEV_1: 2 L ▪ Sputum culture: ⊕ for *S pneumoniae* sensitive to levofloxacin ▪ Blood culture: ⊖ **Rx** ▪ Change to PO levofloxacin ▪ Change to PO prednisone	▪ Taper prednisone over the next two weeks ▪ Smoking cessation ▪ Consider pneumococcal vaccine and flu shot

Final Dx: Chronic obstructive pulmonary disease (COPD) exacerbation/pneumonia

INITIAL MGMT	CONTINUING MGMT	F/U
Emergency room W/U ▪ CXR: Infiltrate/nodules in upper lobes ▪ AFB sputum/culture × 3 days: ⊕ stain ▪ Sputum Gram stain and culture ▪ PPD: 16 mm ▪ CBC ▪ Chem 14 ▪ HIV testing ▪ CT–chest: Infiltrates and cavity consistent with TB **Rx** ▪ Respiratory isolation ▪ Transfer to the ward	**Ward W/U** ▪ Social worker consult **Rx** ▪ INH + rifampin + pyrazinamide + ethambutol ▪ Vitamin B_6	▪ Sputum culture and smear at three months ▪ LFTs ▪ Ophthalmology consult ▪ Family education ▪ Family PPD placement ▪ Report case to the local public health department

Final Dx: Tuberculosis (TB)

CASE 24

HX	PE	DDX
55 yo M presents with cough that is exacerbated when he lies down at night and improves when he props his head up on three pillows. He also reports worsening exertional dyspnea for the past two months (he now has dyspnea at rest). He has had a 25-pound weight gain since his symptoms began. His past medical history is significant for hypertension, an MI five years ago, hyperlipidemia, and smoking.	VS: P 70, BP 120/70, RR 28, O_2 sat 86% room air Gen: Moderate respiratory distress Neck: JVD Lungs: Bibasilar crackles CV: S1/S2/S3 RRR, 3/6 systolic murmur at apex Abd: WNL Ext: +2 bilateral pitting edema	■ CHF ■ COPD exacerbation ■ MI ■ Pericardial tamponade ■ Pulmonary embolism ■ Pulmonary fibrosis ■ Renal failure

CASE 25

HX	PE	DDX
5 yo F presents with shortness of breath. She has a history of recurrent pulmonary infection and fatty, foul-smelling stool. She has also shown failure to thrive and has a history of meconium ileus.	VS: T 38°C (101°F), BP 110/65, HR 110, RR 24 Gen: Pallor, mild respiratory distress, low weight and height for age, dry skin HEENT: Nasal polyps Lungs: Barrel-shaped chest, rales, dullness and ↓ breath sounds over lower lung fields CV: WNL Abd: Abdominal distention, hepatosplenomegaly	■ Asthma ■ Cystic fibrosis ■ Failure to thrive ■ Malabsorption syndrome ■ Sinusitis

INITIAL MGMT	CONTINUING MGMT	F/U
Emergency room STAT ▪ O_2 ▪ IV ▪ IV furosemide ▪ CXR: Pulmonary edema ▪ ECG: Old Q wave in anterior leads **Emergency room W/U** ▪ Cardiac/BP monitoring ▪ CPK-MB, troponin q 8 h ▪ CBC ▪ Chem 8: K 3.4 ▪ Serum calcium, magnesium, phosphate **Rx** ▪ IV KCl ▪ Daily weight ▪ Discontinue any β-blockers ▪ SQ heparin ▪ Low-fat, low-sodium diet	**Ward W/U** ▪ TSH ▪ Lipid profile ▪ Echocardiography: Hypokinesia in anterior wall; EF 20% ▪ Chem 8: K 3.7 **Rx** ▪ Fluid restriction ▪ Lisinopril ▪ Atorvastatin ▪ ASA ▪ Digoxin ▪ Spironolactone ▪ Change IV furosemide ▪ Restart β-blockers (when euvolemic)	▪ Cardiac rehabilitation ▪ Counsel patient re smoking cessation, hypertension, exercise, relaxation, and lipids ▪ Follow up in one week ▪ Refer to cardiology; with ischemic cardiomyopathy and EF < 30%, patients may benefit from an automatic implantable cardiac defibrillator (AICD)

Final Dx: Congestive heart failure (CHF) exacerbation

INITIAL MGMT	CONTINUING MGMT	F/U
Emergency room W/U ▪ CBC: ↓ hemoglobin ▪ Chem 8: ↑ sugar, ↓ albumin ▪ ABG: Hypoxia ▪ CXR: Hyperinflation ▪ Sputum Gram stain and culture ▪ O_2	**Ward W/U** ▪ PFTs ▪ Sweat chloride test: ⊕ ▪ Pancreatic enzymes ▪ 24-hour fecal fat ▪ Dietary consult ▪ Genetics consult ▪ Cystic fibrosis specialist ▪ Pulmonary medicine, pediatrics consults **Rx** ▪ IV normal saline ▪ O_2 ▪ IV piperacillin ▪ Albuterol, inhalation	▪ Follow up in two months ▪ Chest physical therapy ▪ Regular multiple vitamins ▪ Influenza vaccine ▪ Pneumococcal vaccine ▪ Family counseling

Final Dx: Cystic fibrosis (CF)

CASE 26

HX	PE	DDX
65 yo F with a history of hypertension and diabetes mellitus presents with LUQ pain accompanied by fever and a productive cough with purulent yellow sputum.	VS: T 38°C (101°F), P 105, BP 130/75, RR 22, O_2 sat 95% room air Gen: NAD Neck: WNL Lungs: ↓ breath sounds and rhonchi on left side CV: Tachycardia Abd: Tenderness in LUQ	▪ Bronchitis ▪ Infectious mononucleosis ▪ Lung abscess ▪ Lung cancer ▪ Pneumonia ▪ Pyelonephritis ▪ Spleen abscess

CASE 27

HX	PE	DDX
25 yo HIV-⊕ M presents with shortness of breath, malaise, dry cough, fatigue, and fever.	VS: T 38°C (101°F), BP 110/65, HR 110, RR 24 Gen: Pallor, mild respiratory distress, generalized lymphadenopathy HEENT: Oral thrush Lungs: Intercostal reaction; rales and ↓ breath sounds over both lung fields CV: WNL Abd: Soft, nontender; hepatosplenomegaly Ext: Reddish maculopapular rash	▪ CMV ▪ Interstitial pneumonia ▪ Kaposi's sarcoma ▪ Legionellosis ▪ *Mycobacterium avium–intracellulare* ▪ *Pneumocystis jiroveci* pneumonia ▪ TB

INITIAL MGMT	CONTINUING MGMT	F/U
Office W/U ▪ CBC: ↑ WBC count ▪ Chem 8 ▪ UA ▪ Sputum Gram stain: Gram-⊕ cocci ▪ Sputum culture: Pending ▪ CXR: Left lower lobe infiltrate ▪ U/S—abdomen	**Ward W/U** ▪ Sputum culture: ⊕ for *S pneumoniae* **Rx** ▪ IV normal saline ▪ PO levofloxacin ▪ Chest physiotherapy ▪ Acetaminophen ▪ SQ heparin	▪ Discharge home ▪ Continue PO levofloxacin × 14 days

Final Dx: Pneumonia

INITIAL MGMT	CONTINUING MGMT	F/U
Office W/U ▪ CBC ▪ CD4: 200 ▪ Chem 8 ▪ ABG: Hypoxia ▪ Sputum Gram stain and culture ▪ Sputum AFB smear ▪ Bronchial washings—*Pneumocystis* stain (bronchoscopy is a prerequisite along with thoracic surgery consult): ⊕ ▪ CXR: Bilateral interstitial infiltrate ▪ PPD: ⊖	**Office W/U** ▪ LFTs ▪ VDRL ▪ Anti-HCV ▪ HBsAg ▪ Anti-HBc ▪ Serum *Toxoplasma* serology **Rx** ▪ TMP-SMX or pentamidine (if patient cannot tolerate TMP-SMX) ▪ Prednisone ▪ Begin highly active antiretroviral therapy (HAART)	▪ Regular follow-up visits ▪ LFTs ▪ Influenza vaccine ▪ Pneumococcal vaccine ▪ Counsel patient re safe sex practices ▪ HIV support group ▪ Patient counseling ▪ Family counseling

Final Dx: *Pneumocystis jiroveci* pneumonia (PCP)

CHEST PAIN

CASE 28

HX	PE	DDX
40 yo F presents with sudden onset of 8/10 substernal chest pain that began at rest, has lasted for 20 minutes, and radiates to the jaw. The pain is accompanied by nausea. The patient has a prior history of hypertension, hyperlipidemia, and smoking.	VS: P 80, BP 130/60, RR 14, O_2 sat 99% room air Gen: Moderate distress Lungs: WNL CV: WNL Abd: WNL Ext: WNL	▪ Angina ▪ Aortic dissection ▪ Costochondritis ▪ GERD ▪ MI ▪ Pericarditis ▪ Pneumothorax ▪ Pulmonary embolism

CASE 29

HX	PE	DDX
58 yo M was working in his office 30 minutes ago when he suddenly developed right-sided chest discomfort and shortness of breath. He has a prior history of asthma and emphysema.	VS: P 123, BP 101/64, RR 28, O_2 sat 91% room air Gen: Cyanosis, severe respiratory distress Trachea: Deviated to left Lungs: No breath sounds on right side with hyperresonance on percussion CV: Tachycardia; apical impulse displaced to the left Abd: WNL	▪ Angina ▪ Aortic dissection ▪ Asthma exacerbation ▪ Pneumothorax ▪ Pulmonary embolism ▪ Tension pneumothorax

INITIAL MGMT	CONTINUING MGMT	F/U
Emergency room STAT ▪ O_2 ▪ Chewable aspirin ▪ SL nitroglycerin ▪ IV normal saline ▪ IV morphine ▪ ECG: T-wave inversions **Emergency room W/U** ▪ Cardiac/BP monitoring ▪ CPK-MB, troponin q 8 h: ⊖ ▪ CBC ▪ Chem 14 ▪ PT/PTT ▪ CXR ▪ Cardiac catheterization	**ICU W/U** ▪ ECG ▪ Lipid profile ▪ TSH ▪ Echocardiography: 60% ▪ Stress test: ⊕ **Rx** ▪ Enoxaparin ▪ ASA ▪ Clopidogrel ▪ β-blocker (atenolol) ▪ ACEI (enalapril) ▪ Atorvastatin ▪ Cardiology consult	▪ Cardiac rehabilitation ▪ Counsel patient re smoking cessation, hypertension, exercise, relaxation, and lipids ▪ Advise patient to rest at home ▪ Low-fat, low-sodium diet

Final Dx: Unstable angina

INITIAL MGMT	CONTINUING MGMT	F/U
Emergency room STAT ▪ IV normal saline ▪ O_2 ▪ Needle thoracostomy ▪ Chest tube ▪ CXR: Collapsed right lung, mediastinal shift to left ▪ IV morphine **Emergency room W/U** ▪ Cardiac/BP monitoring ▪ ECG: Sinus tachycardia ▪ CBC ▪ Chem 14 ▪ PT/PTT	**Ward W/U** ▪ Thoracic surgery consult ▪ CXR: Inflated right lung **Rx** ▪ Morphine ▪ Chest tube to water seal and vacuum device	**Ward** ▪ Pleurodesis if indicated

Final Dx: Tension pneumothorax

CASE 30

HX	PE	DDX
34 yo F presents with stabbing retrosternal chest pain that radiates to the back. The pain improves when she leans forward and worsens with deep inspiration. She had a URI one week ago.	VS: T 37°C (99.2°F), P 80, BP 130/70, RR 16, O_2 sat 98% room air Gen: NAD Neck: WNL Lungs: WNL CV: S1/S2, pericardial friction rub Abd: WNL Ext: WNL	■ Angina/MI ■ Aortic dissection ■ Costochondritis ■ Esophageal rupture ■ GERD ■ Pericarditis ■ Pneumothorax ■ Pulmonary embolism

CASE 31

HX	PE	DDX
48 yo F presents with palpitations and anxiety. She reports that she feels hot and has to run the air conditioner all the time. She also reports hand tremors. She has lost 10 pounds over the past few months despite her good appetite.	VS: P 113, BP 145/85, RR 20 Gen: Mild respiratory distress, dehydration, sweaty palms and face, warm skin, hand tremor HEENT: Exophthalmos with lid lag, generalized thyromegaly, thyroid bruit Lungs: WNL CV: Tachycardia Abd: WNL Ext: Edema over the tibia bilaterally	■ Anxiety ■ Atrial fibrillation ■ Early menopause ■ Hyperthyroidism ■ Mitral valve prolapse ■ Panic attack ■ Withdrawal syndrome

INITIAL MGMT	CONTINUING MGMT	F/U
Emergency room W/U ▪ Continuous cardiac and BP monitoring ▪ Stat ECG: Diffuse ST elevation, PR depression ▪ CPK-MB, troponin × 3 ▪ CBC ▪ Chem 8 ▪ CXR: No cardiomegaly ▪ ESR **Rx** ▪ ASA or NSAIDs ▪ Start IV ▪ O_2	**Ward W/U** ▪ Discontinue continuous monitoring ▪ Echocardiography: Minimal pericardial effusion **Rx** ▪ Reassure patient ▪ ASA	▪ Discharge home ▪ Follow up in two weeks

Final Dx: Pericarditis

INITIAL MGMT	CONTINUING MGMT	F/U
Office W/U ▪ CBC ▪ BMP ▪ Thyroid studies (T_4, T_3RU, T_3, TSH): ↑ T_3/T_4, ↓ TSH ▪ Serum thyroid autoantibodies: ⊕ ▪ ECG ▪ CXR ▪ Nuclear scan—thyroid: ↑ uptake **Rx** ▪ Propranolol ▪ Methimazole ▪ PTU	**Office W/U** ▪ Endocrinology consult	▪ Check thyroid studies in one month ▪ Patient counseling

Final Dx: Hyperthyroidism

CASE 32

HX	PE	DDX
65 yo M presents with sudden onset of severe tearing anterior chest pain that radiates to the back. He is anxious and diaphoretic. He has a history of long-standing hypertension.	VS: T 36°C (97°F), BP 195/110 right arm, 160/80 left arm, HR 100, RR 30, O_2 sat 98% room air Gen: Acute distress Lungs: WNL CV: Tachycardia, S4, diastolic decrescendo heard best at left sternal border Abd: WNL Ext: Unequal pulse in both arms **Limited PE**	■ Aortic dissection ■ MI ■ Pericarditis ■ Pulmonary embolism

CASE 33

HX	PE	DDX
34 yo F is brought to the ER after a car accident. She is gasping for air and complains of weakness, chest pain, and dizziness.	VS: Afebrile, BP 100/50, HR 115, RR 22, pulsus paradoxus Gen: Confusion, cyanosis, respiratory distress Neck: ↑ JVP, engorged neck veins, Kussmaul's sign Lungs: WNL CV: Muffled heart sounds, ↓ PMI Abd: WNL Ext: WNL	■ Aortic dissection ■ Cardiogenic shock ■ MI ■ Pericardial tamponade ■ Pericarditis ■ Pneumothorax ■ Pulmonary embolism

INITIAL MGMT	CONTINUING MGMT	F/U
Emergency room STAT ▪ ASA ▪ O_2 ▪ IV normal saline ▪ SL nitroglycerin ▪ CXR: Widened mediastinum ▪ IV β-blockers ▪ ECG: LVH ▪ IV morphine **Emergency room W/U** ▪ Cardiac/BP monitoring ▪ CPK-MB, troponin × 3: ⊖ ▪ CBC ▪ Chem 8 ▪ TEE: Aortic dissection type A or ▪ CT–chest with IV contrast: Aortic dissection **Rx** ▪ Thoracic surgery consult	**ICU W/U** ▪ Continuous cardiac and BP monitoring ▪ Blood type and cross-match ▪ PT/PTT, INR **Rx** ▪ Continuing IV β-blockers ▪ Emergent surgery	▪ Diet and lifestyle modifications ▪ Lipid/BP management

Final Dx: Aortic dissection

INITIAL MGMT	CONTINUING MGMT	F/U
Emergency room W/U ▪ O_2 ▪ IV normal saline ▪ NPO ▪ Pulse oximetry ▪ ECG: Tachycardia, low voltage, nonspecific ST- and T-wave changes ▪ CPK-MB ▪ CBC ▪ Chem 8 ▪ ABG ▪ Coagulation profile ▪ Blood type and cross-match ▪ CXR: Cardiomegaly ▪ Echocardiography: Tamponade ▪ Pericardiocentesis	**ICU W/U** ▪ Continuous cardiac and BP monitoring ▪ ECG ▪ Echocardiography ▪ CXR ▪ Cardiac surgery consult ▪ ABG **Rx** ▪ NPO to liquid ▪ O_2 ▪ Follow up in two weeks	▪ CXR ▪ Echocardiography ▪ Patient counseling

Final Dx: Pericardial tamponade

CASE 34

HX	PE	DDX
28 yo F presents with palpitations, chest pain, nausea, and dizziness that last for almost 5–6 minutes. She has had several attacks over the past few weeks. During these episodes, she becomes diaphoretic and occasionally has diarrhea. In the course of some of her attacks, she describes feeling as if she might die.	VS: P 90, BP 125/75, RR 20 Gen: Mild respiratory distress, dehydration, sweating, cold hands HEENT: WNL Lungs: WNL CV: WNL Abd: WNL Ext: WNL	■ Anxiety ■ Asthma attack ■ Atrial fibrillation ■ Early menopause ■ Hyperthyroidism ■ Hyperventilation ■ Hypoglycemia ■ Mitral valve prolapse ■ Panic attack ■ Pheochromocytoma ■ Pulmonary embolus ■ Substance abuse

CASE 35

HX	PE	DDX
32 yo F presents with occasional palpitations, chest pain, and dizziness. She also reports shortness of breath and chest tightness during her attacks.	VS: P 90–200 (variable), BP 125/75, RR 20 Gen: Mild cyanosis HEENT: WNL Lungs: Bibasilar crackles CV: Irregularly irregular, tachycardia Abd: WNL Ext: WNL	■ Anxiety ■ Atrial fibrillation ■ Hyperthyroidism ■ Hyperventilation ■ Mitral valve prolapse ■ Panic attack

INITIAL MGMT	CONTINUING MGMT	F/U
Office W/U		▪ Outpatient follow-up in four weeks
▪ CBC		▪ Psychiatry consult
▪ Chem 8		▪ Patient counseling
▪ UA		▪ Behavioral modification program
▪ Urine toxicology: ⊖		▪ Relaxation exercises
▪ TFTs		
▪ ECG		
▪ CXR		
Rx		
▪ Reassure patient		
▪ Benzodiazepines (eg, alprazolam, lorazepam, clonazepam) or		
▪ SSRIs		

Final Dx: Panic attack

INITIAL MGMT	CONTINUING MGMT	F/U
Emergency room W/U	**ICU W/U**	▪ Follow up in two weeks
▪ IV normal saline	▪ ECG	▪ Patient counseling
▪ O_2	▪ Continuous cardiac monitoring	
▪ CBC	▪ Continuous BP monitoring	
▪ Chem 8	▪ Warfarin	
▪ TFTs	▪ ASA	
▪ ECG: Atrial fibrillation		
▪ CXR: Pulmonary vascular congestion		
▪ Echocardiography: Enlarged left atrium		
Rx		
▪ Synchronous cardioversion		
▪ Amiodarone (give prior to DC cardioversion if possible)		
▪ Propranolol		
▪ Heparin		

Final Dx: Atrial fibrillation

ABDOMINAL PAIN

CASE 36

HX	PE	DDX
38 yo M presents with RUQ abdominal pain of 48 hours' duration. The pain radiates to his right groin and scrotal area and comes in waves of severe intensity that prevent him from finding a comfortable resting position.	VS: T 36°C (96°F), BP 130/85, HR 110, RR 22 Gen: In pain Lungs: WNL CV: Tachycardia Abd: Soft, nontender, no distention, tenderness in right flank, no peritoneal signs, normal BS Rectal exam: WNL, guaiac ⊖	▪ Gastroenteritis ▪ Nephrolithiasis ▪ Pancreatitis ▪ Perforated duodenal ulcer ▪ Retrocecal appendicitis

CASE 37

HX	PE	DDX
60 yo M presents with generalized weakness, left flank discomfort, nausea, and constipation of two weeks' duration. He has lost 20 pounds over the past four months.	VS: T 37°C (99.2°F), P 90, BP 120/60, RR 18 Gen: NAD Lungs: WNL CV: WNL Abd: ↓ BS, left flank tenderness with deep palpation Rectal exam: WNL Ext: WNL Neuro: WNL	▪ Colorectal cancer ▪ Renal abscess ▪ Renal cell carcinoma

CASE 38

HX	PE	DDX
32 yo F presents with two days of progressive flank pain, urinary frequency, and a burning sensation during urination. She also reports associated fever and shaking chills.	VS: T 39.1°C (102°F), BP 130/85, HR 86, RR 18 Gen: Mild discomfort with exam Lungs: WNL CV: Tachycardia Abd: ⊕ BS, mild suprapubic tenderness, no peritoneal signs Back: Mild CVA tenderness on the left Pelvic: WNL Rectal exam: WNL, guaiac ⊖	▪ Acute cervicitis ▪ Acute cystitis ▪ Acute PID ▪ Acute pyelonephritis ▪ Acute urethritis ▪ Ectopic pregnancy ▪ Nephrolithiasis

INITIAL MGMT	CONTINUING MGMT	F/U
Emergency room W/U - CBC: Normal WBC count - Chem 8 - Serum amylase, lipase - UA: Microscopic hematuria - Urine culture - KUB: Radiopaque 3-mm stone - CT—kidney: Stone visualized in distal ureter **Rx** - Analgesia: Narcotics and NSAIDs - Counsel patient re oral hydration	- Serum calcium, magnesium, phosphate - Serum uric acid - Urine strain - Stone analysis: Calcium oxalate	- ↑ fluid intake - Follow up in four weeks - Patient counseling - Counsel patient to limit alcohol intake - Counsel patient to limit caffeine intake - Smoking cessation

Final Dx: Nephrolithiasis

INITIAL MGMT	CONTINUING MGMT	F/U
Office W/U - CBC: Hemoglobin 9.0 - Chem 14: Ca 15, BUN 40, creatinine 2.0 - UA: ⊕ for RBCs - CXR - U/S—complete abdominal: Left renal mass - Admit to ward **Rx** - IV normal saline - Bisphosphonate (pamidronate)	**Ward W/U** - Intact PTH: ↓ - Chem 7: Ca 10, BUN 20, creatinine 1.5 - CT—abdomen and chest: Left renal mass - Renal mass biopsy - Bone scan - CT—head - Ferritin, TIBC, serum iron **Rx** - Oncology consult - Surgery consult	

Final Dx: Renal cell carcinoma

INITIAL MGMT	CONTINUING MGMT	F/U
Office W/U - CBC: ↑ WBC count - Chem 8 - UA: WBC, bacteria, nitrite ⊕ - Urine culture: Pending - Urinary β-hCG: ⊖ - U/S—renal **Rx** - Ciprofloxacin (fluoroquinolone)	**Office W/U** - Urine culture: ⊕ for *E coli*	- Follow up in 3–5 days - Patient counseling - Counsel patient re medication compliance - Counsel patient to limit alcohol intake

Final Dx: Pyelonephritis

CASE 39

HX	PE	DDX
10 yo African-American M presents with sudden onset of jaundice, dark-colored urine, back pain, and fatigue. He was started on TMP-SMX for an ear infection a few days ago. He has a family history of blood disorders.	VS: T 38°C (99.8°F), P 90, BP 110/50, RR 14 Gen: NAD Skin: Jaundice HEENT: Icterus, pallor Lungs: WNL CV: WNL Abd: WNL Ext: WNL	■ Autoimmune hemolytic anemia ■ DIC ■ G6PD deficiency ■ Sickle cell anemia ■ Spherocytosis ■ Thalassemias ■ TTP

CASE 40

HX	PE	DDX
58 yo alcoholic M presents with a one-day history of sharp epigastric pain that radiates to his back. He is nauseated and has vomited several times. He also complains of anorexia. The patient reports heavy alcohol use over the past 2–3 days. He has no previous history of peptic ulcer disease.	VS: T 38.2°C (101°F), BP 138/68, HR 110, RR 22 Gen: WD/WN but agitated, lying on bed with knees drawn up Lungs: ↓ breath sounds over left lower lung CV: Tachycardia Abd: Tender and distended with ↓ BS	■ Acute cholecystitis ■ Acute gastritis ■ Acute pancreatitis ■ Aortic dissection ■ Cholelithiasis ■ Intestinal perforation ■ MI ■ Perforated duodenal ulcers ■ Pneumonia

INITIAL MGMT	CONTINUING MGMT	F/U
Office W/U ▪ CBC stat and q 12 h: ↓↓ hemoglobin, ↓↓ hematocrit ▪ Peripheral smear: Bite cells, fragment cells ▪ Chem 14: ↑ indirect bilirubin ▪ PT/PTT, INR **Rx** ▪ Discontinue TMP-SMX	**Ward W/U** ▪ Reticulocyte count: Elevated ▪ LDH: ↑ ▪ Haptoglobin: ↓ ▪ UA: Hemoglobinuria ▪ G6PD assay: Consistent with G6PD deficiency ▪ Type and cross two units of packed RBCs **Rx** ▪ Start IV ▪ IV normal saline ▪ Transfuse two units of packed RBCs	▪ Discharge home ▪ Follow up in two months ▪ Educate patient/family

Final Dx: G6PD deficiency

INITIAL MGMT	CONTINUING MGMT	F/U
Emergency room W/U ▪ IV normal saline ▪ NPO ▪ Monitor, continue BP cuff ▪ NG tube suction ▪ ECG: No evidence of ischemia ▪ CBC ▪ Chem 14 ▪ Serum amylase, lipase: ↑ ▪ ABG ▪ O_2 ▪ Pulse oximetry ▪ LFTs ▪ Serum calcium ▪ AXR, upright ▪ CXR **Rx** ▪ NG tube ▪ IV meperidine	**Ward W/U** ▪ Monitor, continue BP cuff ▪ Continue NPO ▪ U/S—liver, gallbladder and bile duct, pancreas ▪ PT/PTT ▪ CT—abdomen ▪ Surgery consult ▪ GI consult ▪ Advance diet as tolerated	▪ Follow up in seven days ▪ Patient counseling ▪ Counsel patient to cease alcohol intake ▪ Smoking cessation

Final Dx: Acute pancreatitis

CASE 41

HX	PE	DDX
1-day-old M born at home is brought to the ER because of bilious vomiting, irritability, poor feeding, lethargy, and an acute episode of rectal bleeding.	VS: T 38°C (100°F), P 170, BP 69/44, RR 43, O_2 sat 89% room air Skin: Evidence of poor perfusion Chest: WNL CV: WNL Abd: Distention; evidence of intestinal obstruction **Limited PE**	▪ Duodenal web ▪ Intestinal atresia ▪ Malrotation with volvulus ▪ Meconium plug/ileus ▪ Necrotizing enterocolitis

CASE 42

HX	PE	DDX
21-month-old M is brought to the ER because of intermittent abdominal pain that causes him to become still while drawing up his legs. He also presents with irritability and vomiting that initially was clear but then became bilious. The child seemed lethargic between the pain episodes. In the ER, the child passes some dark red stool.	VS: T 38.5°C (101°F), P 157, BP 81/59, RR 35, O_2 sat 93% room air Skin: No evidence of purpura Chest: WNL CV: WNL Abd: Soft and mildly tender; examination of RUQ fails to identify presence of bowel; ill-defined mass in the RUQ **Limited PE**	▪ Intoxication ▪ Intussusception ▪ Metabolic disease ▪ Neurologic disease ▪ Small bowel obstruction ▪ Volvulus

INITIAL MGMT	CONTINUING MGMT	F/U
Emergency room STAT ■ IV normal saline ■ O_2 ■ ABG: Metabolic acidosis **Emergency room W/U** ■ CBC: ↑ WBC count, mildly ↓ hemoglobin ■ Chem 8 ■ AXR: Airless rectum; large gastric bubble ■ CXR: No evidence of diaphragmatic hernia **Rx** ■ NG tube suction ■ IV bicarbonate (to correct acidosis if pH < 7.0) ■ Pediatric surgery consult	**Ward W/U** ■ Upper GI series: Bird's beak, corkscrew appearance of proximal jejunum ■ Barium enema: Cecum in RUQ **Rx** ■ NG tube suction ■ IV normal saline	■ Follow up in 48 hours ■ Family counseling

Final Dx: Malrotation with volvulus

INITIAL MGMT	CONTINUING MGMT	F/U
Emergency room STAT ■ IV normal saline ■ O_2 **Emergency room W/U** ■ CBC: ↑ WBC count ■ Chem 14 ■ ABG: Metabolic acidosis ■ AXR: Distended bowel with air-fluid levels; mass in right abdomen ■ U/S—abdomen: Compatible with intussusception **Rx** ■ NG tube suction ■ Barium enema: Coiled-spring appearance; disorder is relieved by air insufflation ■ Pediatric surgery consult	**Ward W/U** ■ AXR: Gastric bubble; no air-fluid levels ■ ABG: Derangements being resolved **Rx** ■ D/C NG tube suction ■ IV normal saline ■ Advance diet	■ Follow up in 48 hours ■ Family counseling

Final Dx: Intussusception

CASE 43

HX	PE	DDX
27-month-old M presents to the ER with seizures, irritability, anorexia, altered sleep patterns, emotional lability, and vomiting. His mother states that the family has been living for about a year in an old, poorly maintained building that has only recently begun to undergo renovation. Since she was laid off at the battery plant, the family has been considering moving out of town.	VS: T 37°C (99°F), P 129, BP 89/61, RR 20, O_2 sat 92% room air Neuro: Lethargy, ataxia, seizures. Remainder of physical examination is noncontributory (except for some conjunctival pallor)	▪ Lead toxicity ▪ Metabolic disease ▪ Neurologic disease ▪ Nonmetal intoxication ▪ Other heavy metal toxicity

CASE 44

HX	PE	DDX
7-day-old alert M presents to a clinic with jaundice that started two days ago. The baby was born at term via an uneventful vaginal delivery and started breast-feeding after some delay. The mother states that she took the baby to the doctor's office at that time and that the baby's bilirubin was 14 mg/dL. The mother does not take any drugs. She is very concerned that the baby's jaundice is not improving and asks if the baby has kernicterus.	VS: T 37°C (99°F), P 129, BP 80/51, RR 29, O_2 sat 94% room air PE: WNL except for jaundice Neuro: WNL	▪ Breast-feeding jaundice ▪ Hereditary spherocytosis ▪ Physiologic hyperbilirubinemia ▪ Unconjugated hyperbilirubinemia (Gilbert's/Crigler-Najjar)

CASE 45

HX	PE	DDX
31 yo M comes to the office complaining of midepigastric pain that usually begins 1–2 hours after eating and sometimes awakens him at night. He also has occasional indigestion. He is taking an antacid for his problem. He denies melena or hematemesis.	VS: T 37.1°C (99°F), BP 130/75, HR 100, RR 16 Gen: Pallor, no distress Lungs: WNL CV: WNL Abd: Epigastric tenderness Rectal exam: WNL	▪ Acute gastritis ▪ Diverticulitis ▪ GERD ▪ Mesenteric ischemia ▪ Pancreatic disease ▪ Peptic ulcer disease

INITIAL MGMT	CONTINUING MGMT	F/U
Emergency room W/U ▪ CBC: Hemoglobin 9 g/dL, MCV 75, blood smear reveals coarse basophilic stippling in RBCs ▪ Chem 8 ▪ Serum lead: 80 μg/dL ▪ UA: Glycosuria ▪ Free erythrocyte protoporphyrin: ↑ ▪ Serum toxicology: ↑ lead levels **Rx** ▪ IV normal saline ▪ IM EDTA	**Ward Rx** ▪ IV normal saline ▪ Serum lead ▪ IM EDTA (if necessary) ▪ Family counseling	▪ Follow up in seven days ▪ Family counseling ▪ Lead paint assay in home

Final Dx: Lead intoxication with encephalopathy

INITIAL MGMT	CONTINUING MGMT	F/U
Office W/U ▪ CBC: WNL, smear WNL ▪ Direct Coombs' test: Noncontributory ▪ Serum bilirubin: ↑ indirect bilirubin ▪ TSH: WNL	**Office W/U** ▪ Breast-feeding suppression test: Bilirubin levels ↓ on cessation of breast-feeding; levels ↑ again when breast-feeding restarted **Rx** ▪ Continue breast feedings ▪ Consider phototherapy (if bilirubin levels do not ↓)	▪ Follow up in seven days ▪ Family counseling

Final Dx: Breast-feeding neonatal jaundice

INITIAL MGMT	CONTINUING MGMT	F/U
Office W/U ▪ CBC ▪ Chem 8 ▪ Serum amylase, lipase ▪ Serum *H pylori* antibody ▪ Stool *H pylori* antibody **Rx** ▪ Proton pump inhibitor ▪ Clarithromycin (Biaxin) ▪ Metronidazole		▪ Follow up in four weeks; patient reports that he is feeling better (if symptoms persist or if *H pylori* is still present, may proceed to endoscopy) ▪ Patient counseling ▪ Counsel patient to limit alcohol intake ▪ Smoking cessation

Final Dx: Gastritis (*H pylori* infection)

CASE 46

HX	PE	DDX
45 yo M presents with a six-week history of jaundice, pale stools, tea-colored urine, and epigastric pain that radiates to the back. He also reports that he has bilateral lower extremity swelling.	VS: T 37°C (98°F), BP 130/70, HR 90, RR 16 Gen: Jaundice Lungs: WNL CV: WNL Abd: Palpable epigastric mass Ext: Lower extremity swelling with pain on dorsiflexion of ankle	▪ Cholangiocarcinoma ▪ Colon/stomach cancer with metastases in the porta hepatis region causing biliary obstruction ▪ Pancreatic cancer

CASE 47

HX	PE	DDX
60 yo F G0 presents with a two-month history of ↑ abdominal girth, ↓ appetite, and early satiety. She also has mild shortness of breath.	VS: T 36°C (97°F), BP 140/60, HR 90, RR 23 Gen: Pallor Breast: WNL Lungs: WNL CV: WNL Abd: Distended, nontender, normal BS, no palpable hepatosplenomegaly Pelvic: Solid right adnexal mass Rectal exam: Solid right adnexal mass; no involvement of rectovaginal septum	▪ CHF ▪ Liver cirrhosis ▪ Ovarian cancer

CASE 48

HX	PE	DDX
32 yo F presents with sudden onset of left lower abdominal pain that radiates to the scapula and back and is associated with vaginal bleeding. Her last menstrual period was five weeks ago. She has a history of pelvic inflammatory disease and unprotected intercourse.	VS: T 37°C (99°F), P 90, BP 120/50, RR 14 Gen: Moderate distress 2° to pain Lungs: WNL CV: WNL Abd: RLQ tenderness, rebound, and guarding Pelvic: Slightly enlarged uterus with small amount of dark bloody discharge from cervix; right adnexal tenderness	▪ Ectopic pregnancy ▪ Ovarian torsion ▪ PID ▪ Ruptured ovarian cyst

INITIAL MGMT	CONTINUING MGMT	F/U
Office W/U ▪ CBC ▪ Chem 14 ▪ Bilirubin, ALT, AST, alkaline phosphatase ▪ CT—abdomen: Large necrotic pancreatic mass in head ▪ ERCP/EUS: Biopsy to obtain histology	**Ward Rx** ▪ Medical oncology consult; palliative care ▪ Surgery is not an option owing to advanced disease	

Final Dx: Pancreatic cancer

INITIAL MGMT	CONTINUING MGMT	F/U
Office W/U ▪ CBC ▪ Chem 14 ▪ CA-125: 900 ▪ CT—abdomen and pelvis: 10- × 12-cm right complex ovarian cyst; severe ascites ▪ CXR: Right moderate pleural effusion ▪ ECG ▪ Pap smear ▪ Mammogram ▪ Colonoscopy ▪ Gynecology consult	**Ward Rx** ▪ Blood type and cross-match ▪ PT/PTT, INR ▪ Exploratory laparotomy ▪ TAH-BSO, laparotomy ▪ Staging, laparotomy	▪ Carboplatin ▪ CA-125 ▪ CBC ▪ Chem 14

Final Dx: Ovarian cancer

INITIAL MGMT	CONTINUING MGMT	F/U
Emergency room W/U ▪ Urinary β-hCG: ⊕ ▪ Quantitative serum β-hCG: 2500 ▪ CBC ▪ Chem 8 ▪ Cervical Gram stain and G&C culture ▪ U/S—transvaginal: 2-cm right adnexal mass, no intrauterine pregnancy, free fluid in cul-de-sac **Rx** ▪ IV normal saline	▪ Blood type and cross-match ▪ PT/PTT, INR ▪ Gynecology consult ▪ Laparoscopy ▪ Rh IgG (RhoGAM) if Rh-⊖	▪ Counsel patient on contraception ▪ Counsel patient re safe sex practices

Final Dx: Ectopic pregnancy

CASE 49

HX	PE	DDX
74 yo M presents with LLQ abdominal pain, fever, and chills for the past three days. He also reports recent-onset episodes of alternating diarrhea and constipation. He consumes a low-fiber, high-fat diet.	VS: T 38°C (101°F), BP 130/85, HR 100, RR 22 Gen: Pallor, diaphoresis Lungs: WNL CV: Tachycardia Abd: LLQ tenderness, no peritoneal signs, sluggish BS Rectal exam: Guaiac ⊖	■ Crohn's disease ■ Diverticular abscess ■ Diverticulitis ■ Gastroenteritis ■ Ulcerative colitis

CASE 50

HX	PE	DDX
41 yo F presents with sudden-onset RUQ abdominal pain of six hours' duration. She also reports nausea and emesis. The pain started after lunch and has become more severe and constant. She reports that the pain is exacerbated by deep breathing and that it radiates to her shoulder. She had a similar attack almost one year ago. She is taking OCPs and has three children.	VS: T 39.0°C (102°F), BP 130/82, HR 80, RR 16 Gen: WD, slightly obese, moderate distress Lungs: WNL CV: WNL Abd: Obesity, tenderness and guarding to palpation on RUQ, ⊕ Murphy's sign, ↓ BS Rectal exam: WNL, guaiac ⊖	■ Acute appendicitis ■ Acute cholangitis ■ Acute cholecystitis ■ Acute hepatitis ■ Acute pancreatitis ■ Acute peptic ulcer disease with or without perforation ■ Biliary atresia ■ Cardiac ischemia ■ Cholelithiasis ■ Fitz-Hugh–Curtis syndrome (gonococcal perihepatitis) ■ Gastritis ■ Renal colic ■ Right-sided pneumonia ■ Small bowel obstruction

INITIAL MGMT	CONTINUING MGMT	F/U
Emergency room W/U ▪ CBC: ↑ WBC count ▪ Chem 14 ▪ Serum amylase, lipase ▪ UA ▪ Urine culture: Pending ▪ Blood culture: Pending ▪ Stool culture and sensitivity ▪ Stool for ova and parasites ▪ CXR ▪ KUB ▪ CT—abdomen: Diverticulitis **Rx** ▪ NPO ▪ IV normal saline ▪ IV metronidazole + ciprofloxacin	**Ward W/U** ▪ Urine culture: Pending ▪ Blood culture: Pending **Rx** ▪ NPO or clear liquid diet ▪ Surgery consult ▪ Metronidazole + ciprofloxacin × 7–10 days ▪ Discharge home in 3–4 days	▪ High-fiber diet ▪ Colonoscopy four weeks after recovery

Final Dx: Diverticulitis

INITIAL MGMT	CONTINUING MGMT	F/U
Emergency room W/U ▪ IV normal saline ▪ NPO ▪ Monitor, continue BP cuff ▪ ECG ▪ CBC ▪ Chem 14 ▪ Serum amylase, lipase ▪ LFTs ▪ Blood/urine cultures ▪ AXR/CXR ▪ Pregnancy test—urine ▪ U/S—abdomen: Gallstones with gallbladder edema **Rx** ▪ IM prochlorperazine ▪ IV morphine ▪ IV cefuroxime	**Ward W/U** ▪ Blood type and cross-match ▪ PT/PTT, INR ▪ Surgery consult for cholecystectomy ▪ Vitals q 4 h ▪ CBC next day ▪ Chem 8 next day **Rx** ▪ NPO → advance diet as tolerated ▪ Continue antibiotic therapy	▪ Follow up in two weeks ▪ Patient counseling ▪ Counsel patient to limit alcohol intake

Final Dx: Acute cholecystitis

CASE 51

HX	PE	DDX
24 yo F presents with bilateral lower abdominal pain that started with the first day of her menstrual period. The pain is associated with fever and a thick, greenish-yellow vaginal discharge. She has had unprotected sex with multiple sexual partners.	VS: T 38°C (100.4°F), P 90, BP 110/50, RR 14 Gen: Moderate distress 2° to pain Lungs: WNL CV: WNL Abd: Diffuse tenderness (greatest in the lower quadrants), no rebound, no distention, ↓ BS Pelvic: Purulent, bloody discharge from cervix; cervical motion and bilateral adnexal tenderness Rectal exam: WNL Ext: WNL	▪ Dysmenorrhea ▪ Endometriosis ▪ PID ▪ Pyelonephritis ▪ Vaginitis

CASE 52

HX	PE	DDX
25 yo M is brought to the ER because of abdominal pain and ↓ appetite for four days. This episode was preceded by ↑ urinary frequency, nausea, and vomiting.	VS: T 37°C (98°F), P 120, BP 100/60, RR 25 Gen: Moderate distress Skin: Poor skin turgor HEENT: Dry mucous membranes, "fruity breath" Lungs: WNL CV: Tachycardia Abd: Generalized tenderness Ext: WNL Neuro: WNL **Limited PE**	▪ Acute intestinal obstruction ▪ Alcoholic ketoacidosis ▪ Appendicitis ▪ DKA ▪ Drug intoxication ▪ Gastroenteritis ▪ Pancreatitis ▪ Pyelonephritis

INITIAL MGMT	CONTINUING MGMT	F/U
Emergency room W/U ▪ Urinary β-hCG: ⊖ ▪ CBC: ↑ WBC count ▪ Chem 14 ▪ Cervical Gram stain and G&C culture ▪ U/S—pelvis ▪ UA and urine culture **Rx** ▪ IV normal saline ▪ IV ceftriaxone + PO doxycycline or PO azithromycin ▪ Acetaminophen	**Ward W/U** ▪ Cervical culture: *N gonorrhoeae* **Rx** ▪ Discontinue **IV** ceftriaxone when symptoms improve (usually in 24–48 hours) ▪ Switch to doxycycline or clindamycin	▪ Counsel patient re safe sex practices ▪ Treat partners

Final Dx: Pelvic inflammatory disease (PID)

INITIAL MGMT	CONTINUING MGMT	F/U
Emergency room STAT ▪ Glucometer: 480 mg/dL ▪ IV normal saline **Emergency room W/U** ▪ Continuous monitoring ▪ Chem 14: Normal K, normal Na, ↑ anion gap ▪ CBC: ↑ WBC count ▪ Serum amylase, lipase ▪ UA and urine culture: ⊕ glucose, ⊕ ketone ▪ Urine/serum toxicology ▪ Phosphate: ↓ ▪ ECG ▪ ABG: Metabolic acidosis (pH = 7.1) ▪ Quantitative serum ketones: ↑ ▪ Serum osmolality: Normal ▪ CXR/AXR **Rx** ▪ IV regular insulin, continue ▪ Phosphate therapy	**ICU W/U** ▪ Continuous monitoring ▪ Random glucose q 1 h ▪ Chem 8 q 4 h: ↓ K, glucose < 250 **Rx** ▪ Switch IV fluid to D_5W ▪ IV potassium ▪ SQ insulin NPH ▪ SQ insulin regular ▪ Discontinue IV insulin two hours after starting long-acting insulin (NPH or Lantus)	▪ Diabetic diet ▪ Diabetic teaching ▪ HbA_{1c} q 3 months ▪ Follow up in two weeks in the office ▪ Diabetic foot care ▪ Ophthalmology consult ▪ Lipid profile ▪ Instruct patient in home sugar monitoring ▪ Home sugar monitoring, glucometer

Final Dx: Diabetic ketoacidosis (DKA)

CONSTIPATION/DIARRHEA

CASE 53

HX	PE	DDX
67 yo M presents with constipation, ↓ stool caliber, and blood in his stool for the past eight months. He also reports unintentional weight loss. He is on a low-fiber diet and has a family history of colon cancer.	VS: P 85, BP 140/85, RR 14, O_2 sat 98% room air Gen: NAD HEENT: Pale conjunctivae Lungs: WNL CV: WNL Abd: WNL Pelvic: WNL Rectal exam: Hemoccult ⊕	▪ Angiodysplasia ▪ Colorectal cancer ▪ Diverticulosis ▪ GI parasitic infection (ascariasis, giardiasis) ▪ Hemorrhoids ▪ Hypothyroidism ▪ Inflammatory bowel disease ▪ Irritable bowel syndrome

CASE 54

HX	PE	DDX
28 yo M presents with diffuse abdominal pain, loose stools, perianal pain, mild fever, and weight loss over the past four weeks. He denies any history of travel or recent use of antibiotics.	VS: T 37°C (99°F), BP 130/65, HR 70, RR 14 Gen: NAD Lungs: WNL CV: WNL Abd: WNL Rectal exam: Perianal skin tags, hemoccult ⊕	▪ Crohn's disease ▪ Diverticulitis ▪ Gastroenteritis ▪ Infectious colitis ▪ Irritable bowel syndrome ▪ Ischemic colitis ▪ Lactose intolerance ▪ Pseudomembranous colitis ▪ Small bowel lymphoma ▪ Ulcerative colitis

CASE 55

HX	PE	DDX
30 yo F presents with periumbilical crampy pain of six months' duration. The pain never awakens her from sleep. It is relieved by defecation and worsens when she is upset. She has alternating constipation and diarrhea but no nausea, vomiting, weight loss, or anorexia.	VS: Afebrile, P 85, BP 130/65, RR 14 Gen: NAD Lungs: WNL CV: WNL Abd: WNL Pelvic: WNL Rectal exam: Guaiac ⊖	▪ Celiac disease ▪ Chronic pancreatitis ▪ Colorectal cancer ▪ Crohn's disease ▪ Diverticulosis ▪ Endometriosis ▪ GI parasitic infection (ascariasis, giardiasis) ▪ Hypothyroidism ▪ Inflammatory bowel disease ▪ Irritable bowel syndrome

INITIAL MGMT	CONTINUING MGMT	F/U
Office W/U ▪ CBC: ↓ hematocrit, ↓ MCV ▪ Chem 8: Normal ▪ Ferritin: ↓ ▪ Serum iron: ↓ ▪ TIBC: ↑ ▪ TSH: Normal ▪ Stool for ova and parasites ▪ ESR: Normal ▪ Stool guaiac: ⊕	**Office W/U** ▪ GI consult ▪ Colonoscopy: Polyp with adenocarcinoma ▪ CT—abdomen and pelvis with contrast ▪ CEA **Rx** ▪ Iron sulfate ▪ General surgery consult ▪ Plan partial colectomy	

Final Dx: Colorectal cancer

INITIAL MGMT	CONTINUING MGMT	F/U
Office W/U ▪ CBC ▪ Chem 14 ▪ Serum amylase, lipase ▪ Stool for ova and parasites ▪ Stool *C difficile* ▪ AXR ▪ Colonoscopy: Crohn's disease **Rx** ▪ 5-ASA ▪ Metronidazole (for perianal abscess or fistula)		▪ Follow up in two weeks ▪ Counsel patient re medication compliance and adherence

Final Dx: Crohn's disease

INITIAL MGMT	CONTINUING MGMT	F/U
Office W/U ▪ CBC ▪ Chem 14 ▪ TSH ▪ Stool for ova and parasites ▪ Stool for WBCs ▪ Stool culture and sensitivity ▪ Transglutaminase antibody **Rx** ▪ Educate patient ▪ Reassurance ▪ High-fiber diet ▪ Lactose-free diet		▪ Follow up in four weeks ▪ Call with questions

Final Dx: Irritable bowel syndrome

CASE 56

HX	PE	DDX
8 yo M is brought to the clinic by his mother for intermittent diarrhea alternating with constipation together with vomiting and cramping abdominal pain. His mother also reports that he has had progressive anorexia.	VS: T 37°C (98°F), BP 110/65, HR 90, RR 16 Gen: Pale and dry mucosal membranes; lack of growth Lungs: WNL CV: WNL Abd: WNL Ext: Muscle wasting, especially in gluteal area	▪ Bacterial gastroenteritis ▪ Celiac disease ▪ Food allergy ▪ Giardiasis ▪ Protein intolerance ▪ Viral gastroenteritis

CASE 57

HX	PE	DDX
28 yo M reports intermittent episodes of vomiting and diarrhea along with cramping abdominal pain for the past two days. He describes his stool as watery. He returned from Mexico three days ago.	VS: T 39°C (101.9°F), BP 135/85, HR 100, RR 22 Gen: Mild dehydration Lungs: WNL CV: WNL Abd: Mild tenderness, no peritoneal signs, hyperactive BS Rectal exam: WNL, guaiac ⊖	▪ *Campylobacter* infection ▪ Cholera ▪ *C difficile* colitis ▪ Crohn's disease ▪ Gastroenteritis ▪ Giardiasis ▪ Salmonellosis ▪ Shigellosis

CASE 58

HX	PE	DDX
40 yo F presents with fever, anorexia, nausea, profuse and watery diarrhea, and diffuse abdominal pain. Last week she was on antibiotics for a UTI.	VS: T 38°C (100.4°F), BP 100/50, HR 100, RR 22, orthostatic hypotension Gen: WNL Lungs: WNL CV: Tachycardia Abd: Diffuse tenderness, no peritoneal signs, ⊕ BS Rectal exam: Guaiac ⊕	▪ Amebiasis ▪ Food poisoning ▪ Gastroenteritis ▪ Giardiasis ▪ Hepatitis A ▪ Infectious diarrhea (bacterial, viral, parasitic, protozoal) ▪ Inflammatory bowel disease ▪ Pseudomembranous (*C difficile*) colitis ▪ Traveler's diarrhea

INITIAL MGMT	CONTINUING MGMT	F/U
Office W/U ▪ CBC ▪ Chem 14 ▪ UA ▪ Stool for ova and parasites ▪ Stool occult blood ▪ Stool Gram stain ▪ Stool fat stain ▪ Barium enema ▪ CT—abdomen ▪ Ferritin ▪ Serum folate ▪ Serum B_{12} ▪ Serum endomysial antibody: ⊕ titers ▪ Serum transglutaminase antibody: ⊕ titers	**Ward W/U** ▪ CXR: Normal ▪ KUB: Normal ▪ CT—abdomen: Normal ▪ D-xylose tolerance test: Carbohydrate malabsorption ▪ Peroral duodenal biopsy: Villi are atrophic or absent ▪ Dietary consult **Rx** ▪ Gluten-free diet ▪ Prednisone ▪ Vitamin D ▪ Calcium	▪ Follow up in one week ▪ Patient counseling ▪ Pneumococcal vaccine

Final Dx: Celiac disease

INITIAL MGMT	CONTINUING MGMT	F/U
Emergency room W/U ▪ CBC ▪ Chem 14 ▪ Stool culture ▪ Fecal leukocyte stain ▪ Stool for *C difficile* ▪ Stool Gram stain ▪ Stool for ova and parasites ▪ Stool occult blood ▪ Stool fat stain ▪ UA and urine culture	**Emergency room W/U** ▪ Stool culture: ⊕ for *E coli* ▪ Stool Gram stain: ⊕ for gram-⊖ rods and ↑ leukocytes **Rx** ▪ Oral hydration ▪ Ciprofloxacin	▪ Follow up in one week ▪ Patient counseling ▪ Counsel patient to limit alcohol intake ▪ Smoking cessation

Final Dx: Gastroenteritis

INITIAL MGMT	CONTINUING MGMT	F/U
Emergency room W/U ▪ Stool culture ▪ Stool *Giardia* antigen ▪ Stool for ova and parasites ▪ Stool WBCs: ⊕ ▪ Stool for *C difficile:* ⊕ ▪ CBC: ↑ WBC count ▪ Chem 14 **Rx** ▪ IV normal saline ▪ Metronidazole	**Ward W/U** ▪ No orthostatic hypotension **Rx** ▪ Send home on metronidazole (when diarrhea improves); no Lomotil/Imodium	▪ Counsel patient re oral hydration

Final Dx: Pseudomembranous (*C difficile*) colitis

CASE 59

HX	PE	DDX
33 yo M presents with foul-smelling, watery diarrhea together with diffuse abdominal cramps and bloating that began yesterday. He also vomited once. He was recently in Mexico.	VS: T 37°C (98°F), BP 110/50, HR 85, RR 22, no orthostatic hypotension Gen: WNL Lungs: WNL CV: WNL Abd: No tenderness, no peritoneal signs, active BS Rectal exam: Guaiac ⊖	▪ Amebiasis ▪ Food poisoning ▪ Gastroenteritis ▪ Giardiasis ▪ Hepatitis A ▪ Infectious diarrhea (bacterial, viral, parasitic, protozoal) ▪ Inflammatory bowel disease ▪ Pseudomembranous (*C difficile*) colitis ▪ Traveler's diarrhea

GI BLEEDING

CASE 60

HX	PE	DDX
38 yo M presents with intermittent hematemesis of two weeks' duration. He has a history of epigastric pain for almost two years that occasionally worsens when he eats food or drinks milk. He also reports melena of three weeks' duration. His social history is significant for alcohol and tobacco use.	VS: T 37°C (98.9°F), BP 90/65, HR 110, RR 24 Gen: Pallor Lungs: WNL CV: WNL Abd: No tenderness, no peritoneal signs, normal BS Rectal exam: WNL, guaiac ⊕ **Limited PE**	▪ Duodenal ulcers ▪ Esophageal tear ▪ Gastric carcinoma ▪ Gastric ulcer ▪ Portal hypertension

INITIAL MGMT	CONTINUING MGMT	F/U
Office W/U ■ Stool culture ■ Stool *Giardia* antigen: ⊕ ■ Stool for ova and parasites ■ Stool WBCs ■ Stool for *C difficile* ■ CBC ■ Chem 8 **Rx** ■ Metronidazole		■ Counsel patient re oral hydration

Final Dx: Giardiasis

INITIAL MGMT	CONTINUING MGMT	F/U
Emergency room STAT ■ IV normal saline ■ O_2 ■ Orthostatic vitals: Drop on standing ■ Type and cross-match **Emergency room W/U** ■ CBC: Hematocrit 24 ■ Chem 14 ■ Upper GI series: Gastric antral lesion with adherent clot ■ PT/PTT, INR ■ CXR ■ ECG **Rx** ■ NPO ■ NG tube, iced saline lavage: Clears with 1 L of normal saline ■ IV pantoprazole ■ IV cimetidine	**ICU W/U** ■ CBC q 4 h until hematocrit is stable; then frequency can be ↓ **Rx** ■ GI consult ■ Combination therapy with epinephrine injection followed by thermal coagulation ■ Octreotide for varices ■ Advance diet ■ Ranitidine ■ Pantoprazole ■ Transfer to wards if patient remains stable ■ *H pylori* serology and eradication if ⊕	■ Follow up in one week ■ Patient counseling ■ Counsel patient to cease alcohol intake ■ Smoking cessation ■ Dietary consult

Final Dx: Bleeding gastric ulcer

CASE 61

HX	PE	DDX
67 yo F presents with acute crampy abdominal pain, weakness, and black stool. She reports diffuse abdominal pain of three months' duration. Eating worsens the pain. She has had a five-pound weight loss over the last three months.	VS: T 37°C (98.9°F), BP 90/65, HR 100, RR 24 Gen: Mild dehydration Lungs: WNL CV: WNL Abd: Tender and mildly distended; no rigidity or rebound tenderness Rectal exam: WNL, guaiac ⊕ **Limited PE**	▪ Adenocarcinoma of the colon ▪ Crohn's disease ▪ Diverticular bleed ▪ Infectious colitis ▪ Ischemic colitis ▪ Peptic ulcer disease ▪ Ulcerative colitis

CASE 62

HX	PE	DDX
30 yo M presents with loose, watery stools that are streaked with blood and mucus. He has also had colicky abdominal pain and weight loss over the past three weeks. He denies any history of travel, radiation, or recent medication use (antibiotics, NSAIDs).	VS: T 37°C (99°F), BP 130/65, HR 70, RR 14 Gen: NAD Lungs: WNL CV: WNL Abd: WNL Rectal exam: Blood-stained stool	▪ Crohn's disease ▪ Diverticulitis ▪ Gastroenteritis ▪ Infectious colitis ▪ Internal hemorrhoid ▪ Ischemic colitis ▪ Pseudomembranous colitis ▪ Radiation colitis ▪ Ulcerative colitis

INITIAL MGMT	CONTINUING MGMT	F/U
Emergency room STAT ▪ IV normal saline ▪ O_2 **Emergency room W/U** ▪ CBC ▪ Chem 14 ▪ Serum amylase: Normal ▪ LDH: ↑ ▪ PT/PTT ▪ CXR ▪ ECG ▪ AXR ▪ CT–abdomen: Pneumatosis coli ▪ Blood type and cross-match **Rx** ▪ NPO ▪ Surgery consult (for bowel resection) ▪ Broad-spectrum antibiotics ▪ NG tube suction	**Ward W/U** ▪ Hemoglobin and hematocrit q 4 h **Rx** ▪ Advance diet ▪ Monitor carefully for persistent fever, leukocytosis, peritoneal irritation, diarrhea, and/or bleeding	▪ Follow up in four weeks ▪ Patient counseling ▪ Counsel patient to cease alcohol intake ▪ Smoking cessation ▪ Dietary consult

Final Dx: Ischemic colitis

INITIAL MGMT	CONTINUING MGMT	F/U
Office W/U ▪ CBC: Mild anemia ▪ Chem 14 ▪ Serum amylase, lipase ▪ Stool culture and sensitivity ▪ Stool for ova and parasites ▪ Stool WBCs ▪ PT/PTT ▪ Flexible sigmoidoscopy and rectal biopsy: Consistent with ulcerative colitis involving rectum and distal sigmoid colon **Rx** ▪ IV steroids (for attack) or ▪ 5-ASA enema/suppositories ▪ Sulfasalazine		▪ Follow up in two weeks ▪ Counsel patient re medication compliance and adherence

Final Dx: Ulcerative colitis

CASE 63

HX	PE	DDX
58 yo M presents with painless bright red blood in his stool. He reports that his diet is low in fiber.	VS: T 37°C (98°F), BP 130/85, HR 90, RR 20 Gen: Pallor, diaphoresis Lungs: WNL CV: WNL Abd: Soft, nontender, no peritoneal signs, ⊕ BS Rectal exam: Bloody stool	■ Colon cancer ■ Crohn's disease ■ Diverticulitis ■ Diverticulosis ■ Ulcerative colitis

HEMATURIA

CASE 64

HX	PE	DDX
71 yo Asian M presents with a three-month history of low back pain that is 3/6 in severity and steady with no radiation. He has BPH and denies any history of trauma.	VS: T 37°C (98.5°F), P 76, BP 140/75, RR 14 Gen: NAD Neck: WNL Back: Tenderness along lumbar spine (L4, L5) Lungs: WNL CV: WNL Abd: WNL Rectal exam: Irregular, enlarged prostate; hemoccult ⊖ Ext: WNL Neuro: WNL	■ Disk herniation ■ Lumbar muscle strain ■ Muscular spasm ■ Osteoporosis ■ Prostate cancer ■ Sciatic irritation ■ Spinal stenosis ■ Tumor in the vertebral canal

CASE 65

HX	PE	DDX
40 yo M complains of a slow-onset dull pain in his left flank and blood in his urine. His father died of a stroke.	VS: T 37°C (98°F), P 98, BP 150/95, RR 18 Gen: WD/WN HEENT: WNL Lungs: WNL CV: WNL (no pericardial rub) Abd: Palpable, nontender mass on both flanks Ext: WNL	■ Polycystic kidney disease ■ Renal cell carcinoma ■ Renal dysplasia ■ Simple renal cysts ■ Tuberous sclerosis ■ Wilms' tumor

INITIAL MGMT	CONTINUING MGMT	F/U
Emergency room W/U - NPO - IV normal saline - CBC: ↓ hemoglobin - Chem 14 - PT/PTT - Serum amylase, lipase - UA - CXR - CT—abdomen: Diverticulosis	**Ward W/U** - Colonoscopy: Diverticulosis, no other source **Rx** - NPO → clear liquid diet - Surgery consult - GI consult	- Follow up in four weeks - Patient counseling - Counsel patient to cease alcohol intake - Smoking cessation - Dietary consult - High-fiber diet

Final Dx: Diverticulosis

INITIAL MGMT	CONTINUING MGMT	F/U
Office W/U - CBC - Chem 14 - UA: Hematuria - ESR: ↑ - PSA: ↑↑ - XR—back: Metastatic lesions in L4 and L5 - CT—lumbar spine: Mets to L4 and L5 - Echo—rectal: Multinodular enlarged prostate - Prostate biopsy: Pending **Rx** - Acetaminophen - Morphine or codeine if pain persists	**Office W/U** - Bone scan: Diffuse metastases - Prostate biopsy: Adenocarcinoma - CT—abdomen and pelvis: ⊕ for lymphatic involvement above aortic bifurcation **Rx** - Flutamide (antiandrogen therapy) or - Urology consult - Radiation oncology consult	- Patient counseling

Final Dx: Prostate cancer

INITIAL MGMT	CONTINUING MGMT	F/U
Office W/U - CBC - Chem 8 - UA: Hematuria - U/S—renal or CT—abdomen: Bilateral renal cysts, enlarged kidneys, no liver cysts - CT—head: No berry aneurysms **Rx** - ACEIs (eg, captopril, enalapril, lisinopril)	**Office W/U** - Nephrology consult (to look for evidence of renal insufficiency)—creatinine > 2 mg/dL - Urology consult (for nephrectomy, cyst decompression, or unroofing)	- Follow up in eight weeks with blood testing and ultrasound - Patient counseling - Counsel patient to cease alcohol intake - Smoking cessation - Dietary consult - Low-sodium diet - Counsel patient to avoid sports

Final Dx: Polycystic kidney disease

CASE 66

HX	PE	DDX
10 yo M presents with tea-colored urine and periorbital edema. He had a fever and sore throat one week ago. He also complains of malaise, weakness, and anorexia.	VS: T 36°C (97.5°F), BP 140/85, HR 88, RR 18 Gen: Periorbital edema, pallor Lungs: WNL CV: WNL Abd: WNL Ext: Edema around ankles	- Cryoglobulinemia - IgA nephropathy - Membranoproliferative glomerulonephritis - Poststreptococcal glomerulonephritis (PSGN)

OTHER URINARY SYMPTOMS

CASE 67

HX	PE	DDX
70 yo M complains of waking up 4–5 times a night to urinate. He also has urgency, a weak stream, and dribbling, and he needs to strain to initiate urination. He denies any weight loss, fatigue, or bone pain. He also has a sensation of incomplete evacuation of urine from the bladder.	VS: T 37°C (98.5°F), P 78, BP 140/85, RR 14 Gen: NAD Neck: WNL Lungs: WNL CV: WNL Abd: WNL Rectal exam: Enlarged, nodular, nontender, rubbery prostate gland Ext: WNL	- Benign prostatic hypertrophy - Bladder cancer - Bladder stones - Bladder trauma - Chronic pelvic pain - Cystitis - Neurogenic bladder - Prostate cancer - Prostatitis - Urethral strictures - UTI

CASE 68

HX	PE	DDX
39 yo M complains of sudden-onset fever and chills, urgency and burning on urination, and perineal pain. His symptoms started after he underwent urethral dilation for stricture.	VS: T 37.3°C (99°F), P 65, BP 101/64, RR 16 Gen: No acute distress Lungs: WNL CV: WNL Abd: Suprapubic tenderness GU: Genitalia WNL Rectal exam: Asymmetrically swollen, firm, markedly tender, hot prostate	- Acute cystitis - Anal fistulas and fissures - Epididymitis - Obstructive calculus - Orchitis - Prostatitis - Pyelonephritis - Reiter's syndrome - Urethritis

INITIAL MGMT	CONTINUING MGMT	F/U
Emergency room W/U ▪ CBC ▪ Chem 8 ▪ UA: Hematuria, proteinuria, RBC casts ▪ 24-hour urine protein: Proteinuria ▪ ASO titer: Normal ▪ Throat culture: Pending ▪ Total serum complement: ↓ **Rx** Furosemide Captopril Penicillin	**Office W/U** ▪ U/S—renal ▪ Throat culture: ⊕ **Rx** ▪ Furosemide ▪ Captopril ▪ Nephrology consult	▪ Follow up in three weeks with UA and periodic BP monitoring ▪ Family counseling ▪ Dietary consult ▪ Low-sodium diet ▪ Restrict fluid intake

Final Dx: Acute glomerulonephritis (PSGN)

INITIAL MGMT	CONTINUING MGMT	F/U
Office W/U ▪ CBC ▪ BMP: Creatinine ▪ UA ▪ Urine culture ▪ U/S—prostate ▪ ESR ▪ Total serum PSA ▪ Residual urinary volume **Rx** ▪ Finasteride ▪ Prazosin (selective short-acting α-blockers)	**Office W/U** ▪ Urology consult ▪ Urodynamic studies	▪ Follow up in six months with digital rectal examination and PSA ▪ Patient counseling ▪ Dietary consult

Final Dx: Benign prostatic hypertrophy (BPH)

INITIAL MGMT	CONTINUING MGMT	F/U
Office W/U ▪ UA ▪ Urine Gram stain and culture ▪ CBC ▪ Chem 8 ▪ VDRL **Rx** ▪ TMP-SMX or fluoroquinolone	**Office W/U** ▪ Urology consult ▪ Cystoscopy	▪ Follow up in four weeks ▪ Patient counseling ▪ Counsel patient to cease alcohol intake ▪ Smoking cessation ▪ Counsel patient re safe sex practices ▪ Treat sexual partner

Final Dx: Prostatitis

CASE 69

HX	PE	DDX
21 yo M complains of a burning sensation during urination and urethral discharge. He recently began having unprotected sex with a new partner. He denies urinary frequency, urgency, fever, chills, sweats, or nausea.	VS: T 37.3°C (98.9°F), P 65, BP 101/64, RR 14 Gen: NAD Lungs: WNL CV: WNL Abd: Mild suprapubic tenderness GU: Erythema of urethral meatus, no penile lesions, pus expressed from urethra	■ Acute cystitis ■ Epididymitis ■ Foreign body ■ Nephrolithiasis ■ Orchitis ■ Prostatitis ■ Pyelonephritis ■ Reiter's syndrome ■ Urethritis

CASE 70

HX	PE	DDX
20 yo F presents with a two-day history of dysuria, ↑ urinary frequency, and suprapubic pain. She is sexually active only with her husband. She has no flank pain, fever, or nausea.	VS: P 65, BP 101/64, RR 16 Gen: NAD Lungs: WNL CV: WNL Abd: Mild suprapubic tenderness Pelvic: WNL	■ Acute cystitis ■ Nephrolithiasis ■ PID ■ Pyelonephritis ■ Urethritis ■ Vaginitis

INITIAL MGMT	CONTINUING MGMT	F/U
Office W/U ▪ UA and urine culture ▪ Urethral Gram stain: Many WBCs/hpf without bacteria ▪ Urethral G&C culture (for *Neisseria gonorrhoeae* and *Chlamydia trachomatis*) ▪ CBC ▪ VDRL **Rx** ▪ Azithromycin (single dose) ▪ Ceftriaxone (single dose)		▪ Follow up in four weeks ▪ Patient counseling ▪ Treat partner ▪ Counsel patient re safe sex practices

Final Dx: Urethritis

INITIAL MGMT	CONTINUING MGMT	F/U
Office W/U ▪ UA: ↑↑ WBCs, +4 bacteria, ⊕ nitrites, ⊕ esterase ▪ Urine culture ▪ CBC ▪ Chem 8 ▪ Pregnancy test—urinary **Rx** TMP-SMX × 3 days	**Office W/U** ▪ Urine culture: ⊕ for *E coli* sensitive to TMP-SMX **Rx** ▪ TMP-SMX	

Final Dx: Acute cystitis

AMENORRHEA

CASE 71

HX	PE	DDX
21 yo F complains of irregular menstrual periods every 3–5 months since menarche at age 15. She also complains of facial hair, weight gain, acne, and darkening of the skin in her axillae.	VS: T 36°C (97°F), P 80, BP 120/80, RR 14 Gen: Obese Skin: Thick hair on face, chest, and buttocks; thickened skin in axillae Lungs: WNL CV: WNL Abd: WNL Pelvic: WNL	■ Adrenal tumor ■ Cushing's syndrome ■ Idiopathic hirsutism ■ Late-onset congenital adrenal hyperplasia ■ Ovarian neoplasm ■ Polycystic ovarian syndrome

CASE 72

HX	PE	DDX
50 yo F presents with hot flashes and dyspareunia. Her last menstrual period was six months ago.	VS: T 36°C (97°F), BP 120/60, HR 70, RR 13 Gen: NAD HEENT: WNL Breast: WNL Lungs: WNL CV: WNL Abd: WNL Pelvic: Atrophy of vaginal mucosa	■ Hyperthyroidism ■ Hypothyroidism ■ Menopause ■ Pregnancy ■ Prolactinoma

INITIAL MGMT	CONTINUING MGMT	F/U
Office W/U ▪ DHEAS ▪ Testosterone: ↑ ▪ U/S—pelvis: Ovaries with multiple small cysts ▪ Serum 17-hydroxyprogesterone ▪ LH/FSH: ↑ ▪ Prolactin ▪ TSH/free T_4 ▪ Insulin/fasting glucose **Rx** ▪ Weight loss ▪ Exercise program ▪ OCPs ▪ Spironolactone ▪ Smoking cessation		▪ Follow up in six months

Final Dx: Polycystic ovarian syndrome (PCOS)

INITIAL MGMT	CONTINUING MGMT	F/U
Office W/U ▪ Urine pregnancy test ▪ Prolactin ▪ TSH ▪ FSH: ↑ ▪ Wet mount ▪ Pap smear ▪ Mammogram ▪ DEXA scan **Rx** ▪ Calcium ▪ Vitamin D ▪ SSRI (venlafaxine) for hot flashes ▪ Premarin (vaginal estrogen) ▪ Vaginal jelly for lubrication		▪ Follow up in 12 months ▪ Counsel patient re HRT—not recommended unless only short-term treatment is planned and if the patient has no CAD, breast cancer, or thromboembolic risk factors

Final Dx: Menopause

CASE 73

HX	PE	DDX
14 yo F is brought into the office by her mother. The mother is concerned because her daughter is considerably shorter than her classmates and because her daughter has not yet had her menses. The girl's parents are of normal height, and her sisters had their menses at age 13.	VS: Afebrile, BP 110/70, HR 70, RR 12 Gen: Short stature HEENT: Low posterior hairline, high-arched palate Neck: Short and wide Lungs: Widely spaced nipples CV: Tachycardia, irregular	■ Constitutional growth delay ■ Familial short stature ■ Hypopituitarism ■ Hypothyroidism ■ Turner's syndrome

VAGINAL BLEEDING

CASE 74

HX	PE	DDX
21 yo F complains of prolonged and excessive menstrual bleeding and menstrual frequency for the past six months.	VS: T 36°C (97°F), P 65, BP 120/60, RR 14 Gen: NAD HEENT: WNL Lungs: WNL CV: WNL Abd: WNL GU: WNL	■ Bleeding disorder ■ Dysfunctional uterine bleeding ■ Fibroids ■ Hyperthyroidism ■ Hypothyroidism ■ Pregnancy

INITIAL MGMT	CONTINUING MGMT	F/U
Office W/U ▪ TSH ▪ FSH: ↑ ▪ LH: ↑ ▪ Karyotyping: Consistent with Turner's syndrome ▪ Lipid panel ▪ Fasting glucose **Rx** ▪ Growth hormone therapy ▪ Estrogen + progestin ▪ Psychiatry consult for IQ estimation ▪ Vitamin D ▪ Calcium	**Office W/U** ▪ 2D echocardiography ▪ U/S—renal ▪ U/S—pelvis: Streaked ovaries ▪ Skeletal survey: Short fourth metacarpal ▪ Chem 13 ▪ CBC ▪ UA ▪ Lipid profile ▪ Hearing test **Rx** ▪ Continue growth hormone therapy until epiphysis is closed ▪ Combination estrogen and progestin ▪ Encourage weight-bearing exercises	▪ Stop growth hormone when bone age > 15 years ▪ Audiogram every 3–5 years ▪ Check yearly for hypertension ▪ Monitor aortic root diameter every 3–5 years

Final Dx: Turner's syndrome

INITIAL MGMT	CONTINUING MGMT	F/U
Office W/U ▪ Qualitative urine pregnancy test ▪ TSH ▪ CBC: Hypochromic microcytic anemia ▪ Bleeding time ▪ PT/aPTT, INR ▪ U/S—pelvis ▪ Pap smear **Rx** Iron sulfate NSAIDs OCPs		▪ Follow up in six months ▪ Counsel patient re safe sex practices

Final Dx: Dysfunctional uterine bleeding

CASE 75

HX	PE	DDX
27 yo F whose last menstrual period was seven weeks ago presents with lower abdominal cramping and heavy vaginal bleeding.	VS: T 36°C (97°F), BP 120/60, HR 80, RR 12 Gen: NAD Lungs: WNL CV: WNL Abd: Suprapubic tenderness with no rebound or guarding Pelvic: Active bleeding from cervix, cervical os open, seven-week-size uterus, mildly tender, no cervical motion tenderness, no adnexal masses or tenderness	▪ Cervical or vaginal pathology (polyp, infection, neoplasia) ▪ Cervical polyp ▪ Ectopic pregnancy ▪ Menstrual period with dysmenorrhea ▪ Spontaneous abortion

CASE 76

HX	PE	DDX
60 yo F G0 who had her last menstrual period 10 years ago presents with mild vaginal bleeding for the last two days. Her medical history is significant for type 2 diabetes, hypertension, and infertility.	VS: T 36°C (97°F), BP 120/60, HR 80, RR 14 Gen: NAD HEENT: WNL Lungs: WNL CV: WNL Abd: WNL Pelvic: WNL	▪ Atrophic endometritis ▪ Cervical cancer ▪ Endometrial cancer ▪ Endometrial polyp

CASE 77

HX	PE	DDX
32 yo F G2P1011 presents with vaginal bleeding after intercourse for the last month. She has no history of abnormal Pap smears or STDs and has had the same partner for the last eight years. She uses OCPs.	VS: WNL Gen: NAD Abd: WNL Pelvic: Visible cervical lesion Rectal exam: ⊖, guaiac ⊖	▪ Cervical cancer ▪ Cervical polyp ▪ Cervicitis ▪ Ectropion ▪ Vaginal cancer ▪ Vaginitis

INITIAL MGMT	CONTINUING MGMT	F/U
Emergency room W/U ▪ Qualitative urine pregnancy test: ⊕ ▪ Quantitative serum β-hCG: 3000 ▪ CBC: Hemoglobin 9 ▪ Blood type and cross-match ▪ Rh factor ▪ U/S—pelvis: Intrauterine pregnancy sac, fetal pole, no fetal heart tones ▪ Gynecology consult **Rx** ▪ Fluids, IV normal saline ▪ D&C	**Ward W/U** ▪ CBC **Rx** ▪ Methylergonovine ▪ Doxycycline ▪ Counsel patient re birth control ▪ Grief counseling ▪ Pelvic rest for two weeks	▪ Follow up in three weeks

Final Dx: Spontaneous abortion

INITIAL MGMT	CONTINUING MGMT	F/U
Office W/U ▪ CBC ▪ Chem 14 ▪ PT/PTT, INR ▪ Bleeding time ▪ Pap smear ▪ Endometrial biopsy: Poorly differentiated endometrioid adenocarcinoma ▪ U/S—pelvis: 10-mm endometrial stripe ▪ Gynecology consult	**Ward W/U** ▪ CXR ▪ ECG ▪ CA-125 **Rx** ▪ Exploratory laparotomy ▪ TAH-BSO ▪ Depending on staging, patient may benefit from adjuvant therapy (radiation vs. chemo vs. hormonal therapy)	

Final Dx: Endometrial cancer

INITIAL MGMT	CONTINUING MGMT	F/U
Office W/U ▪ UA ▪ Pap smear: HGSIL ▪ Pelvic: Visible cervical lesion ▪ G&C culture or PCR ▪ Wet mount ▪ Gynecology consult	**Office W/U** ▪ Colposcopy ▪ Cervical biopsy: Invasive squamous cell carcinoma of the cervix	▪ Radical hysterectomy vs. radiation therapy ▪ +/– adjuvant chemoradiotherapy ▪ Console patient

Final Dx: Cervical cancer

MUSCULOSKELETAL PAIN

CASE 78

HX	PE	DDX
28 yo F complains of multiple facial and bodily injuries. She claims that she fell on the stairs. She was hospitalized for some physical injuries seven months ago. She denies any abuse.	VS: P 90, BP 120/64, RR 22, O_2 sat 95% room air Gen: Moderate distress with shallow breathing HEENT: 2.5-cm bruise on forehead; 2-cm bruise on left cheek Chest/lungs: Severe tenderness on left fifth and sixth ribs; CTA bilaterally CV: WNL Abd: WNL Ext: WNL Neuro: WNL	▪ Accident proneness ▪ Domestic violence ▪ Substance abuse

CASE 79

HX	PE	DDX
28 yo F presents with joint pain and swelling along with a butterfly-like rash over her nasal bridge and cheeks that worsens after exposure to the sun. She also reports pleuritic chest pain, shortness of breath, myalgia, and fatigue over the past few months. She says that her joint pain tends to move from joint to joint and primarily involves her hands, wrists, knees, and ankles. She also has weight loss, loss of appetite, and night sweats.	VS: T 38°C (101°F), BP 140/95, HR 80, RR 18 Gen: Pallor, fatigue HEENT: Oral ulcers, malar rash Lungs: CTA, pleural friction rub CV: WNL Abd: WNL Ext: Maculopapular rash over arms and chest; effusion in knees, wrists, and ankles	▪ Dermatomyositis ▪ Drug reaction ▪ Photosensitivity ▪ Polymyositis ▪ SLE

INITIAL MGMT	CONTINUING MGMT	F/U
Emergency room W/U ▪ XR—ribs: Fracture of left fifth and sixth ribs ▪ Urine toxicology ▪ CT—head ▪ Skeletal survey: Old fracture in forearm **Rx** ▪ Ibuprofen ▪ Oxycodone PRN ▪ Splint ▪ Counsel patient re domestic abuse ▪ Counsel patient re safety plan		▪ Support group referral ▪ Social work referral

Final Dx: Domestic abuse

INITIAL MGMT	CONTINUING MGMT	F/U
Office W/U ▪ CBC: ↓ hemoglobin ▪ BMP ▪ PT/PTT ▪ ESR: ↑ ▪ Serum ANA: ⊕ ▪ UA: Proteinuria ▪ CXR ▪ Total complement: ↓ C3 and C4 **Rx** ▪ NSAIDs	**Office W/U** ▪ Anti-dsDNA or SLE prep: ⊕ ▪ Bone densitometry **Rx** ▪ Prednisone ▪ NSAIDs ▪ Rheumatology consult ▪ Nephrology consult	▪ Follow up in four weeks with UA ▪ Patient counseling ▪ Counsel patient to cease alcohol intake ▪ Smoking cessation ▪ Sunblock

Final Dx: Systemic lupus erythematosus (SLE)

CASE 80

HX	PE	DDX
35 yo M with a history of hypertension presents with pain and swelling in his left knee for the last three days. He was recently started on HCTZ for his hypertension. He is sexually active only with his wife and denies any history of trauma or IV drug abuse.	VS: T 38°C (100.7°F), P 80, BP 130/60, RR 12 Gen: In pain Skin: WNL HEENT: WNL Lungs: WNL CV: WNL Abd: WNL Ext: Left knee is swollen, erythematous, and tender with limited range of motion and effusion	▪ Bacterial arthritis ▪ Gout ▪ Infective endocarditis ▪ Lyme disease ▪ Pseudogout ▪ Psoriatic arthritis ▪ Reiter's arthritis

CASE 81

HX	PE	DDX
40 yo M with a history of diabetes mellitus presents with pain, swelling, and discoloration of his right leg for the last week. He denies any trauma.	VS: T 38°C (100.5°F), P 70, BP 120/60, RR 12 Gen: NAD Lungs: WNL CV: WNL Abd: WNL Ext: +2 edema in right lower extremity; warmth, erythematous discoloration of skin, 20-cm ulcer	▪ Calf tear or pull ▪ Cellulitis ▪ Deep venous thrombosis ▪ Lymphedema ▪ Osteomyelitis ▪ Popliteal (Baker's) cyst ▪ Venous insufficiency

CASE 82

HX	PE	DDX
50 yo M complains of a single episode of steady, diffuse, aching pain that affected his skeletal muscles and made it difficult for him to climb stairs. He states that he has never experienced anything like this before and that no one in his family has had a disease similar to his. Because of his ↑ LDL cholesterol, ↓ HDL cholesterol, and ↑ triglycerides, he was started on simvastatin and gemfibrozil about one year ago.	VS: T 37°C (99°F), P 85, BP 127/85, RR 20, O_2 sat 94% room air HEENT and neck: No dysarthria, dysphagia, diplopia, or ptosis; exam WNL Chest: WNL CV: WNL Abd: WNL Ext: Proximal muscle weakness that is more obvious in lower limbs; no evidence of myotonia	▪ Cocaine abuse ▪ Inclusion body myositis ▪ Myopathy due to drugs/toxins ▪ Myotonic dystrophy ▪ Polymyositis

INITIAL MGMT	CONTINUING MGMT	F/U
Office W/U ▪ CBC: ↑ WBC count ▪ Chem 14 ▪ ESR: ↑ ▪ PT/PTT, INR ▪ XR—left knee ▪ Joint aspiration fluid analysis: Gram stain ⊖, culture ⊖, ⊖ birefringent and needle-shaped crystals, WBC 8000 ▪ Urethral Gram stain: ⊖ **Rx** ▪ NSAIDs or corticosteroids ▪ Discontinue HCTZ and start losartan	**Ward W/U** ▪ Blood culture: ⊖ ▪ Urethral culture: ⊖ ▪ Lyme serology: ⊖ ▪ CBC: WBC is trending down **Rx** ▪ Continue NSAIDs and corticosteroids until patient improves ▪ Low-purine diet	▪ Follow up in two weeks in the clinic ▪ Uric acid ↑ ▪ Low-purine diet ▪ Start allopurinol or colchicine (to prevent an attack if serum uric acid > 12 or if the patient has tophaceous gout)

Final Dx: Gout

INITIAL MGMT	CONTINUING MGMT	F/U
Emergency room W/U ▪ CBC: ↑ WBC count ▪ Chem 14 ▪ PT/PTT ▪ U/S—left lower extremity: ⊖ for deep venous thrombosis ▪ ESR ▪ X-ray ▪ Blood culture: Pending **Rx** ▪ IV ampicillin-sulbactam ▪ Surgical consult: Debridement of ulcers	**Ward W/U** ▪ Blood culture: ⊖ ▪ Blood glucose: Controlled on insulin regimen ▪ CBC: WBC is trending down **Rx** ▪ Elevate the leg ▪ Switch to amoxicillin when patient is afebrile and symptoms improve (usually in 3–5 days) ▪ Discharge home	▪ Two weeks later his leg is back to normal ▪ Amoxicillin is discontinued after a course of 14 days

Final Dx: Cellulitis

INITIAL MGMT	CONTINUING MGMT	F/U
Emergency room W/U ▪ IV normal saline ▪ CBC ▪ BMP ▪ Serum CPK: ↑ ▪ LDH: ↑ ▪ EMG: Muscle injury ▪ UA: Myoglobinuria **Rx** ▪ Counsel patient re medication side effects ▪ NSAIDs	**Ward W/U** ▪ CPK, LDH: ↑ ▪ UA: ⊕ for myoglobin **Rx** ▪ Stop the offending simvastatin and gemfibrozil	▪ Follow up in four weeks ▪ Patient counseling ▪ Rest at home ▪ Counsel patient re medication side effects

Final Dx: Myopathy due to simvastatin and gemfibrozil

CASE 83

HX	PE	DDX
21 yo F stripper complains of hot, swollen, painful knee joints following an asymptomatic dermatitis that progressed from macules to vesicles and pustules. She admits using IV drugs, binge drinking, and having sex with multiple partners. She states that about three weeks ago, during a trip to Mexico, she had dysuria, frequency, and urgency during her menses, followed a few days later by bilateral conjunctivitis.	VS: T 39°C (102°F), P 122, BP 138/82, RR 28, O_2 sat 96% room air HEENT and neck: WNL Chest: Four vesicles on thoracic skin CV: WNL Abd: Three vesicles and one pustule on abdominal skin Ext: Knee joints are hot, swollen, and tender; ↓ ROM due to severe pain	▪ *Chlamydia trachomatis* infection ▪ *Neisseria gonorrhoeae* infection ▪ Reactive arthritis ▪ *S aureus* infection ▪ *Streptococcus* infection

CASE 84

HX	PE	DDX
25-month-old M is brought to the ER because of sudden respiratory distress. His mother does not remember the boy's immunization, developmental, or nutritional history. She calmly states that her son fell from a sofa a few days ago, and that this accident explains the boy's reluctance to walk. She adds that her son has been exposed to sick children lately and that she has used coin rubbing and cupping as folk medicine practices.	VS: T 37°C (99°F), P 129, BP 82/59, RR 40, O_2 sat 89% room air Gen: Undernourished HEENT: Circumferential cord marks around neck Lungs: Clear; pain with exam CV: Tachycardia; I/VI systolic murmur Abd: Bruising over nipples Ext: Circumferential burns of both feet and ankles with a smooth, clear-cut border; light brown bruises; pain on palpation of right lower limb Neuro/psych: Withdrawn, apprehensive	▪ Accidental trauma ▪ Child abuse ▪ Deliberate criminal violence (home invasion)

INITIAL MGMT	CONTINUING MGMT	F/U
Emergency room W/U ▪ CBC: ↑ WBC count ▪ GC culture assay: ⊕ ▪ Blood culture: ⊖ ▪ Arthrocentesis ▪ Joint fluid analysis ▪ Joint fluid culture: Pending ▪ Throat culture: Pending ▪ Anorectal culture: Pending ▪ Urine β-hCG: ⊖ **Rx** ▪ NSAIDs ▪ Antibiotics: Azithromycin (for *C trachomatis*), penicillin (if susceptible), ceftriaxone (if not resistant), or fluoroquinolones (if not resistant)	**Ward W/U** ▪ Joint fluid analysis and culture: 60,000 leukocytes/mL, ⊕ for *N gonorrhoeae* ▪ Throat culture ▪ Anorectal culture **Rx** ▪ Azithromycin (for *C trachomatis*), penicillin (if susceptible), ceftriaxone (if not resistant), or fluoroquinolones (if not resistant) ▪ Joint drainage and irrigation (if indicated) ▪ Arthroscopy (if indicated)	▪ Follow up in one week ▪ Patient counseling ▪ Counsel patient re safe sex practices ▪ Treat sexual partner ▪ Counsel patient to cease illegal drug use ▪ Counsel patient to cease alcohol intake ▪ Smoking cessation ▪ Rest at home

Final Dx: Septic arthritis due to *N gonorrhoeae* infection

INITIAL MGMT	CONTINUING MGMT	F/U
Emergency room W/U ▪ CBC ▪ PT/aPTT ▪ Electrolyte panel, BUN, creatinine ▪ CXR: Posterior rib fractures ▪ Skeletal survey: Posterior rib fractures; obliquely oriented callus formation in right femur ▪ CT—head: Short-length skull fractures; small subdural hemorrhages ▪ Ophthalmologic exam: Bilateral retinal hemorrhages **Rx** ▪ Admission to hospital ▪ IV fluids ▪ Neurosurgery consult ▪ Ventilator (if necessary)	**Ward W/U** ▪ Child abuse report ▪ Social work/Child Protective Services evaluation in hospital ▪ Ventilator (if necessary) ▪ IV fluids	▪ Child Protective Services

Final Dx: Nonaccidental trauma (child abuse)

CASE 85

HX	PE	DDX
36 yo F complains of malaise, anorexia, unintended weight loss, and morning stiffness together with swollen and painful wrist, knee, and ankle joints of two years' duration. Initially, she disregarded her symptoms, as they were insidious. However, over time they persisted and ↑ in severity. An acute disabling episode prompted her to visit the office.	VS: T 38°C (100°F), P 95, BP 132/86, RR 20, O_2 sat 95% room air HEENT and neck: Cervical lymphadenopathy Chest: WNL CV: WNL Ext: Symmetric wrist, knee, and ankle joint swelling with tenderness and warmth; subcutaneous nodules over both olecranon prominences; no ulnar deviation of fingers, boutonnière deformity, or swan-neck deformity; no evidence of carpal tunnel syndrome; knee valgus is observed	■ Gout ■ Lyme disease ■ Osteoarthritis ■ Paraneoplastic syndrome ■ Rheumatoid arthritis ■ Sarcoidosis

CASE 86

HX	PE	DDX
45 yo F bus driver comes to the clinic complaining of pain radiating down the leg that followed back pain. The pain is aggravated by coughing, sneezing, straining, or prolonged sitting.	VS: T 37°C (99°F), P 86, BP 128/86, RR 20, O_2 sat 93% room air Trunk: Lumbar spine mobility ↓ due to pain Ext: ⊕ straight leg raising (Lasègue) sign; ⊕ crossed straight leg sign Neuro: Weak plantar flexion of foot; loss of Achilles tendon reflex	■ Cauda equina syndrome ■ Compression fracture ■ Facet joint degenerative disease ■ Lumbar disk herniation ■ Spinal stenosis ■ Tumor involving the spine causing radiculopathy

INITIAL MGMT	CONTINUING MGMT	F/U
Office W/U ▪ CBC: Hypochromic normocytic anemia, thrombocytosis ▪ ESR: ↑ ▪ XR—joints: Soft tissue swelling, juxta-articular demineralization, joint space narrowing, erosions in juxta-articular margin ▪ RF: High titer **Rx** ▪ Ibuprofen or celecoxib ▪ Intra-articular triamcinolone (for acute disabling episodes)	**Office W/U** ▪ RF: High titer ▪ Joint fluid analysis: Abnormalities suggesting inflammation **Rx** ▪ Methotrexate (if unresponsive to NSAIDs) ▪ Etanercept (if unresponsive to methotrexate); place PPD ▪ Hydroxychloroquine for mild disease	▪ Follow up in four weeks ▪ Patient counseling ▪ Physical therapy ▪ Occupational therapy ▪ Rest at home ▪ Exercise program ▪ Splint extremity ▪ Ophthalmologic consult if using hydrochloroquine

Final Dx: Rheumatoid arthritis

INITIAL MGMT	CONTINUING MGMT	F/U
Office W/U ▪ None initially **Rx** ▪ Conservative treatment ▪ Pain control (NSAIDs)	**Office W/U** ▪ MRI—lumbar spine: Disk herniation at L5–S1 level (MRI is not routinely ordered for a disk herniation; it is ordered if conservative treatment fails) **Rx** ▪ Conservative treatment ▪ Orthopedic surgery consult (if conservative treatment fails)	▪ Follow up in two weeks ▪ Patient counseling ▪ Rest at home

Final Dx: Lumbar disk herniation

CHILD WITH FEVER

CASE 87

HX	PE	DDX
40-day-old M is brought to the ER because of irritability and lethargy, vomiting, and ↓ oral intake of three days' duration. Today his parents noted that he had a fever of 101.5°F, and he subsequently had a seizure. The baby's weight at delivery was 2500 grams, and he has been well.	VS: T 39°C (102°F), P 160, BP 77/50, RR 40, O_2 sat 92% room air Gen: Irritable infant Lungs: Clear CV: Tachycardia; I/VI systolic murmur Abd: WNL Neuro/psych: Bulging fontanelle, ↓ responsiveness	▪ CNS fungal infection (in immunocompromised patients) ▪ HIV infection (in immunocompromised patients) ▪ Meningitis (viral or bacterial) ▪ Osteomyelitis ▪ Pneumonia ▪ Sepsis ▪ UTI

CASE 88

HX	PE	DDX
4-month-old M is brought to the ER because of apneic episodes following a runny nose, cough, labored breathing, wheezing, and fever of two days' duration. His asthmatic mother was diagnosed with rubella infection during her pregnancy. The baby was delivered prematurely at 28 weeks. The boy has a history of respiratory difficulty and tachycardia, and he has missed several of his health maintenance appointments.	VS: T 39°C (102°F), P 160, BP 77/50, RR 40, O_2 sat 88% room air Gen: Irritable infant Lungs: Tachypnea, intercostal retractions, nasal flaring, expiratory wheezing, bilateral crackles CV: Tachycardia; continuous II/VI murmur Abd: WNL Neuro/psych: Fontanelle is soft and flat; infant is irritable	▪ Asthma ▪ CHF ▪ Cystic fibrosis ▪ Pneumonia ▪ RSV bronchiolitis

INITIAL MGMT	CONTINUING MGMT	F/U
Emergency room W/U ▪ CBC ▪ Blood cultures ▪ Electrolyte panel, BUN, creatinine, glucose ▪ CXR ▪ UA and urine culture ▪ LP: Cell count, differential, bacterial culture, viral PCR pending ▪ ABG: Metabolic acidosis, hyponatremia **Rx** ▪ Empiric IV antibiotics (ampicillin and cefotaxime) ▪ Admission to the hospital ▪ IV fluid bolus ▪ IV fluids with dextrose	**Ward W/U** ▪ Serum glucose: 75 mg/dL ▪ Urine culture: ⊖ ▪ Blood culture: ⊕ for *S pneumoniae* ▪ Ventilator (if necessary) **Rx** ▪ IV fluids, ($D_{5½}$NS) ▪ IV antibiotics × 10–14 days.	▪ Follow up in 48 hours of discharge from hospital ▪ Family counseling

Final Dx: Meningitis

INITIAL MGMT	CONTINUING MGMT	F/U
Emergency room W/U ▪ CBC: WBC 14,000 ▪ Blood culture ▪ Electrolyte panel, BUN, creatinine, glucose ▪ CXR: Hyperinflation, bilateral patchy interstitial infiltrates, ↑ pulmonary blood flow, prominent left atrium and ventricle ▪ UA and urine culture ▪ ABG: Hypoxemia ▪ RSV PCR: Pending **Rx** ▪ Empiric IV antibiotics ▪ Admission to the ICU ▪ IV fluid bolus ▪ Supplemental O_2 ▪ Nebulized albuterol trial	**ICU W/U** ▪ Serum glucose: 70 mg/dL ▪ Urine culture: ⊖ ▪ CXR: No change ▪ Blood culture: ⊖ ▪ RSV PCR ⊕ ▪ Ventilator (if necessary) ▪ Echocardiogram: Patent ductus arteriosus **Rx** ▪ IV fluids ($D_{5½}$NS) ▪ Supplemental O_2 ▪ Nebulized albuterol (if effective) ▪ Cardiology consult	▪ Follow up in 48 hours of discharge from hospital ▪ Family counseling

Final Dx: Bronchiolitis with patent ductus arteriosus (PDA)

CASE 89

HX	PE	DDX
8-month-old F is brought to the urgent care clinic because of abrupt onset of fever that lasted a couple of days with one seizure episode (the girl and her parents were camping in a remote area). The fever resolved after a rash appeared on the girl's chest and abdomen. Her parents did not notice any lethargy, poor feeding, or vomiting. She has no history of seizures.	VS: T 37°C (100°F); other vital signs WNL HEENT and neck: Bilateral cervical lymphadenopathy, ears WNL, ophthalmologic exam WNL Trunk: Macular rash Neuro: Alert and active; no abnormalities	■ Fifth disease ■ Measles ■ Meningitis ■ Roseola infantum ■ Rubella

CASE 90

HX	PE	DDX
3-day-old M presents to the ER with ↑ temperature, lethargy, respiratory distress, and poor feeding for the past 24 hours. His Apgar scores at birth were 6 and 8. His mother had a prolonged rupture of membranes (30 hours).	VS: T 39°C (102°F), P 170, BP 74/51, RR 70, O_2 sat 90% room air Lungs: Grunting respiration, chest indrawing with breathing, ↓ air entry CV: No murmurs or rubs Abd: Distended; ⊖ BS Neuro: Lethargy	■ *Bordetella* lung infection ■ *Chlamydia* lung infection ■ Complicated congenital lung abnormalities (eg, sequestration) ■ Foreign body causing obstruction ■ Group B streptococcus bacterial pneumonia

INITIAL MGMT	CONTINUING MGMT	F/U
Office W/U - CBC: WNL **Rx** - Hydrate - Acetaminophen		- Follow up in seven days or as needed - Family counseling

Final Dx: Roseola infantum (exanthem subitum)

INITIAL MGMT	CONTINUING MGMT	F/U
Emergency room W/U - CBC: ↑ WBC count - Random serum glucose: 60 mg/dL - CXR: Patchy infiltrates, pleural effusion, gastric dilation - Blood cultures: Pending - Viral culture ABG: Po_2 50 mm Hg, Pco_2 55 mm Hg **Rx** - O_2 - Fluids, $D_{5\frac{1}{4}}$NS - Empiric IV antibiotics - Respiratory and hemodynamic support (if necessary)	**Ward W/U** - Random serum glucose: 65 mg/dL - Blood cultures: Group B streptococcus - ABG: Po_2 60 mm Hg, Pco_2 50 mm Hg **Rx** - Antibiotics - Ventilatory and hemodynamic support (if necessary) - Antiviral drugs (if appropriate) - Bronchoscopy (if indicated)	- Follow up in 48 hours - Family counseling

Final Dx: Pneumonia

FEVER

CASE 91

HX	PE	DDX
49 yo F presents to the ER with fever of three days' duration. Since she turned 49 (about seven months ago), she has had recurrent infections that have been treated with antibiotics. She has also been treated with anthracyclines and alkylating agents for another disease for the past 18 months. However, she has not seen a doctor lately. She works in a manufacturing plant that produces cosmetics.	VS: T 39°C (102°F), P 132, BP 108/77, RR 29, O_2 sat 88% room air Lungs: No evidence of consolidation CV: WNL Abd: WNL Ext: WNL Neuro: WNL	▪ Deep abscess (unknown location) ▪ Pneumonia ▪ Pyelonephritis ▪ Sepsis ▪ Severe infection (unknown location)

CASE 92

HX	PE	DDX
43 yo F presents to the ER with fever, fatigue, malaise, and diffuse musculoskeletal pain of two days' duration. She complains of difficulty moving her right eye. The patient has a history of diabetes mellitus and mitral valve prolapse with regurgitation.	VS: T 40°C (104°F), P 134, BP 113/83, RR 31, O_2 sat 93% room air Ophthalmology: Visual field defects, conjunctival hemorrhage Funduscopy: Abnormal spots Lungs: WNL CV: Regurgitant murmur Abd: WNL Ext: Petechiae on feet Neuro: CN III palsy	▪ Complicated pyelonephritis ▪ Infective endocarditis ▪ Infective process (undetermined location) ▪ Intracranial infection ▪ Sepsis

INITIAL MGMT	CONTINUING MGMT	F/U
Emergency room W/U ▪ CT—abdomen: WNL ▪ CBC: Neutropenia ▪ CXR: Bilateral infiltrates in both lungs ▪ Sputum cultures: ⊕ for several bacterial species, including *Klebsiella* ▪ Blood cultures: ⊕ for *Klebsiella* ▪ UA: WNL ▪ Urine cultures: ⊖ **Rx** ▪ IV antibiotics (empiric cefepime or quinolone) ▪ Acetaminophen ▪ IV normal saline	**Ward W/U** ▪ Bone marrow biopsy, needle: Low myelogenous progenitor cell lines ▪ CT—chest, spiral: Widespread bilateral infiltrates in both lungs **Rx** ▪ IV antibiotics (appropriate for *Klebsiella*); tailor antibiotics to sensitivities ▪ IV normal saline ▪ G-CSF (for neutropenia)	▪ Follow up in four weeks ▪ Patient counseling ▪ Counsel patient to cease alcohol intake ▪ Smoking cessation ▪ Chest physical therapy

Final Dx: Multilobar pneumonia in a neutropenic patient

INITIAL MGMT	CONTINUING MGMT	F/U
Emergency room W/U ▪ ESR: 59 mm/hr ▪ CBC : ↑ WBC ▪ CXR: Some areas of patchy consolidation ▪ Blood cultures: Pending ▪ Echocardiography: Mobile mass attached to a valve ▪ ECG: RBBB ▪ UA: Microscopic hematuria **Rx** ▪ IV normal saline ▪ O_2 ▪ Empiric IV antibiotics (oxacillin and gentamicin) ▪ Acetaminophen	**Ward W/U** ▪ Blood cultures: ⊕ for *S viridans* **Rx** ▪ IV antibiotics ▪ Acetaminophen ▪ IV normal saline	▪ Follow up in four weeks ▪ Patient counseling ▪ Counsel patient to cease alcohol intake ▪ Smoking cessation

Final Dx: Infective endocarditis

CASE 93

HX	PE	DDX
60 yo M presents with fever and altered mental status eight hours after undergoing a diverticular abscess drainage.	VS: T 39°C (102°F), P 110, BP 60/35, RR 22, O_2 sat 92% on 2-L NC Gen: Acute distress HEENT: WNL Lungs: WNL CV: Tachycardia Abd: Lower abdominal tenderness Neuro: WNL	▪ Cardiogenic shock ▪ Hypovolemic shock ▪ Septic shock

CASE 94

HX	PE	DDX
17 yo F G0 whose last menstrual period was two days ago presents with fever, vomiting, myalgia, and a generalized skin rash.	VS: T 39°C (102°F), BP 75/30, HR 120 Gen: NAD Skin: Diffuse macular erythema; hyperemic mucous membranes Lungs: WNL CV: WNL Pelvic: Menstrual flow; foul-smelling tampon **Limited PE**	▪ Meningococcemia ▪ Rocky Mountain spotted fever ▪ Streptococcal toxic shock syndrome ▪ Toxic shock syndrome ▪ Typhoid fever

INITIAL MGMT	CONTINUING MGMT	F/U
Emergency room STAT ▪ O_2 ▪ IV normal saline/central line ▪ Blood culture: Pending ▪ Wound culture ▪ UA and urine culture **Emergency room W/U** ▪ CBC: ↑ WBC count ▪ Chem 14 ▪ ABG: Metabolic acidosis ▪ ECG ▪ Serum amylase, lipase ▪ Serum lactate: 6 ▪ Cardiac enzymes ▪ CXR ▪ CT–abdomen: Persistent diverticular abscess **Rx** ▪ Ampicillin-gentamicin-metronidazole or piperacillin-tazobactam or ticarcillin-clavulanate	**ICU W/U** ▪ Urine output q 1 h ▪ 2D echocardiography ▪ Blood culture: ⊕ for *E coli* sensitive to gentamicin and ceftriaxone ▪ Wound culture: ⊕ for *E coli* sensitive to gentamicin and ceftriaxone **Rx** ▪ Tailor antibiotics to sensitivities ▪ Surgery consult	

Final Dx: Septic shock

INITIAL MGMT	CONTINUING MGMT	F/U
Emergency room STAT ▪ O_2 inhalation ▪ IV normal saline ▪ Tampon removal **Emergency room W/U** ▪ CBC with differential ▪ Chem 14 ▪ UA ▪ Blood culture: Pending ▪ Urine culture: Pending **Rx** ▪ IV clindamycin + vancomycin ▪ Methylprednisolone	**ICU W/U** ▪ Blood culture: ⊖ ▪ Urine culture: ⊖ **Rx** ▪ Continue IV clindamycin and vancomycin ▪ Wound care	

Final Dx: Toxic shock syndrome

OUTPATIENT POTPOURRI

CASE 95

HX	PE	DDX
50 yo F presents with a painless lump in her right breast. She first noted this mass one month ago. There is no nipple discharge.	VS: Afebrile, P 70, BP 110/50, RR 12 Gen: NAD Skin: WNL HEENT: WNL Lymph nodes: ⊖ Breast: 3-cm, hard, immobile, nontender mass with irregular borders; no nipple discharge Lungs: WNL CV: WNL Abd: WNL	▪ Breast cancer ▪ Fibroadenoma ▪ Fibrocystic disease ▪ Mastitis ▪ Papillomas

CASE 96

HX	PE	DDX
62 yo F complains of vaginal itching, painful intercourse, and a clear discharge.	VS: WNL Gen: NAD Lungs: WNL CV: WNL Pelvic: Vulvar erythema, thin and pale mucosa with areas of erythema, clear discharge, mucosa bleeds easily during exam	▪ Atrophic vaginitis ▪ Bacterial vaginosis ▪ Candidal vaginitis ▪ Cervicitis (chlamydia, gonorrhea) ▪ Trichomonal vaginitis

CASE 97

HX	PE	DDX
33 yo Rh-negative F who currently lives in a battered-women's shelter calls the on-call physician because she noticed ↓ fetal movements. She is a G1P0 pregnant F at 36 weeks' gestational age. She states that fetal growth has been normal and that her obstetric ultrasound at 18 weeks showed a single normal fetus. The patient has no known preexisting diseases and does not smoke, drink alcohol, or take medications or illicit drugs. She received a dose of anti-D at 28 weeks.	VS: T 37°C (99°F), P 96, BP 141/91, RR 26, O_2 sat 93% room air Gen: No jaundice Eyes: Normal vision Lungs: No rales CV: No gallops or murmurs Pelvic: Fundal height in centimeters is appropriate for gestational age; cephalic presentation; speculum exam reveals unripe cervix, no ferning, Nitrazine ⊖ Ext: Slight pedal edema	▪ Preeclampsia ▪ Pregnancy-induced hypertension

INITIAL MGMT	CONTINUING MGMT	F/U
Office W/U ▪ Mammography: Suspicious of tumor ▪ FNA biopsy: Malignancy **Rx** ▪ Surgery consult		

Final Dx: Breast cancer

INITIAL MGMT	CONTINUING MGMT	F/U
Office W/U ▪ Vaginal pH: 6 ▪ Chlamydia PCR ▪ Gonorrhea PCR ▪ Wet mount ▪ Pap smear **Rx** ▪ Vaginal jelly for lubrication ▪ Counsel patient re local HRT ▪ Premarin (vaginal estrogen)		▪ Follow up as needed

Final Dx: Atrophic vaginitis

INITIAL MGMT	CONTINUING MGMT	F/U
Office W/U ▪ BUN, creatinine, ALT, AST ▪ CBC ▪ Chem 8 ▪ UA: ⊕ protein ▪ Random serum glucose ▪ Serum uric acid **Rx** ▪ Complete bed rest ▪ Monitor, continue BP cuff ▪ Fetal monitoring	**Ward W/U** ▪ UA: Protein 0.3 g/L/24 hrs; normal sediment ▪ LFTs: WNL **Rx** ▪ Complete bed rest ▪ Monitor, continue BP cuff ▪ Fetal monitoring	▪ Patient counseling ▪ Admit to labor and delivery for induction of labor ▪ Obstetric consult

Final Dx: Antenatal disorder: Pregnancy-induced hypertension

CASE 98

HX	PE	DDX
30 yo F presents for her regular checkup. She denies any complaints but is concerned about her BP, as it has been high on both of her previous visits over the past two months.	VS: P 75, BP 160/90 (no difference in BP between both arms), RR 12 Gen: WNL HEENT: WNL Breast: WNL Lungs: WNL CV: WNL Abd: WNL Pelvic: WNL Ext: WNL Neuro: WNL	▪ Cushing's disease ▪ Essential hypertension ▪ Hyperaldosteronism ▪ Hyperthyroidism ▪ Pheochromocytoma ▪ Renal artery stenosis ▪ White coat hypertension/anxiety

CASE 99

HX	PE	DDX
6 yo M is brought by his mother with continuous oozing of blood from the site of a tooth extraction he underwent two days ago. The bleeding initially stopped but restarted spontaneously a few hours later. His mother denies any history of epistaxis, easy bruising, petechiae, or bleeding per rectum. The patient's mother has a brother with hemophilia.	VS: Afebrile, P 80, BP 80/50, RR 14 Gen: NAD Skin: WNL HEENT: Blood oozing from site of extracted tooth Lungs: WNL CV: WNL Abd: WNL Ext: WNL	▪ DIC ▪ Hemophilia ▪ ITP ▪ Liver disease ▪ TTP ▪ Vitamin K deficiency ▪ von Willebrand's disease

CASE 100

HX	PE	DDX
27 yo F complains of pain during intercourse. She has a long history of painful periods.	VS: WNL Gen: NAD Lungs: WNL CV: WNL Pelvic: Normal vaginal walls, normal cervix, mild cervical motion tenderness; uterus tender, retroverted, and fixed; right adnexa slightly enlarged and tender	▪ Endometriosis ▪ PID ▪ Vaginismus ▪ Vaginitis

INITIAL MGMT	CONTINUING MGMT	F/U
Office W/U ▪ Lipid profile ▪ Chem 14 ▪ CBC ▪ UA: +1 protein ▪ ECG: LVH ▪ Echocardiography: LVH ▪ TSH **Rx** ▪ Lisinopril ▪ Exercise program ▪ Low-sodium diet	**Office W/U** ▪ Consider workup for 2° hypertension given the patient's young age (MRI/MRA renal arteries, urine catecholamines, urine cortisol)	▪ Follow up in one month

Final Dx: Essential hypertension

INITIAL MGMT	CONTINUING MGMT	F/U
Office W/U ▪ CBC ▪ Peripheral smear ▪ Bleeding time ▪ PTT: Prolonged ▪ PT, INR ▪ Plasma factor VIII: 3% ▪ Plasma factor IX **Rx** ▪ Factor VIII therapy ▪ Genetics consult ▪ Counsel parents		▪ Console and reassure patient ▪ Patient counseling ▪ Family counseling

Final Dx: Hemophilia

INITIAL MGMT	CONTINUING MGMT	F/U
Office W/U ▪ Wet mount ▪ Chlamydia DNA probe ▪ Gonorrhea DNA probe ▪ U/S—pelvis: Retroverted uterus of normal size; 2- × 3-cm cyst on the right adnexa that may represent a hemorrhagic corpus luteum or endometrioma **Rx** ▪ NSAIDs ▪ OCPs		▪ If initial treatment with OCPs and NSAIDs does not relieve pain, refer to a gynecologist for a trial of GnRH analogs, progestins, or danazol. ▪ Follow up as needed

Final Dx: Endometriosis

APPENDIX

ACRONYMS AND ABBREVIATIONS

Abbreviation	Meaning
A-a	alveolar-arterial (oxygen gradient)
AAA	abdominal aortic aneurysm
ABC	airway, breathing, circulation
ABG	arterial blood gas
AC	alternating current
ACA	anterior cerebral artery
ACEI	angiotensin-converting enzyme inhibitor
ACh	acetylcholine
ACL	anterior cruciate ligament
ACLS	advanced cardiac life support (protocol)
ACTH	adrenocorticotropic hormone
ADA	American Diabetes Association
ADH	antidiuretic hormone
ADHD	attention-deficit hyperactivity disorder
AED	antiepileptic drug
AF	atrial fibrillation
AFB	acid-fast bacillus
AFI	amniotic fluid index
AFP	α-fetoprotein
AHI	apnea-hypopnea index
AICD	automatic implantable cardiac defibrillator
AIDS	acquired immunodeficiency syndrome
ALL	acute lymphocytic leukemia
ALS	amyotrophic lateral sclerosis
ALT	alanine aminotransferase
AMA	antimitochondrial antibody
AML	acute myelogenous leukemia
ANA	antinuclear antibody
ANCA	antineutrophil cytoplasmic antibody
AP	anteroposterior
APC	activated protein C
aPTT	activated partial thromboplastin time
ARB	angiotensin receptor blocker
ARDS	acute respiratory distress syndrome
ARF	acute renal failure
ARR	absolute risk reduction
5-ASA	5-aminosalicylic acid
ASA	acetylsalicylic acid
ASCA	anti–*Saccharomyces cerevisiae* antibody
ASD	atrial septal defect
ASMA	anti–smooth muscle antibody
ASO	antistreptolysin O
AST	aspartate aminotransferase
ATN	acute tubular necrosis
AV	arteriovenous, atrioventricular
AVM	arteriovenous malformation
AVN	avascular necrosis
AVNRT	atrioventricular nodal reentrant tachycardia
AXR	abdominal x-ray
AZT	zidovudine
BAL	British anti-Lewisite
BCG	bacille Calmette-Guérin
BID	twice daily
BMI	body mass index
BMP	basic metabolic panel
BMT	bone marrow transplantation
BP	blood pressure
BPH	benign prostatic hyperplasia
BPP	biophysical profile
BPPV	benign paroxysmal positional vertigo
BS	bowel sounds
BSA	body surface area
BSO	bilateral salpingo-oophorectomy
BUN	blood urea nitrogen
CABG	coronary artery bypass graft
CAD	coronary artery disease
CAH	congenital adrenal hyperplasia
CALLA	common acute lymphocytic leukemia antigen
CAP	community-acquired pneumonia
CBC	complete blood count
CBT	cognitive-behavioral therapy
CCB	calcium channel blocker
CCP	cyclic citrullinated peptide
CD	cluster of differentiation
CEA	carcinoembryonic antigen
CF	cystic fibrosis
CH_{50}	total hemolytic complement
CHF	congestive heart failure
CI	confidence interval
CIN	cervical intraepithelial neoplasia
CK	creatine kinase
CKD	chronic kidney disease
CK-MB	creatine kinase, MB fraction
CLL	chronic lymphocytic leukemia
CML	chronic myelogenous leukemia
CMV	cytomegalovirus
CN	cranial nerve

Abbreviation	Meaning
NAD	no acute distress
NC	nasal cannula
NCS	nerve conduction study
NE	norepinephrine
NEC	necrotizing enterocolitis
NG	nasogastric
NHL	non-Hodgkin's lymphoma
NICU	neonatal intensive care unit
NK	natural killer (cells)
NNRTI	non-nucleoside reverse transcriptase inhibitor
NNT	number needed to treat
NPO	nil per os (nothing by mouth)
NPV	negative predictive value
NRTI	nucleoside reverse transcriptase inhibitor
NS	normal saline
NSAID	nonsteroidal anti-inflammatory drug
NSCLC	non–small cell lung cancer
NST	nonstress test
NTD	neural tube defect
O&P	ova and parasites
OA	osteoarthritis
OCD	obsessive-compulsive disorder
OCP	oral contraceptive pill
17-OHP	17-hydroxyprogesterone
OR	odds ratio, operating room
OSA	obstructive sleep apnea
P	pulse
PA	posteroanterior
PAC	premature atrial contraction
p-ANCA	perinuclear antineutrophil cytoplasmic antibody
Pa_{O_2}	partial pressure of oxygen in arterial blood
PCL	posterior cruciate ligament
P_{CO_2}	partial pressure of carbon dioxide
PCOS	polycystic ovarian syndrome
PCP	phencyclidine hydrochloride, *Pneumocystic carinii* (now *jiroveci*) pneumonia
PCR	polymerase chain reaction
PCV	polycythemia vera
PCWP	pulmonary capillary wedge pressure
PD	Parkinson's disease
PDA	patent ductus arteriosus
PDE-5a	phosphodiesterase type 5a
PE	physical exam, pulmonary embolism
PEA	pulseless electrical activity
PEEP	positive end-expiratory pressure
PEG	polyethylene glycol
PET	positron emission tomography (scan)
PF	platelet factor
PFT	pulmonary function test
$PGF_{2\alpha}$	prostaglandin F2-α
PI	protease inhibitor
PID	pelvic inflammatory disease
PIP	proximal interphalangeal (joint)
PIV	parainfluenza virus
PMI	point of maximal impulse
PMN	polymorphonuclear (leukocyte)
PNH	paroxysmal nocturnal hemoglobinuria
PNS	peripheral nervous system
PO	per os (by mouth)
POC	product of conception
P_{osm}	plasma osmolarity
PPD	purified protein derivative (of tuberculin)
PPH	postpartum hemorrhage
PPI	proton pump inhibitor
PPROM	preterm premature rupture of membranes
PPV	positive predictive value
PR	progesterone receptor
PRN	pro re nata (as needed)
PROM	premature rupture of membranes
PSA	prostate-specific antigen
PSGN	poststreptococcal glomerulonephritis
PT	prothrombin time
PTH	parathyroid hormone
PTHrP	parathyroid hormone–related peptide
PTSD	post-traumatic stress disorder
PTT	partial thromboplastin time
PTU	propylthiouracil
PUD	peptic ulcer disease
PUVA	psoralen and ultraviolet A
PVC	premature ventricular contraction
PVS	persistent vegetative state
PWI	perfusion-weighted imaging
RA	rheumatoid arthritis
RAST	radioallergosorbent testing
RBBB	right bundle branch block
RBC	red blood cell
RCT	randomized controlled trial
RDS	respiratory distress syndrome
RDW	red cell distribution width
REM	rapid eye movement
RF	rheumatoid factor
RIBA	recombinant immunoblot assay
RLQ	right lower quadrant
ROM	rupture of membranes
RPR	rapid plasma reagin
RR	relative risk, respiratory rate
RRR	regular rate and rhythm, relative risk reduction
RS	Reed-Sternberg (cells)
RSV	respiratory syncytial virus
RTA	renal tubular acidosis
RUQ	right upper quadrant
RV	residual volume
RVH	right ventricular hypertrophy
SAAG	serum-ascites albumin gradient
SAB	spontaneous abortion
SAD	seasonal affective disorder

Abbreviation	Meaning
SAH	subarachnoid hemorrhage
SBFT	small bowel follow-through
SBI	serious bacterial infection
SBP	systolic blood pressure
SCLC	small cell lung cancer
SERM	selective estrogen receptor modulator
SES	socioeconomic status
SIADH	syndrome of inappropriate secretion of antidiuretic hormone
SIDS	sudden infant death syndrome
SIRS	systemic inflammatory response syndrome
SLE	systemic lupus erythematosus
SMA	superior mesenteric artery
SMX	sulfamethoxazole
SNRI	serotonin-norepinephrine reuptake inhibitor
SPEP	serum protein electrophoresis
SPN	solitary pulmonary nodule
SQ	subcutaneous
SSRI	selective serotonin reuptake inhibitor
STD	sexually transmitted disease
SVT	supraventricular tachycardia
T_3	triiodothyronine
T_4	thyroxine
TAH	total abdominal hysterectomy
TB	tuberculosis
3TC	lamivudine
Tc	technetium
TCA	tricyclic antidepressant
Td	tetanus and diphtheria toxoid
TD	traveler's diarrhea
TdT	terminal deoxynucleotidyl transferase
TEE	transesophageal echocardiography
TGA	transposition of the great arteries
TIA	transient ischemic attack
TIBC	total iron-binding capacity
TID	three times daily
TIG	tetanus immune globulin

Abbreviation	Meaning
TIPS	transjugular intrahepatic portosystemic shunt
TLC	total lung capacity
TLS	tumor lysis syndrome
TMP	trimethoprim
TMP-SMX	trimethoprim-sulfamethoxazole
TNF	tumor necrosis factor
TNV	tenofovir
tPA	tissue plasminogen activator
TPN	total parenteral nutrition
TSH	thyroid-stimulating hormone
TTP	thrombotic thrombocytopenic purpura
TURP	transurethral resection of the prostate
UA	urinalysis
UMN	upper motor neuron
U_{osm}	urine osmolarity
UPEP	urine protein electrophoresis
UPPP	uvulopalatopharyngoplasty
URI	upper respiratory infection
USPSTF	United States Preventive Services Task Force
UTI	urinary tract infection
UV	ultraviolet
VCUG	voiding cystourethrography
VDRL	Venereal Disease Research Laboratory
VF	ventricular fibrillation
VIP	vasoactive intestinal peptide
VMA	vanillylmandelic acid
V/Q	ventilation-perfusion (ratio)
VRE	vancomycin-resistant enterococcus
VS	vital signs
VSD	ventricular septal defect
VTE	venous thromboembolism
vWD	von Willebrand's disease
vWF	von Willebrand's factor
VZV	varicella-zoster virus
WBC	white blood cell
WD/WN	well developed, well nourished
WNL	within normal limits

NOTES

Index

NOTES

NOTES

NOTES

NOTES

NOTES

NOTES

NOTES

NOTES